W9-ANJ-453

Family Communication
About Genetics

Family Communication About Genetics

Theory and Practice

Edited by

Clara L. Gaff, PhD

Carma L. Bylund, PhD

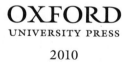

OXFORD

UNIVERSITY PRESS

2010

OXFORD
UNIVERSITY PRESS

Oxford University Press, Inc., publishes works that further
Oxford University's objective of excellence
in research, scholarship, and education.

Oxford   New York
Auckland   Cape Town   Dar es Salaam   Hong Kong   Karachi
Kuala Lumpur   Madrid   Melbourne   Mexico City   Nairobi
New Delhi   Shanghai   Taipei   Toronto

With offices in
Argentina   Austria   Brazil   Chile   Czech Republic   France   Greece
Guatemala   Hungary   Italy   Japan   Poland   Portugal   Singapore
South Korea   Switzerland   Thailand   Turkey   Ukraine   Vietnam

Library of Congress Cataloging-in-Publication Data

Family communication about genetics : theory and practice / edited by Clara L. Gaff,
Carma L. Bylund.
p. ; cm.
Includes bibliographical references
ISBN 978-0-19-536982-3
1. Genetic Counseling.   2. Communication in families.   I. Gaff, Clara L.
II. Bylund, Carma L.
[DNLM: 1. Genetic Counseling — ethica.   2. Genetic Counseling—methods.
3. Family Relations.   4. Professional-Family Relations–ethics.
QZ 50 F1977 2010]
RB155.7.F36 2010
616'.042–dc22
2009044746

1 3 5 7 9 8 6 4 2
Printed in the United States of America
on acid-free paper.

ACKNOWLEDGMENTS

We gratefully acknowledge the following people for their contribution to this book project:

Maggie Gregory, PhD, for suggesting a book on family communication and genetics and early work on developing the proposal.

Our advisory committee of Angus Clarke, PhD, Allyn McConkie-Rosell, PhD, Paul Atkinson, DSc (Econ), and Kathleen Galvin, PhD, who contributed and advised us throughout the project.

Jan Hodgson, PhD, and Mrs. Margaret Sahhar for formative discussions.

Ms. Sherice Davis for her assistance in referencing.

Our own families for their support and patience through this project.

Finally, the authors of the chapters for their patience and diligence in writing and for their willingness to work with co-authors whom they had never met. We believe these international and interdisciplinary collaborations make this book unique.

CONTENTS

CONTRIBUTORS

Paul Atkinson, DScEcon, AcSS
Distinguished Research Professor
School of Social Sciences
Cardiff University
Cardiff, United Kingdom

Carma L. Bylund, PhD
Director
Communication Skills Training and Research Laboratory
Assistant Attending Behavioral Scientist
Department of Psychiatry and Behavioral Sciences
Memorial Sloan-Kettering Cancer Center
New York, New York

James Dillard, PhD
Professor of Communication Arts & Sciences
The Pennsylvania State University
University Park, Pennsylvania

Laura Forrest, PhD
Genetics Education and Health Research
Murdoch Childrens Research Institute
Melbourne, Australia and
Department of Paediatrics
The University of Melbourne
Melbourne, Australia

CLARA L. GAFF, PhD
Senior Genetic Counsellor
Genetic Health Services
Victoria and
Departments of Paediatrics and Medicine
University of Melbourne
Melbourne, Australia

KATHLEEN M. GALVIN, PhD
Professor
Communication Studies Department
Northwestern University
Evanston, Illinois

MAGGIE GREGORY, PhD
Director
Chordata Research
Mark, United Kingdom

JODY KOENIG KELLAS, PhD
Associate Professor
Department of Communication Studies
University of Nebraska-Lincoln
Lincoln, Nebraska

ASCAN F. KOERNER, PhD
Associate Professor
Department of Communication Studies
University of Minnesota
Minneapolis, Minnesota

SAMANTHA J. LEONARD, MBBS, MA, MRCPCH
Clinical Geneticist and PhD Scholar
Centre for Ethics in Medicine
Department of Community-Based Medicine
University of Bristol
Bristol, United Kingdom

BONNIE LEROY, MS, CGC
Associate Professor
Department of Genetics
   Cell Biology and Development
University of Minnesota
Minneapolis, Minnesota

MARION F. MCALLISTER, PhD
Genetic Counsellor and MRC Research Fellow
Genetic Medicine
Manchester Academic Health Science Centre
University of Manchester
United Kingdom

PATRICIA MCCARTHY VEACH, PhD
Professor
Department of Educational Psychology
University of Minnesota
Minneapolis, Minnesota

ALLYN MCCONKIE-ROSELL, PhD, CGC
Associate Research Professor
Division of Medical Genetics
Department of Pediatrics
Duke University Medical Center
Durham, North Carolina

SYLVIA METCALFE, PhD
Group Leader
Genetics Education and Health Research
Murdoch Childrens Research Institute
and
Associate Professor in Medical Genetics
Department of Pediatrics
The University of Melbourne
Royal Children Hospital
Melbourne, Australia

ANNA MIDDLETON, PhD, MSc, RGC
Consultant Research Genetic Counsellor
Institute of Medical Genetics
Cardiff University
Cardiff, United Kingdom

MICHELLE MILLER-DAY, PhD
Associate Professor of Communication
    Arts and Sciences
The Pennsylvania State University
University Park, Pennsylvania

AINSLEY J. NEWSON, LLB(HONS), PhD
Senior Lecturer in Biomedical Ethics
Centre for Ethics in Medicine
Department of Community-Based Medicine
University of Bristol
Bristol, United Kingdom

ROXANNE PARROTT, PhD
Professor
Department of Communication Arts and Sciences
The Pennsylvania State University
University Park, Pennsylvania

KATHRYN PETERS, MS, CGC
Senior Research Assistant and Genetic Counselor
Penn State Institute for Diabetes and Obesity
The Pennsylvania State University
University Park, Pennsylvania

SANDRA PETRONIO, PhD
Professor, Senior Affiliate Faculty Member
Charles Warren Fairbanks Center for Medical Ethics
IUPUI Department of Communication Studies
Indiana University School of Medicine
Clarian Health Partners
Indianapolis, Indiana

MYRA I. ROCHE, MS, CGC
Associate Professor in Pediatrics
and
Director, Genetic Counseling Services
Division of Genetics and Metabolism
Department of Pediatrics
University of North Carolina-Chapel Hill
Chapel Hill, North Carolina

CHRISTINA M. SABEE, PhD
Assistant Professor
Communication Studies
San Francisco State University
San Francisco, California

JENNIFER A. SAMP, PhD
Associate Professor and Graduate Coordinator
Department of Speech Communication
University of Georgia
Athens, Georgia

LOANE SKENE, LLD, LLM, LLB
Professor
Melbourne Law School
University of Melbourne
Melbourne, Australia

HEATHER SKIRTON, PhD, RGN, REG GC,
    QUAL MW, DIP COUNSELLING
Professor of Applied Health Genetics
Faculty of Health
University of Plymouth
Plymouth, United Kingdom

AMANDA STRICKLAND
Graduate Assistant
Department of Speech Communication
University of Georgia
Athens, Georgia

JENNIFER SULLIVAN, MS, CGC
Senior Genetic Counselor
Division of Medical Genetics
Department of Pediatrics
Duke University Medical Center
Durham, North Carolina

APRIL R. TREES, PhD
Assistant Professor
Department of Communication
Saint Louis University
St Louis, Missouri

MELANIE WATSON, RGN, BA(HONS), MSc
Principal Genetic Counsellor
Wessex Clinical Genetics Service
Southampton University Hospitals Trust
Princess Anne Hospital
Southampton, United Kingdom

MARY-ANNE YOUNG, MHSc
Senior Genetic Counsellor
Familial Cancer Centre
Peter MacCallum Cancer Centre
Melbourne, Australia

INTRODUCTION

Clara L. Gaff and Carma L. Bylund

By virtue of their common ancestors, relatives share genes and, consequently, health risks. Rapid improvement in our understanding of the genetic basis of disease has allowed more information and options to become available to families with genetic conditions. Although only some family members may receive this information directly from health services, it often has implications for other family members. Over the past 30 or so years, there has been a steady increase in research investigating the communication of genetic test results and information about genetic conditions within families, reflecting genetics practitioners' concern for the health and well-being of families beyond the clients they see in clinic. Concurrently, in the academic discipline of communication studies, family communication was established, first as an area of teaching and secondly as an area of research [1]. Interest in family communication began with scholarly attention to long-term relationships, including marriage, but then broadened to include the study of everyday family life [1]. Over the past decade, there has been increased interest from family communication scholars in the intersection between family communication and health [2].

Although the realms of genetics and family communication intersect naturally in people's lives, opportunities for family communication researchers and genetics practitioners to come together and explore common interests have been relatively limited. In developing this book, we sought to provide a meeting point where these disciplines could consider the ways in which theory and empirical insights from communication research may inform practice. Equally, the difficulties that arise in communication within families about inherited traits—especially genetic disease—present opportunities and challenges for the research community to develop and test out their theoretical understanding. Almost all chapters have been written collaboratively by at least one author with a theory perspective and another with a genetics practice perspective.

Each theory was selected for its value as a useful lens through which to examine the processes families undergo when responding to and dealing with genetic issues. Our selection of theories was based on the belief that understanding family communication is central to understanding and addressing the implications of genetic conditions with families affected by them.[1] We draw on theory, rather than empirical data or clinical experience alone, as theories in the social sciences "help us understand or explain phenomena that we observe in the social world" [3] (p. 20). Miller [3] lays out different types of problems that may be solved by theory: the empirical problem, the conceptual problem, and the practical problem. Whereas solving empirical problems and conceptual problems lead to increased explanations and a more sophisticated understanding of the interrelated concepts of theories, theories as solutions to practical problems are a major focus of this book.

The "practical problems" that are the raison d'être of this book require some description and explanation. From the perspective of genetics practitioners, the thorniest problem is nondisclosure—that is, when news about a genetic condition is not passed on to at-risk relatives by the person who was seen at the genetics service. Although it is rare for people to directly tell genetics practitioners that they do not intend to pass information on to one or more family members [4], in fact weak social, emotional, or biological links mean that there are usually a significant number of at-risk relatives who are not informed [5]. A tension between practitioners' respect for an individual's privacy and confidentiality and concern for relatives, who may be unaware of their risk, has led to debate about practitioners' responsibility to warn and what courses of action can or should be taken [6, 7]. The predominant view among families with genetic conditions is that they themselves are responsible for telling family members about a genetic condition, with variable views about how active doctors and genetic specialists should be in this process [8, 9]. For families, the practical problems appear to lie in planning communication and coping with the reactions of those with whom they communicate, particularly if the relative rejects the information or its personal relevance or fails to pass the news on to offspring [5, 10].

We see the challenge—and opportunity—more broadly than simply facilitating the transmission of information from people seen in clinic to relatives who may not be aware of the family history or its implications for themselves. Family communication about genetic conditions is not simply defined by a "sender-receiver" model of deliberately transmitted information. Family communication is a part of life; families establish patterns and rules of communication through their interactions that both influence and are influenced by the presence of a genetic condition or inherited health risk in a family. Families may discuss the day-to-day life events that are a result of the condition, though not necessarily its genetics, during their usual conversation. A genetic condition or concern about an apparently inherited health risk may impact communication as well as be impacted by the ways families relate. In addition, family communication forms a context and pattern for subsequent communication of information received by the clinics. Our aims are then three-fold: to raise health-care practitioners' awareness of the ways families communicate normally, to encourage consideration of the way in which communication about genetics and normal family communication patterns intersect, and finally to explore ways that practitioners may work with families to address issues that arise in family communication about genetics.

To these ends, we have drawn predominantly on a particular body of communication theory: theories in family communication. As Braithwaite and Baxter point out in the introduction to their edited book, *Family Communication Theories* (2006), theories that are used in the study of family communication come from both within and without the discipline of communication studies [11]. The theories presented in this book have multiple origins, including communication studies, psychology, cognitive psychology, mass media theory, and family therapy [11]. Chapters 4–7 and 11 discuss ways in which particular theories can raise awareness of these issues. Chapters 8–10 move toward action-oriented and practical considerations in facilitating communication within families, with a focus on attributions, uncertainty, and planning communication.

SOME EXPLANATIONS

Some of our choices of terminology require explanation. First, we predominantly use the term *health-care practitioner* rather than the more specific term *genetic counselor*. Although most counseling about family communication of genetic information currently takes place in genetics services, we chose to use the less specific term for several reasons. First of all, we believe that many health professions will increasingly face similar issues as management on the basis of genetic makeup (genotype) becomes integrated into their area of specialization. This book is intended to assist all health-care practitioners to think about the ways families communicate and about their own practice in relation to this. Second, in many countries, specialist genetic services are in their early stages and do not necessarily include genetic counselors. *Genetic counselor* is also a term that is applied to people of different training internationally. Despite our use of the more inclusive term *health-care practitioner*, we recognize and acknowledge that specially trained genetics professionals have a different skill set than many other practitioners. In the cases where we do use the term *genetic counselor*, we are referring specifically to these trained genetics specialists, including genetic nurses.

Secondly, the use of the term *patient* is a thorny one in genetics. *Patient* tends to imply a person with or being treated for a condition, whereas many people seeking information about genetic conditions are healthy and wish to maintain their health. *Client* is a term commonly generally used in genetic counseling; however, many of the issues discussed in the book relate to individuals more broadly than only clients of genetic services. Further, terms such as *consultand* and *proband* have little meaning to those outside genetics. We have attempted to use the term most appropriate to the context of the issue being discussed.

PREVIEW OF CHAPTERS

The book begins with three chapters that provide a foundation for the rest of the book. Chapter 1 introduces core concepts related to the study of family communication and will be particularly helpful for readers who are unfamiliar with family communication as an area of study. Chapter 2 provides an introduction to genetics and genetic health care, an essential background chapter for readers who are not genetic practitioners. Chapter 3 takes a "big picture" approach, describing and analyzing the ways in which the multiple discourses about genetics (e.g., from society, experts, and lay individuals) may affect family members' perceptions of and communication about genetic issues.

As indicated earlier, Chapters 4–11 in this book are centered around a particular theory or body of theoretical work that helps us to better understand family communication. These theory chapters begin in Chapter 4 with narrative theory, which offers insight into the ways in which family narratives about genetics can affect adjustment and family communication. In Chapter 5, we turn to a theoretical understanding about time and how genetic information impacts individuals and families over a life span and generations. We explore family systems theory in Chapter 6, the most widely adopted theory by family communication scholars. Chapter 7 examines genetic information (which some may consider private information) through the lens of Communication Privacy Management Theory. In Chapter 8, a theory of uncertainty management is used to explain how managing uncertainty about genetics may result in a variety of outcomes, including seeking and avoiding information and adaptation. In Chapter 9, we explore how attributions and personal theories might help explain some family communication practices and look at how practitioners can use this knowledge to help clients understand or even reframe their attributions if necessary. Chapter 10 explores how goals, plans, and action theories may inform a health-care practitioner wishing to facilitate the family member's process of communication with relatives. Chapter 11 focuses on families' predictable and stable communication cultures. In addition, this chapter focuses on how a family's communication patterns may actually affect how family members interact with a genetics practitioner. Each of these theories brings a unique perspective to the issues surrounding family communication and genetics. It is our hope that readers will be able to appreciate the contributions of individual theories, while also recognizing important areas of overlap.

The final chapters of the book move from theory toward some of the practical considerations of helping families communicate about genetics. Chapters 12 and 13 describe ethical and legal perspectives on the debate about practitioners' roles and responsibilities in relation to the communication of genetic information within families. The final two chapters specifically address clinical practice. Chapter 14 focuses on enabling practitioners to prepare parents for talking to their children about genetic issues, a constant concern raised in counseling sessions and which, as previous chapters emphasize, is important for the way in which children will communicate and manage genetic information in the future. The last chapter draws on previous chapters and on genetic counseling literature to consider how these theories might be incorporated into practice. Fictionalized cases are used throughout this book to illustrate points of theory and practice. Although these cases reflect situations often encountered by genetic counselors in clinical practice, any resemblance to an individual or family is coincidental.

Health-care practitioners with a solid understanding of families' communication processes are well equipped to guide individuals and families as they integrate genetic risk into their lives. This is a role that is likely to have greater prominence as understanding of the genetic contribution to disease increases and health outcomes are improved through prevention or treatment based on the genetic constitution of the patient (their genetic makeup) or of their tumor (if they are being treated for a cancer). It is our hope that this book will help to guide health-care practitioners in their work as well as spark new ideas for research in the areas of family communication and genetics.

NOTE

1. Although we recognize the reality of cultural influence on family communication, we chose not to explicitly address culture in this book. We believe these family communication theories transcend cultural differences (e.g., family narratives are present in all families, though they may manifest differently and serve different functions).

REFERENCES

1. Galvin KM. Family communication instruction: A brief history and call. *Journal of Family Communication* 2001;1(1):15–20.
2. Bylund CL, Duck S. The everyday interplay between family relationships and family members' health. *Journal of Social and Personal Relationships* 2004;21(1):5–7.
3. Miller K. *Communication Theories: Perspectives, Processes, and Contexts.* Boston: The McGraw-Hill Companies; 2002.

4. Clarke A, Richards M, Kerzin-Storrar L, Halliday J, Young MA, Simpson SA, et al. Genetic professionals' reports of nondisclosure of genetic risk information within families. *Europern Journal of Human Genetics* 2005;13(5):556–562.

5. Gaff CL, Clarke AJ, Atkinson P, Sivell S, Elwyn G, Iredale R, et al. Process and outcome in communication of genetic information with families: A systematic review. *European Journal of Human Genetics* 2007;15:999–1011.

6. Dugan RB, Wiesner GL, Juengst ET, O'Riordan M, Matthews AL, Robin NH. Duty to warn at-risk relatives for genetic disease: Genetic counselors' clinical experience. American *Journal of Medical Genetics Part C: Seminars in Medical Genetics* 2003;119C(1):27–34.

7. Offit K, Groeger E, Turner S, Wadsworth EA, Weiser MA. The "duty to warn" a patient's family member about hereditary disease risks. *JAMA* 2004;292:1469–1473.

8. Kerzin-Storrar L, Wright C, Williamson PR, Fryer A, Njindou A, Quarrell O, et al. Comparison of genetic services with and without genetic registers: Access and attitudes to genetic counseling services among relatives of genetic clinic patients. *Journal of Medical Genetics* 2002;39(12):e85.

9. Kohut K, Manno M, Gallinger S, Esplen MJ. Should healthcare providers have a duty to warn family members of individual with an HNPCC-causing mutation? A survey of patients from the Ontario Familial Colon Cancer Registry. *Journal of Medical Genetics* 2007;44(6):404–407.

10. Wilson BJ, Forrest K, van Teiglingen ER, McKee L, Haites N, Matthews E, et al. Family communication about genetic risk: The little that is known. *Community Genetics* 2004;7(1):15–24.

11. Baxter LA, Braithwaite DO. Introduction: Meta-theory and theory in family communication research. In: Braithwaite DO, Baxter LA, eds. *Engaging Theories in Family Communication: Multiple Perspectives.* Thousand Oaks, CA: Sage; 2006.

Family Communication
About Genetics

1

PRINCIPLES OF FAMILY COMMUNICATION

Carma L. Bylund, Kathleen M. Galvin, & Clara L. Gaff

Communication in families has been of interest to researchers for many years. In this chapter, we explain some core principles of family communication and how these principles provide a foundation for understanding family communication about genetics.

Genetic disease affects entire families, not just individual members. A focus on communication is critical for truly understanding family dynamics and how members manage genetic information. Family interactions both construct and reflect family relationships, as well as support family members' management of everyday life. A family's relational ties and identity also are established and managed through communication practices. One perspective on family communication suggests that families are actively engaging in *meaning making*, creating shared worldviews for their members. These shared meanings and views are developed over time through continual interpretation and response regarding interpersonal messages, as well as the reactions of family members to life events. Family meanings serve to establish family identity as they are woven into interaction patterns over time. Unless deliberately rejected, each generation, consciously or unconsciously, teaches the next generation patterns and strategies for managing intimacy, conflict, and stress.

The importance of understanding principles of family communication as a way to improve the way in which families manage their communication about genetic information cannot be understated. From a biomedical perspective, a definitive genetic diagnosis in one individual may not only reveal information about that person but also about potential risks to his or her relatives and their offspring, effectively presenting other members with "deterministic predictions of their fate." [1] (p. 1). Here, "fate" may encompass the family member's own health and/or the possibility of having a child with a genetic condition. The presence of a genetic condition in families impacts family systems and their members' communication patterns regardless of the genetic status of an individual family member. A key issue in managing a family's genetic health involves the disclosure and discussion of genetic information, as well as handling the emotions that accompany these discussions.

Communicating about genetics within a family may or may not occur during a time of stress. For example, family communication about the new diagnosis of a previously unknown genetic condition in the family, such as the life-shortening respiratory disorder cystic fibrosis (CF), occurs in a context of severe stress on the family. Alternatively, during a low stress period, new information may become available that adds to existing family knowledge and understanding of their genetic situation; this information has the potential to become a stressor on the family. For example, the availability of a genetic test for hereditary breast and ovarian cancer (HBOC) in a family enables individuals to make welcome or unwelcome choices about how to use this information. In other cases, information may be sought about the condition and related health risk, such as a pregnant woman seeking details from her mother about a cousin with a disability, in order to learn her chances of having a child with the same condition. Regardless of the precise situation, communication generally occurs in accordance with existing family communication patterns and impacts the short- and long-term communication between family members [2].

From a clinical standpoint, "the most important communication function ... may be to accurately exchange health risk and disease information among family members" [3] (p. 629). Informing family members of their potential genetic risks may be viewed as the responsibility of all members, but health-care practitioners rely heavily on the proband, or first medically diagnosed member. Many factors influence the *enactment* of such disclosure messages, where enactment refers to both whether disclosure occurs and how it occurs. These factors include (*1*) interpersonal histories, (*2*) family structures, (*3*) members' roles, (*4*) gender, (*5*) communication privacy rules, (*6*) the nature of the disorder, and (*7*) cultural patterns [4].

When well-functioning families engage in open communication, this exchange of information may take place relatively easily. However, for many other families, such an exchange can disrupt normal family communication patterns and lead to distress. Sometimes, individuals will be confronted with the task of communicating to relatives lost or rejected through family estrangement, or through interpersonal or geographic distance. In other cases, testing results will challenge the understanding of family as certain members know it, as concealed pregnancies, hidden paternity, and unacknowledged adoptions or births involving surrogates or sperm donors are revealed. Individuals who are unrelated biologically or legally but are considered family (sometimes called "fictive kin") may feel excluded from the family concerns. In certain cases, individual family members will confront the need to reconsider their understanding of "family." Eventually, subsequent conversations will occur regarding the ongoing implications of the genetic diagnosis. Family communication patterns and practices will interface directly with members' ability to cope with issues of genetic disease.

This chapter provides the groundwork for understanding families and communication. First, we present an overview of the changing definitions and demographics of families. Next, we describe some fundamental concepts to understanding interpersonal communication and family communication, followed by an explanation of current thinking on communication in functional families.

FAMILY DEFINITIONS AND DEMOGRAPHICS

Today's extraordinary advances in genetics are occurring in a period when the concept of family is increasingly fluid. Therefore, a description of who incurs genetic risk in the family does not predictably overlap with a description of who is in the family. The implications of genetic findings, increasingly available as a result of the Human Genome Project and related research, will serve to reinforce the traditional and biomedical concepts of family as biologically and genetically linked. Yet contemporary families reflect a world of "normative instability and definitional crisis" [5] (p. 489) as the conception of family membership becomes increasingly variable. Although all cultures and societies witness changing kinship patterns, Western families lie at the forefront of familial redefinition. This is due to the multiplicity of emerging and shifting kinship patterns that rely less on biological/genetic or traditional legal ties and increasingly on nontraditional legal ties, medical advances in fertility research, and interpersonal commitments. Addressing the complexities of family definitions, Floyd, Mikkelson, and Judd [6] offer three generally accepted approaches for defining a family: a role lens, a sociolegal lens, and a biogenetic lens. These contrast with the emerging *constitutive perspective*, which asserts that "our families and our images of families are constituted through social interaction" [7] (p. xiii). Today's families may be described on a continuum ranging from traditional (biologically/legally linked) to constitutive (linked through communication or how they define themselves). Therefore, health-care practitioners face the challenge of adapting and responding to a range of family types, which might not fit with a biomedical perspective, when dealing with genetic information such as clinical diagnosis, test results, risk, and prognostic data.

A brief overview of current family forms will establish the landscape of contemporary families, although every family has its own variations. Some of the traditional family categories include *two-parent biological family*—consisting of parents and children from the union of those parents. This traditional form, tied by blood and marriage, remains more common in the British Isles, New Zealand, and Australia, whereas it no longer represents the majority family form in the United States. Other family forms tend to be variable in their definition and composition. The *blended* family, for example, an adoptive or stepfamily, traditionally consists of remarried parents and children whom are not all biologically related and is usually formed through remarriage. In the United States committed cohabiters form approximately 25% of stepfamilies. In addition, divorce rates are high for second marriages, leading to subsequent marriages for one or both partners. Increasingly single mothers are marrying eventually, and same-sex partners are forming stepfamilies with their children from earlier relationships. Cohabiting pairs, heterosexual or homosexual, are increasing in many parts of the globe. In 2003, 60% of nonmarried U.S. family groups included a child under 18 years [8]. Increasingly same-sex partners are jointly entering parenthood through adoption, foster care, and new reproductive technologies.

The number of *single-parent* families continues to rise. In Australia the number of one-parent families increased by 53% between 1986 and 2001 [9], while in New Zealand this family form is predicted to increase 26% from 2001 to 2021 [10]. In the United States, the proportion of all births to unmarried women ages 15 to 44 years increased to 50.7% in 2006 [11]. Many of these single parents will partner eventually, whereas other women will divorce and live as single parents at a later date. In 2005, 26% of children in the United States lived with one custodial parent [12].

More families are forming through adoption and reproductive technologies. The United States contains over 2 million adoptees, whereas adoption is growing, but not as rapidly, in other Western nations such as Australia, in which adoption rose 6% in 2003–2004 [9]. Across Western nations the practice of international adoption has become increasingly common, often involving transracial or transcultural connections. In addition, the development of reproductive technologies has provided heterosexual couples, homosexual couples, and single persons with the opportunity to parent children who may or may not be biologically related to both of the parents. Essentially "nontraditional families" are emerging as normative family forms [13], without biological or traditional legal ties, and are given labels such as "social kin" and "fictive kin." Given longer life spans, many people will experience a variety of family forms before they die—this may involve minor or major variations from what used to be the norm. The current complexity of family forms complicates any generalizations about the best practices for working with families.

Family structure changes result in communication challenges. "As families become increasingly diverse, *their definitional processes expand exponentially, rendering their identity highly discourse-dependent*" [14] (p. 3). In other words, family members increasingly rely on talk to create their family identity; how they talk about their family in turn defines their family. Such discourse may be directed to those outside the family or may involve those inside the family reaffirming their family connection. For example, families may represent themselves as biologically related, although this is not fully accurate. Consider the case in which a health-care practitioner is collecting a family history from a mother and her teenage daughter, after the daughter has been diagnosed with a genetic condition. After the consultation, the mother calls to inform the practitioner that her daughter was in fact adopted but is unaware of this.

The significant changes in family composition are reflected in changes in communication patterns. For example, in many families formed after divorce or other painful circumstances, distance or cutoffs may develop between former family members. The choice to create families though same-sex partnering or adoption may create rifts among disapproving extended family members. The traditional secrecy surrounding adoption has diminished dramatically as open adoption and transracial adoption renders secrecy useless. Concurrently, secrecy emerges as a common pattern in families formed through reproductive technologies.

COMMUNICATION AS TRANSACTIONAL

The genetics literature commonly places an emphasis on the "act" of communication as one family member conveys a piece of news, such as a new diagnosis or the availability of genetic testing, to at-risk, biological relatives. This perspective is known in communication as a "sender–receiver" model. In contrast, our approach to family communication reflects the belief that communication is "transactional." This means that interpersonal communication mutually impacts on each participant. Thus, in communicative relationships, participants simultaneously affect and are affected by others. When persons interact with each other, they create a context for each other and relate to each other within that context. For example, one sibling may grow to see a father as warm, understanding, and approachable; their interactions may be openly expressive, including hugs, smiles, and direct eye contact. Another sibling may see him as unpredictable, judgmental, and distant; this sibling may rarely self-disclose and disengage from the father. In turn, the father may experience one sibling as open and agreeable and the other as distant and cautious; their interactions may be distant and more formal. Such differences may reflect a wide range of issues such as gender, birth order, personality, intelligence, physical capacities, and so on. What matters is that over time, predictable patterns emerge and, unless directly or indirectly challenged, are likely to define the interpersonal relationship of these family members indefinitely.

In some families there is greater congruence of members' perceptions of each other, whereas in other families there is great diversity.

For example, imagine three adult siblings: Melanie, Jonathan, and Daniel. Melanie is 6 years older than Jonathan and 8 years older than Daniel and acted in many ways as a second parent to them. Over the years, through their communication, Melanie and each of her younger brothers have created a relationship that positions Melanie in an authoritative role. When Melanie would give them instructions, they would follow them, thus creating a power differential. This relationship continued as they grew older. As an adult, Jonathan was diagnosed with an iron accumulation disorder, hereditary hemochromatosis (HH). He was advised by his physician to encourage his siblings to be tested, as they each had a 25% chance of also having the condition. Melanie did so immediately, but Daniel showed little interest when Jonathan originally told him. However, because of the relationship they had co-constructed through communication, Daniel did have testing after Melanie told him he should.

FAMILY COMMUNICATION CONCEPTS

In order to provide a foundation for the family communication theories that will be explained later in the book, we introduce five concepts that are fundamental to understanding family communication. Each of these concepts provides a lens for answering important questions about families and how they communicate. We will organize this section around these questions: *(1)* How do families see themselves? *(2)* How do families regulate their communication? *(3)* How do families socialize their members? *(4)* How do families set boundaries? *(5)* How do families make decisions?

How Do Families See Themselves?

Family systems tend to develop unique images and themes that influence how they deal with change and stress. Family images may be thought of as root metaphors for a family's relational patterns; they reflect the family worldview as they represent the family's collective experience [15]. A root metaphor captures the overarching image of family identity. For example, a family may see itself as a *nest, corporation, jazz combo*, or a *soccer team*. Whereas the nest image conjures up visions of warmth, support, nurturing, and safety, the soccer team image depicts competition, teamwork, discipline, and toughness. Each member develops images of what the family unit and other family members are like—images that affect how individuals, pairs, and the group deals with stress. For example, one family faced with a child's diagnosis of CF may enact their implicit nest metaphor by hovering and nurturing each other. Extended family members may look after the other children, bring food, or listen to parental concerns for hours. In contrast, another family may enact their soccer team metaphor by assigning family members to key roles or tasks and strategizing ways to fight this condition. In addition, families develop themes or statements that reflect their beliefs and values. Most families may live by two to three core themes. Themes represent a fundamental view of reality and answer questions such as, Who are we and what do we stand for? Family themes are represented in statements such as the following: "We have responsibility for those less fortunate than us"; "You can always depend on your family"; "Seize the moment"; "Think for yourself"; and "You can always do better" [2].

Themes bear a direct relation to family actions. In fact, family members' behaviors serve as indicators of the overall family themes. The same family theme may be played out differently across families. For example, in one family, serving to the less fortunate may create individuals who are sensitive to others' needs as well as their own. In another family, this theme may result in young adults who cannot even identify their own needs because they can always find others who are less well off and need assistance. The theme "You can always depend on your family" may cause a member with HBOC to feel guilty about revealing this news due to its negative effects on others; it could "harm" or "upset" those who depend on each other. In another family, this theme may convince a member to alert others immediately to a possible health risk because dependable family members act responsibly. A theme of "The Atkinsons play to win" may be reflected in family members marshalling resources to "beat" a disease and its potential impact on other relatives. Some members may scour the Internet for the latest information, others may sign up to be tested to inform or protect themselves and other family members, and others may join self-help groups to stay informed. Family themes play a critical role in how families manage stress.

How Do Families Regulate Their Communication?

Communication patterns and rules serve to regulate family communication. Patterns develop in family relationships as a result of family members' coordinating their actions. Such patterns become reciprocal and repetitive over time. These verbal and nonverbal communication patterns significantly affect their health-related behavior. As an example, a wife may act as the health manager, taking charge of health-care visits and preventative screenings, giving constant reminders to her husband of what he should be doing. Her husband may in fact view this as nagging, and he may resist it by not carrying through with her directions. This pattern of demand–withdraw [16] is seen frequently in family relationships. If the husband is found to be at genetic risk for colon cancer, this demand–withdraw pattern may be so firmly entrenched in their relationship that it is difficult to overcome, and he may be slow to get tested.

Over time many family patterns transform into family rules, usually reflecting patterns that have become "oughts" or "shoulds."

Communication rules are shared understandings of what communication means and what kinds of communication are appropriate in various situations [17]. Every family enacts communication rules, helping members to coordinate their joint meanings and creating a sense of predictability. Some rules are explicit, such as "Don't ask Aunt Janet about her cancer" or "Nathan's diabetes is discussed only within the family." Other rules are implicit, such as those a child who learns by observing the behavior of other family members.

Rules may be categorized as *constitutive* and *regulative*. Constitutive rules establish what serves as acceptable or unacceptable communication. Family members model and instruct other members in what counts as being "respectful" or "nosy" or "caring." In one family it may be respectful to ask about an aunt's colitis every time you see a member of her family; in another family it may be considered as nosy to keep raising the subject. Regulative rules specify behavior—how, when, where and with whom to talk. For example, in one family the rule may be "Only ask about Jenny's chemotherapy treatments when you are alone with her." This may signal that you respect her privacy. In another family the rule may be "Never ask Jenny about her chemotherapy treatments. It upsets her to talk about it." Rules represent taken-for-granted ways of interacting until there are reasons to reconsider them. Rules may be challenged or varied as members age and as families are changed through circumstances such as adding in-laws or becoming a stepfamily. Health-related rules may be affected by a member's experience with a genetic disease that challenges the family's rules about privacy. For example, after being diagnosed with early-onset breast cancer, Jane was found to have a mutation in the breast-ovarian cancer predisposition gene *BRCA2*. Such a condition may challenge a rule about "not upsetting" Sara, Jane's sister, because it is deemed critical that she learn of her possible risk. It may also challenge the implicit rules related to cross-gender conversations. Whereas in the past breast cancer may have been a topic of discussion only for women in the family, a man's potential to be a carrier may move a female relative to urge him to be tested.

How Do Families Socialize Their Members?

The family is a primary source of gender identity [18], and a family's culture will impact any socialization practices. Children learn what it means to be masculine or feminine at an early age. Usually it is more acceptable for girls to act masculine than it is for boys to act feminine, leading to the claim that "overall, boys are more intensively and rigidly pushed to become masculine than girls are to become feminine" [18] (p. 168). Traditionally health-related responsibilities fall to female family members. Gender frequently impacts familial disclosure of genetic disease because women tend to be viewed as gatekeepers of such knowledge and as links to relatives in older generations. A study of Lynch syndrome (a hereditary cancer syndrome formerly called hereditary nonpolyposis colorectal cancer) found that women felt normal talking about health issues, whereas men did not. Men expressed a greater need for guidance or support in communicating with relatives about the disease [19]. This is particularly the case when the disease is perceived as feminine, such as HBOC, although males may be affected [4]. Frequently, women hold the power to set rules for disclosing health information.

The family also serves as a source for cultural identity. Ethnic heritage may dictate norms for communication, which may be maintained across generations. Research on Irish families indicates a strong privacy boundary [20], creating unwillingness to openly discuss private health issues. Similarly, Asian family members may express emotional problems in somatic terms rather than through direct verbal messages [21]. In contrast, members of Jewish families are more likely to prize verbal interaction; members of all ages are invited to make contributions to solving family problems [22], and family members may make health-related decisions to benefit their cultural community. For example, Warner, Curnow, Polglase, and Debinski [23] found that members of the Australian Ashkenazi Jewish community report a very high level of family-related motivation to be tested for colorectal cancer for altruistic reasons. In some cases genetic diseases are found extensively within cultural groups—such as sickle cell anemia within the African American community and Tay-Sachs disease within the Ashkenazi Jewish community—leading to community discussions of such diseases. Across cultural groups, certain family members may serve key roles in health decision making. Thus, the ways people make sense of health and illness varies greatly among cultures.

How Do Families Set Boundaries?

Every family engages in boundary management practices that affect how members deal with the outside world as well as with each other. An external boundary separates the family from its environment; an internal boundary separates individual members or a subgroup from other members or subgroups. Boundaries may be visualized as *(1)* rigid and inflexible, *(2)* permeable or flexible, or *(3)* diffuse or invisible. Boundaries provide access to how open or closed the family system is, and they are reflected in the rules for privacy or discussion of family matters. For example, an inflexible external boundary may be reflected in families that do not talk about their health conditions with outsiders and who resist outside intervention in family business. An inflexible internal boundary may become apparent when subgroups or individuals protect their privacy, even from other family members. Thus, in one family a diagnosis of the fatal neurodegenerative condition Huntington disease (HD) may be shared with members but kept from friends or coworkers; in another family such a diagnosis may be shared only with a partner and kept from children or siblings. In contrast, a diffuse external boundary may be revealed as a diagnosis of HD becomes known to multiple persons outside the family. Boundary management involves the processes used to set, maintain, or change boundaries. Rules, questions, and nonverbal messages represent examples of boundary management practices. According to Petronio [24], "Regulating boundary openness and closedness contributes to balancing the publicness or privacy of individuals. The regulation process is fundamentally communicative in nature" (p. 8).

Multiple factors alter family boundaries and privacy. The visibility or invisibility of a medical condition interacts with a family's ability to set their own boundaries. With certain diseases physical changes over time may force a revelation to others inside or outside the family. Individuals with Marfan syndrome, who tend to be tall and prone to dissection of the aorta, and their family members may not be able to maintain inflexible health boundaries; however, those with HH, which does not have visible manifestations, may be able to maintain personal or family privacy. Developmental life changes, such as when a child leaves home or plans to marry, frequently confront families with boundary management decisions. For example, Forrest and colleagues [4] found that in cases of HD and HBOC, many parents identified the correct time to talk about genetic history with their children was when "the first key life decision affected by the disease needed to be made" (p. 322), such as the point at which a child developed a serious romantic relationship, planned to marry, or was considering becoming a parent. Even marrying into a family with different boundaries may alter a person's boundary management practices because, in some cases, telling one spouse implies telling the couple because their internal boundaries are diffuse.

How Do Families Make Decisions?

Families may be viewed along a continuum ranging from position oriented to person oriented [25]. These concepts refer to the interaction of gender, age, power, and decision making. In position-oriented families, members' gender, age, and title establish expectation and regulations for individuals—essentially one is assigned certain scripts in life and is defined by his or her family label, such as grandmother or youngest son. For example, mothers are advisory to their husbands (who are the breadwinners) and are in charge of family health issues; sons are responsible for outdoor chores and are given more independence, whereas daughters are assigned a different set of chores and are given less independence. Grandparents are treated with respect, expected to be involved in caring for grandchildren, and given any assistance they require. On the other end of the continuum, members of person-oriented families are guided by qualities such as talent, interests, and availability. Therefore, a father may be primarily responsible for health care because he is a paramedic and is around frequently during the day. The middle daughter may be assigned the task of identifying and helping to purchase the family computer because of her extensive computer knowledge and skills. In certain families, when a child is diagnosed with a genetic disorder, the mother becomes the primary health manager and the father abides by her decision. On the other hand, a stepfather may become actively involved in his stepdaughter's health-care decisions because he is a scientist. In one family with a history of hereditary diffuse gastric cancer, a woman may be allowed to make the decision to get tested, whereas in another family, all medical decision making rests with a male adult or a dominant grandmother. Expectations for specific family members will surface when the family is confronted with health concerns.

FUNCTIONAL FAMILIES

Family researchers have struggled with the concept of a "normal" family, only to conclude that such an entity does not exist. Currently there is some agreement that characteristics of well-functioning families include the ability to adapt to *(1)* changes over the family's developmental life course and *(2)* unpredictable stresses and changing contexts. Although some families may adapt to changes rather well over decades, other families may be well functioning during certain periods and less so at other times. Studies of well-functioning families highlight how ethnicity and socioeconomic status may result in variability in what constitutes a well-functioning family. To better understand the well-functioning family, it is important to examine the concepts of cohesion and adaptability.

The *Circumplex Model* of marital and family systems [26, 27] proposes that there are three central dimensions to family communication: cohesion and adaptability as well as communication. These scholars develop the first two in their research and model, treating communication as a facilitating dimension that enables couples and families to move along the cohesion and adaptability dimensions.

Cohesion refers to the degree of emotional closeness between family members, including concepts such as "emotional bonding, boundaries, coalitions, time, space, friends, decision-making, interests and recreation" [26] (p. 145). There are four levels of cohesion that can be thought of as being on a continuum from very low to very high: disengaged, separated, connected, and enmeshed. At the lowest end is the disengaged family, in which family members display individuality and autonomy, with extreme emotional separateness. The next level is separated; these are family members who are primarily independent emotionally but also feel some sense of emotional closeness. Connected families are those that value emotional connectedness and loyalty, while still maintaining some individuality. Enmeshed families are at the highest level of emotional connectedness and are extremely close and loyal to the point that individuality is minimal [28]. In a disengaged family, the discovery of a genetic condition may be discussed factually, without attending to affected family members' emotions or the impact of one person's test results on other family members. For example, Andrew is a son, brother, and uncle, but these ties are quite shallow. He travels constantly for work and seldom appears at the few family events that occur each year. Issues of parental alcoholism dominated his childhood and these stresses resulted in each sibling seeking comfort from peers' families. When Andrew is diagnosed with a melanoma and learns that he has an inherited predisposition to this cancer, he is reluctant to inform the others for two reasons: he fears creating anxiety, a family trigger for drinking, and he feels unprepared for any serious emotional contact that might occur. He rationalizes that his lighter skin is more susceptible to such cancer than the darker skins of his siblings.

An enmeshed family may be so close emotionally that the reactions of one person are also experienced by enmeshed family members or, alternatively, the distinct privacy needs of the affected member are not recognized. For instance, Jade is a member of an enmeshed family, whose members are constantly in each others' lives. There is little privacy or individuality; adult family members socialize frequently, hold daily phone calls if they do not meet in person, and treat each others' homes as their own. When Jade is diagnosed with the hereditary heart condition hypertrophic cardiomyopathy after a series of fainting episodes in her late twenties, she becomes extremely anxious about the possibility that she may have a sudden cardiac arrest. She begins to call the cardiac genetics service frequently requesting an urgent appointment. Although she is given an appointment time, this panic has been transmitted to her immediate family. Jade is living independently, but her mother also begins to call the genetics service to emphasize Jade's situation and needs. Jade's mother and one of her sisters change their vacation plans to attend the session with Jade.

Adaptability is the extent to which a family is flexible in responding to stress and change. Again, four levels on a continuum describe the range of adaptability in families from least to most. Rigid families are those that have inflexible roles and strict rules for operating in an autocratic decision-making environment. The next level is structured; these are families where roles and rules are stable, though not absolutely inflexible. Their decision-making style is highly predictable. Flexible families are those that can easily change rules and roles and use negotiation as a primary decision-making process. At the highest level of adaptability is the chaotic family, in which there is nonexistent leadership, no predictable decision-making processes, and limited structure of rules and roles. Imagine the Marshalls, a rigid family in which Martin, a 66-year-old father and grandfather, is diagnosed with familial hypercholesterolemia, an inherited predisposition to high cholesterol levels. The established roles of the family are such that he would never talk with his adult children about a personal health issue; that is a role that his wife, Margaret, has always assumed. When his health-care provider suggests that he have a conversation with his children and grandchildren about this condition and their risk, he nods, but he never plans to hold such a conversation, as that does not fit with the communicative role he has in the family. If his wife is aware of this recommendation, she is likely to take on the role of communicating with their children. In contrast, when James, the father of the chaotic Morris family, faces a similar situation, communication in the family occurs in a scattergun fashion. Some members of the nuclear and extended family are given information (not always accurately) numerous times by different relatives, while others do not seem to be informed. Clearly cohesion and adaptability interact. If a family adheres to the theme "Think for yourself," it is likely to be a family that evidences moderate to low cohesion and high flexibility. Highly position-oriented families are more likely to be low in adaptability while maintaining strong external boundaries.

Most family scholars believe that well-functioning families are generally located somewhere in between the extremes of these continuums, whereas families that are not functioning well will be found at the extremes. This is not to say that well-functioning families will never move to an extreme point; families dealing with significant loss, shock, and painful change may find themselves at extreme points on the continuum for a period of time without being considered nonfunctional. For instance, news of a fatal genetic condition such as Duchenne muscular dystrophy in a 4-year-old boy may send a connected and structured family toward being enmeshed and rigid as everyone circles around the parents of the affected child and tries to regulate strictly how this news is managed and how the family members are expected to show support. Over the course of the next 12 months, as the family adjusts to their new circumstances, they move away from the enmeshed/rigid extreme back to a level of structure and connectedness closer to their previous level, although the communication patterns may have evolved to accommodate the inevitable changes within family life. However, when a family remains at an extreme point on one of the continuums for a long period, it is considered to be nonfunctional. A family may be nonfunctional before ever receiving genetic information, or the impact of genetic information may push a family to an extreme point on the continuum from which it is unable to return.

The idea that families may shift their patterns over time highlights another important concept of family communication: the management of predictable tensions, or relational dialectics. These dialectics (or opposing pulls) include separateness and connectedness, novelty and predictability, and openness and closedness. This approach contends that families are involved actively in managing constant tensions, and that they develop their meanings from their negotiations on multiple competing issues.

Dialectical tensions raise questions such as: How much openness or privacy works for each of us in this relationship? Family members manage these tensions through a variety of communicative strategies. These strategies include (1) choosing one of the opposing poles (e.g., disclosing everything and rejecting personal privacy), (2) adapting behavior to varying contexts or circumstances, (3) switching between one pole and the other, and (4) reframing the issue. For example, an adaptation may occur when a woman who has recently found out she is pregnant may expect openness from her husband's sibling about a genetic condition affecting his nephew—as she is concerned that her unborn child may be similarly affected—but wishes to maintain closedness about the fact that she is pregnant and how she may use the genetic information to access prenatal testing services. A father and son may reframe their reluctance to discuss genetic health issues as protection of the other's privacy.

CONCLUSION

Families are dynamic, complex, and ever changing. It is within the context of established communication patterns that families manage the communication regarding genetic information. In turn, the introduction of genetic information into a family system also impacts these communication patterns. The way in which families assimilate genetic information into their identity is affected by their meaning making of the information. Recognizing and choosing to work within families' communication cultures allows health-care practitioners to help families manage genetic information more effectively.

REFERENCES

1. Rolland JS. Families and genetic fate: A millenial challenge. *Families, Systems & Health* 1999;17:123–132.
2. Galvin KM, Bylund CL, Brommel BJ. *Family Communication: Cohesion and Change.* 7th ed. Boston: Pearson Education; 2008.
3. Peterson SK. The role of the family in genetic testing: Theoretical perspectives, current knowledge, and future directions. *Health Education & Behavior* 2005;32:627–639.
4. Forrest K, Simpson SA, Wilson BJ, van Teijlingen ER, McKee L, Haites N, et al. To tell or not to tell: Barriers and facilitators in family communication about genetic risk. *Clinical Genetics* 2003;64:317–326.
5. Stacey J. Gay and lesbian families are here: All our families are queer; Let's get used to it. In: Coontz S, Parson M, Raley G, eds. *American Families: A Multicultural Reader.* New York: Routledge; 1996:372–405.
6. Floyd K, Mikkelson AC, Judd J. Defining the family through relationships. In: Turner LH, West R, eds. *The Family Communication Sourcebook.* Thousand Oaks, CA: Sage; 2006:21–39.
7. Vangelisti AL. Introduction. In: Vangelisti AL, ed. *Handbook of Family Communication.* Mahwah, NJ: Erlbaum; 2004:xiii-xx.
8. Fields J. *America's Families and Living Arrangements: 2003.* Washington D.C.: U.S. Census Bureau; 2004.
9. Snapshot on adoption in Australia. Australian Institute of Health and Welfare; 2005. Available at: http://test.community.nsw.gov.au/DOCS/INSIDEOUT/629920809/PC_100722.htm. Accessed October 25, 2008.
10. New Zealand Family and Household Projections: 2001–2021. 2007. Available at: http:///www.stats.govt.nz/rdonlyres/953C3688–0. Accessed October 25, 2008.
11. Martin JA, Kung HC, Mathews TJ, Hoeyrt DM, Strobino B, Guyer B, et al. Annual summary of vital statistics: 2006. *Pediatrics* 2008;121:788–801.
12. Grall TS. Custodial mother and fathers and their child support: 2005. Retrieved from Current Population Reports, US Census Bureau, US Department of Commerce, 2007.

13. Le Poire B. Commentary on Part C. In: Floyd K, Morman MT, eds. *Widening the Family Circle: New Research on Family Communication*. Thousand Oaks, CA: Sage; 2006:189–192.

14. Galvin KM. Diversity's impact on defining the family: Discourse-dependence and identity. In: Turner LH, West R, eds. *The Family Communication Sourcebook*. Thousand Oaks, CA: Sage; 2006:3–19.

15. Pawlowski DR. Jelly beans and yo-yos: Perceptions of metaphors and dialectical tensions within the family. Central State Communication Association; Minneapolis, MN; 1996.

16. Caughlin JP. The demand/withdraw pattern of communication as a predictor of marital satisfaction over time. *Human Communication Research* 2002;28(1):49–85.

17. Wood JT. *Interpersonal Communication: Everyday Encounters*. Belmont, CA: Thomson/Wadsworth; 2007.

18. Wood JT. *Gendered Lives*. Belmont, CA: Thomson/Wadsworth; 2007.

19. Gaff CL, Collins V, Symes T, Halliday J. Facilitating family communication about predictive genetic testing: Probands' perceptions. *Journal of Genetic Counseling* 2005;14:133–140.

20. Galvin KM. It's not all blarney: Intergenerational transmission of communication patterns in Irish-American families. In: Cooper P, Calloway C, Simonds C, eds. *Intercultural Communication: A Text with Readings*. Boston: Allyn & Bacon; 2006.

21. Lee E, Mock MR. Asian families: An overview. In: McGoldrick M, Giordano J, Garcia-Preto N, eds. *Ethnicity and Family Therapy*. New York: The Guilford Press; 2005:269–289.

22. Rosen EJ, Weltman SF. Jewish families: An overview. In: McGoldrick M, Giordano J, Pearce JK, eds. *Ethnicity and Family Therapy*. 2nd ed. New York: Guilford Press; 1996:611–630.

23. Warner BJ, Curnow LJ, Polglase AL, Debinski HS. Factors influencing uptake of genetic testing for colorectal cancer risk in an Australian Jewish population. *Journal of Genetic Counseling* 2005;14:387–394.

24. Petronio S. *Boundaries of Privacy*. Albany, NY: State University of New York Press; 2002.

25. Bernstein B. A sociological approach to socialization: With some references to educability. In: Bernstein B, ed. *Class, Codes and Control*. London: Routledge & Kegan Paul; 1971:143–169.

26. Olson DH, ed. Circumplex model of marital and family systems. Family Focus on Death and Dying; 2000; Minneapolis, MN: National Council on Family Relations.

27. Olson DH, Sprenkle D, Russell C. Circumplex model of marital and family systems: Cohesion and adaptability dimensions, family types, and clinical applications. *Family Process* 1979;18(3–28):3–28.

28. Carnes P. *Contrary to Love*. Center City, MN: Hazelden; 1989.

2

CONCEPTS IN GENETIC HEALTH CARE

Clara L. Gaff & Sylvia A. Metcalfe

An understanding of genetics enables a deeper appreciation of the complex issues faced by families when passing on genetic information. This chapter provides a brief introduction to key aspects of genetic conditions, their impact on individuals and families, and specialist genetic services.

Families and society have long been aware that certain traits or medical conditions are inherited [1]. The work of Mendel and the discovery of the structure of DNA by Watson and Crick have added a scientific dimension to this awareness. (See Chapter 3 for more information about the public's awareness of genetic issues.) The enormous volume of research activity around genetics in the latter half of the twentieth century, including completion of the mapping and sequencing of the human genome [2, 3], has led to a greater understanding of the contribution of individual genes to both complex, multifactorial traits and disease and well-recognized inherited conditions. One of the consequences of this research activity is that individuals and families have greater access to information about the potential genetic basis of health conditions affecting them. For example, the number of clinically available tests for genetic conditions has more than doubled in the last 8 years [4].

The results of genetic tests form one type of information that may be sought or purposively conveyed between relatives. Others include family history information, such as the health of family members and the biological relationships between them; diagnosis of a genetic condition and related information, such as prognosis; and risk of occurrence or recurrence of a genetic condition, including the chance the condition may be passed on to offspring. We use the term *genetic information* here to broadly encompass these different types of information. The extent to which this communication occurs and is successful is likely to be influenced by many variables, including the medical and psychosocial impact of the condition. An appreciation of the diversity of genetic conditions, as well as the nature and ethos of the specialist genetic services in which family communication is often explicitly discussed, provides a context for the rest of the book. Therefore, in this chapter we consider some relevant medical, hereditary, and psychosocial aspects and implications of genetic conditions, as well as present an introduction to genetics services.

GENETIC CONDITIONS

Clinical Aspects

Although all genetic conditions share the characteristic of being inherited to some extent, as a single group they have little else in common medically. Rolland and Williams [5] have attempted to "describe and organize the inherent complexity of the genetic landscape" (p. 46) by developing a psychosocial typology of genetic disorders, based on the Family Systems Illness Model. The typology is based on four biological variables: the likelihood of developing the genetic condition; the overall clinical severity; timing of clinical onset in the lifecycle; and the existence of effective treatment or preventive measures. Although its relevance to family communication specifically has not yet been tested, it seems reasonable to hypothesize that these parameters may interact to influence aspects of family communication and thus may provide insight into the diversity of genetic conditions. For these reasons, each is considered in more detail.

First, the likelihood of developing a genetic condition depends in part upon the chance of inheriting sufficient disease-causing genetic changes, termed *mutations*, at birth. An explanation of the way in which genetic mutations cause conditions and can be inherited is presented below in the section *Inheritance*. The likelihood of developing a genetic condition also depends on (often unknown) genetic, environmental, and lifestyle factors and the interactions between these. Consequently, some genetic conditions show *reduced penetrance* (i.e., only a proportion of those individuals with the mutation(s) will develop clinical features) and/or *variable expressivity* (a range of severity, age of onset, and/or clinical signs and symptoms). These two concepts are exemplified by craniosynostosis (or "cloverleaf skull"), a dominant condition causing premature fusion of the sutures in the skull and resulting in facial deformity. Twenty percent of individuals with a mutation that has the potential to cause craniosynostosis never develop features of the condition (i.e., penetrance is 80%). Of those that do have craniosynostosis, there is variation in the way the condition is expressed, with some individuals having fusion of one suture, while others may have multiple sutures fused.

Variability may exist even within one family. The likelihood of developing a condition therefore depends on the inheritance pattern (determined by mutations) as well as the penetrance of the condition (influenced by genetic, environmental, and lifestyle factors), with further uncertainty arising from variability in the way the condition may manifest.

Second, clinical severity conveys the expected degree of disease burden, based on the onset, course, and outcome of the condition and the degree of disability it causes. This concept is of course not restricted to genetic conditions and the variability and impact of clinical severity are familiar to all, through their own experience of illness as well as their experience of illness in those around them.

The third variable is timing of onset. Rolland and Williams describe three time periods in which genetic conditions typically manifest: childhood and adolescence (0–20 years old), early-middle adulthood (20–60 years), and late onset (older than 60 years of age). These periods correspond to different developmental phases, the completion of which will be affected by the onset of the condition. For instance, the challenges faced by an adolescent diagnosed with a progressive muscle weakness in his early teens will be different from the challenges faced by a 30-year-old woman who is a carrier of fragile X syndrome and consequently has a risk of premature ovarian failure, as well as having a child with intellectual and developmental disability and/or autism.

The fourth variable is prevention and treatment. Some genetic conditions have effective interventions to delay or prevent clinical onset. Hereditary hemochromatosis, caused by iron overload, is an excellent example of such a condition: regular bloodletting or donation is sufficient to prevent clinical disease in individuals with two mutations causing the condition. Surveillance by colonoscopy of people with the hereditary bowel cancer condition Lynch syndrome (formerly known as hereditary nonpolyposis colorectal cancer) has been shown to reduce mortality [6]. In contrast, prevention of neurodegenerative genetic conditions such as Huntington disease (HD) or spinal cerebellar ataxia is not currently possible and treatment options are limited. Such categorizations, however, are not set in stone. Research into the early detection and treatment of many genetic conditions has already led to improvements in life span or outcome of many inherited conditions. The most striking example is perhaps phenylketonuria (PKU), where the identification of affected individuals through newborn screening programs and subsequent treatment by diet modification effectively prevents the mental retardation otherwise caused by the condition.

Psychosocial Aspects

Rolland and Williams' typology proposes that a condition which, for instance, affects only adults, has minor effects which are readily treated, and confers a relatively low risk to other family members is likely to have a different degree of impact on a family than one which is present at birth, life shortening, untreatable, and has a significant risk of recurrence in

Table 2.1   Social and Emotional Effects of Genetic Conditions

Social or Societal Effects

Family tension and conflict

Isolation

Parent–child communication difficulties

Family role adjustment

Stigma

Reduced life choices

Financial burden

Misinformation

Emotional Effects

Anxiety

- Own health
- Ability to cope with family member illness

Worry about risks to children

Guilt

- About passing a condition or mutation on to children
- About not having the condition or risk when other family members are affected

Anger

- Toward family members for disclosing or failing to disclose
- About the existential unfairness of nature

Uncertainty

Redemptive adjustment

- Positive effects of the condition in the longer term

Illness/disability

Early/untimely death and loss

Lack of diagnosis/inappropriate care (modifier)

Variability (modifier)

Adapted from: McAllister M, Payne K, Nicholls S, MacLeod R, Donnai D, Davies LM. Improving service evaluation in clinical genetics: Identifying effects of genetic diseases on individuals and families. *Journal of Genetic Counseling.* 2007 Feb;16(1):71–83.

subsequent pregnancies. McAllister et al. [7] consider the *nature* of the impact of genetic conditions, pointing out that when families "talked about the physical, practical or medical effects of genetic diseases… it seemed their biggest concerns were about the social and emotional consequences of these" (p. 75). A growing body of research documents the social and emotional impact of specific genetic conditions. In Table 2.1 a summary is given of the spectrum of social and emotional effects of genetic diseases on individuals and families identified by McAllister and colleagues. It is clear that many of these effects relate either directly or indirectly to family communication. Effects such as family tension and conflict, parent–child communication difficulties and family role adjustment highlight some of the potentially negative impacts of genetic diseases on family communication generally. Emotional effects, such as anxiety, worry, guilt, and anger may also affect communication within the family.

GENETIC SERVICES

Traditionally, much of the diagnosis, testing, and information provision for genetic conditions have been provided by specialist genetic services. The focus of these services has evolved with advances in the understanding of genetic disease and availability of genetic testing: from a medical preventative model with limited counseling to a more sophisticated approach recognizing that "although families often come to genetic counseling seeking information, they cannot effectively process or act on what they have learnt until they have dealt with the powerful reactions such information can evoke" [8] (p. 4). Clearly, this requires the practitioner to attend to both the cognitive and emotional dimensions, as reflected in the National Society of Genetic Counselors' definition of genetic counseling: "the process of helping people understand and adapt to the medical, psychological and familial implications of genetic contributions to disease" [9]. This definition emphasizes that genetic counseling integrates activities relating to interpretation of family and medical history, education about the condition and its management, and counseling to promote informed choices and adaptation to the risk or condition. It appears that this dual focus is also valued by clients of genetic services [10, 11]. Both face-to-face consultations and telephone counseling are established practice in genetic counseling [12] and telemedicine is increasingly considered as an option for the delivery of genetic services.

Walker [8] suggests that genetic services operate on a number of assumptions and philosophies: voluntary utilization of services; equal access to services; the importance of patient education; the complete disclosure of relevant information; nonprescriptive or nondirective counseling; attention to psychosocial and affective dimensions; and confidentiality and protection of privacy. As she acknowledges, some of these are not always achieved (e.g., equal access), some are open to interpretation and are consequently the subject of debate (e.g., nondirectiveness) while others raise tensions (e.g., respecting one individual's confidentiality may compromise access of their relatives to genetic services). Nonetheless, they serve to illustrate the desire of genetics practitioners to provide equitable, person- and family-centered services. Certainly, Rogers' Person-Centered Counseling is the dominant counseling approach of genetic counselors [13], although in practice some genetic counselors appear to prefer an "education-teaching" approach, focusing on information provision, while others prefer a psychosocial model that recognizes the importance of responding to the client's emotional state [14, 15]. A recent genetic counseling model, The Reciprocal Engagement Model, recognizes the centrality of the relationship between counselor and client [16] and is discussed further in Chapters 11 and 15.

Genetics practice intrinsically involves family communication. First, a key component of genetic evaluation is an accurate family history. This is provided by the client and relies on their knowledge of family members' health and on their ability and willingness to gather from relatives additional information deemed necessary by the health-care practitioner [17].

Second, genetic assessments commonly yield information that is relevant to members of the client's family. The vast majority of genetic practitioners internationally state that discussion about the implications of genetic information for other family members is always a component of their consultations and that they rely on the client to pass this information on [18]. This is consistent with a belief that they have a responsibility that extends beyond the patient to at-risk family members [19]. Certainly clients of genetic services value the potential benefit that a genetic consultation may bring to current and future family members [20, 21].

INHERITANCE

When a person asks if she or other family members are at risk for a particular condition in the family, health-care practitioners determine whether there is likely to be an inherited component to developing the condition and, if so, its inheritance pattern. To give more precise information about an individual's own status, genetic testing may be necessary. The following sections serve as an introduction to genetics, inheritance, and genetic testing, providing an explanation of some of the language and concepts commonly presented to families in these consultations.

Genomes, Genes, and Chromosomes

How a person looks (physical characteristics); how the person's body digests and metabolizes food, medicines, and drugs (biochemical characteristics); how the person's body responds to changes in environment (physiological characteristics), and the person's personality, mood, and so on (behavioral characteristics) are determined to a greater or lesser extent by a person's genes. These characteristics also result from the way in which a person's genes interact with the environment; for example, while the genetic makeup of an individual may predispose him or her to obesity, the individual's weight will be determined by the interaction of these genes and their lifestyle (diet, exercise, drugs, and possibly other factors such as sleep).

A person's genes are contained within his or her *genome*. The *genome* is a term used to describe a person's entire genetic instructions that are coded within that person's DNA. DNA is a long string of specific chemicals with variations to the order or sequence of these chemicals such that each person's DNA sequence is unique. This DNA is divided up into discrete packages called *chromosomes*. These are stored in the nucleus of the majority of cells in the human body. A gene is a region of DNA that controls an inherited characteristic. A single chromosome therefore contains many hundreds or thousands of individual genes. To use an analogy, the genome is like a music collection. Each album in the collection contains many tracks, in the same way that each chromosome contains many genes. Looking at an additional level of detail: the individual notes that are combined to make the tracks are like the individual DNA chemicals which are combined to make the gene sequence.

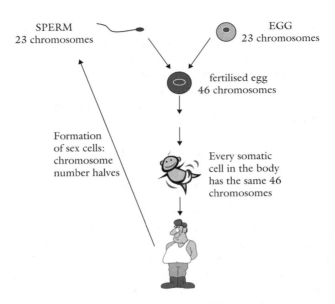

Figure 2.1   Chromosome number and cell type.

Almost all cells in the body contain chromosomes. These cells can be categorized into two types: somatic and sex cells. Sex cells are the sperm and eggs, the cells by which genetic material is passed on from parent to child. The rest of the cells in the body are termed somatic cells. Somatic cells and sex cells have the same genetic information, but in differing amounts.

Looking first at somatic cells, the nucleus in every somatic cell contains 23 matched pairs of chromosomes, or 46 chromosomes in all. Two of these pairs of chromosomes are designated the sex chromosomes (X and Y): males have an X and a Y chromosome, while females have two X chromosomes. The remaining 22 pairs are called autosomal chromosomes. Each pair of autosomal chromosomes has the same genes. So the majority of genes are also present in pairs, although the exact DNA sequence of each of the pair might be different. When the DNA sequence of each of the two genes is identical, we say that the genes are *homozygous*, and when they are different, we say they are *heterozygous*. Typically the information present in both copies of a gene is needed for the cell to make the product of that gene. Therefore, genes act like a recipe and the products of genes contribute to all of the characteristics mentioned above.

The genetic material in somatic cells influences the body's characteristics and functioning, but it is not passed on to future children. Therefore, if a mutation occurs randomly in a somatic cell, it will not be passed on to that person's children. Genetic material is instead passed on to future generations through the sex cells, or the egg and sperm (Fig. 2.1). These contain *one* copy of each of the 23 chromosomes, instead of 23 *pairs* of chromosomes. Therefore, each sex cell contains half the number of chromosomes compared with the somatic cells. At conception, the 23 chromosomes from the egg and 23 chromosomes from the sperm come together to make the pairs which are present in the somatic cells.

Mutations

The sequence of a gene determines the function of each gene. Changes to the sequence of the DNA may simply give rise to normal variation (with no impact on normal function of the gene product), while other changes may be harmful because they can alter how a gene is expressed or how the gene product functions and so can cause genetic conditions. These latter changes are called *mutations*. The nature of the mutation and the location and function of the specific gene(s) involved determine the nature of the genetic condition and also its pattern of inheritance. Many genetic conditions that are well characterized involve mutations in single genes, whereas more complex conditions, such as diabetes, asthma, dementia, and cardiovascular disease, are caused by mutations in multiple genes with additional environmental influences. Some genetic conditions are due to larger changes in the genome that give rise to chromosomal abnormalities, that is, changes to chromosome numbers (aneuploidies) or changes to chromosome structure. The most common aneuploidy is trisomy 21 or Down syndrome, where there are three copies of a particular chromosome (chromosome 21) instead of the usual pair. This extra copy means that there are too many gene products arising from these chromosomes, leading to the clinical features typically seen in Down syndrome. Changes to chromosome structure include rearrangements (often referred to as translocations) as well as deletions and duplications. When these abnormalities involve entire chromosomes or parts of chromosomes, typically many genes along the length of the chromosome(s) are affected, thereby causing more systemic effects, often called syndromes.

Some mutations or chromosomal abnormalities occur spontaneously or sporadically (de novo) early on in development of the embryo or in somatic cells at various stages throughout life. These are not present in the person's parents. Cancer, for instance, occurs as a result of mutations in several genes involved in cell division and cell death pathways, which lead to uncontrolled cell division and the formation of a cancer. These mutations typically occur in somatic cells during the lifetime of the individual. Hence, the cancer is not "passed on" but is sporadic. Only when a mutation in a cancer-predisposing gene, such as *BRCA1*, is passed on through the egg or sperm is the cancer considered familial or inherited.

Patterns of Inheritance

Inherited genetic conditions usually display specific patterns of inheritance in a family. The pattern of inheritance is determined by the location of the gene (on either an autosomal or sex chromosome) and the number

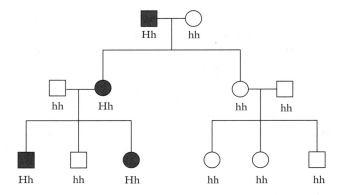

Figure 2.2   Pattern of inheritance of an autosomal dominant condition (e.g., Huntington disease). The square symbols refer to males, and the circle symbols refer to females in the family. Shaded symbols refer to persons who are affected with the condition. Only affected individuals have one copy of the gene with the mutation causing the condition, indicated here by "H," whereas "h" represents the normal gene.

of copies of the gene necessary for normal functioning (one or two). There are three major patterns of inheritance referred to in this book: autosomal dominant, autosomal recessive, and X linked.

For *autosomal dominant* conditions, such as HD, a mutation in a single copy of the specific gene (found on an autosomal chromosome) can cause the condition. Or to put it another way, normal function requires two unaltered copies of the gene to be present. In genetic counseling consultations, this may be explained as needing two workers to get a job done. If one of those workers is making a lot of mistakes, the good worker cannot make up for the mistakes and the job is not done properly. The effects of this may be obvious at birth for some conditions, or it may take many years to take effect. For autosomal dominant conditions, the risk of inheriting the mutation from an affected parent is 50% or 1 chance in 2. As Figure 2.2 shows, there are often multiple affected family members through successive generations.

Autosomal recessive conditions, such as cystic fibrosis (CF), a fatal condition which affects the lungs, or PKU, only develop if two mutations are present (one from each parent) in each copy of the specific gene. Using the worker analogy again, in this case both workers are making mistakes, so the job is not completed. However, if one worker is doing the job correctly, then the job will get done. Therefore, people with only one mutation (called carriers) are usually unaffected. Two healthy carriers each with a single mutation for the condition therefore have a 25% chance (1 chance in 4) in each pregnancy of the child inheriting both mutations and being affected. This is demonstrated on the family tree in Figure 2.3. In autosomal recessive conditions, affected family members

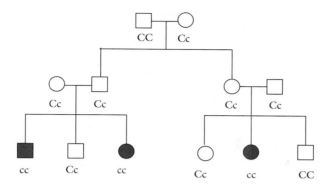

Figure 2.3 Pattern of inheritance of an autosomal recessive condition, such as cystic fibrosis (CF), where "c" represents the copy with the disease-causing mutation and "C" represents the normal gene. Note that parents of children who are affected with an autosomal recessive condition are unaffected, obligate carriers.

may appear to be scattered in the generations and may not show any family history at all, especially where the mutation involved is rare in the population.

Finally, some conditions are due to mutations in specific genes on the X chromosome and these conditions show *X-linked inheritance,* for example, hemophilia (Fig. 2.4). Commonly, these conditions require one copy of the gene to be functional. As females have two copies of the X chromosome, a mutation in one gene copy is unlikely to cause the condition. In contrast, males have only one X chromosome, so inheritance of an X chromosome with a mutated gene is more likely to give rise to symptoms. Affected males can never pass the X chromosome to their sons, only to their daughters. Females with only one affected X chromosome are likely to be unaffected carriers and have a 50% chance of passing on the affected X chromosome to their children.

These different examples of patterns of inheritance of mutated genes in families illustrate the importance of having an accurate family history and the varying risk implications of affected and carrier status for other family members.

Genetic Testing

Essentially, genetic testing in clinical settings aims to identify a mutation or mutations causing a specific inherited condition. However, the context and nature of the testing varies. These are summarized in Table 2.2. The misconception that a simple genetic test is available to definitively answer people's questions about their future risk of disease appears to be common. While there has been a rapid increase in the number of genetic tests available, the information provided by these tests can be limited and the relief from uncertainty sought by some is not necessarily realized [22].

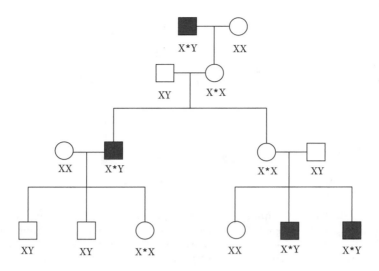

Figure 2.4   Pattern of inheritance of an X-linked condition, such as hemophilia, where "X*" represents X chromosome with the disease-causing gene, "X" represents the chromosome with the normal gene, and Y represents the Y chromosome. Note that fathers who are affected can have carrier daughters but cannot transmit the affected X chromosome to their sons.

Table 2.2   Types of Genetic Testing

Diagnostic testing	Testing of a person who is affected with a genetic condition to identify the causative mutation(s)
Carrier testing	Testing of a healthy person for the presence of a single mutation that is unlikely to be detrimental to his or her health. The healthy person usually has a family history of the condition and the family-specific mutation(s) are tested for. There is a risk of having an affected child with a carrier of the same condition (e.g., cystic fibrosis, or CF)
Carrier screening	Testing of healthy people for mutations that are relatively common within a population, causing a condition which is more frequent in that population. This testing is performed when there is no family history of the condition or the causative mutation in a family is unknown. It usually identifies those more likely to have an affected child (e.g., CF)
Predictive testing	Testing of an apparently unaffected person to determine whether he or she has a genetic mutation(s) that increases the risk of developing a health condition later in life (e.g., hereditary cancer)
Presymptomatic testing	Testing of an apparently unaffected person to determine whether he or she will develop a health condition later in life (e.g., Huntington disease)

Typically, a genetic test can only say if a specific gene mutation is present and cannot provide definitive information about variable aspects of the condition, such as the severity, penetrance, age of onset, and/or specific physical features. Many genetic tests are now available through the

Internet (direct-to-consumer testing), sometimes without the requirement for interpretation of results and counseling by clinicians, with the consequence that accessing information about one's genes is becoming easier. Recently there has been considerable publicity about testing for risk of common conditions such as type 2 diabetes, heart disease (atrial fibrillation), glaucoma, prostate and breast cancer, Alzheimer disease, celiac disease, obesity, osteoarthritis, multiple sclerosis, and Parkinson disease.

Typically companies offer testing to consumers to provide them with information that can help them "detect health conditions early, reduce their effects or even prevent them entirely"[23] (Direct-to-consumer testing is discussed in more depth in Chapter 3). However, there remains much that is still unknown in terms of how genes and the environment interact and combine to influence the health of each person, and this information may not necessarily be clinically useful, either to the individual or to other family members. At the time of writing, there is little evidence to support the value of these tests, as evidenced by the disclaimers given by the companies, which often say that they do not provide medical advice, diagnosis, or treatment. In many instances these companies are testing for variants associated with a condition, rather than known mutations.

Interpretation of genetic testing results requires skilled health-care practitioners. At first glance, a genetic testing result may seem simple: a mutation is either present or not. However, the test results need to be interpreted in the context of the family and what is known about causation of the condition in the family. For instance, the implications of a "mutation negative" result depend on whether a mutation is known to cause a condition in the family. If predictive testing or carrier testing is performed for a known causative mutation, then its absence is effectively definitive. The person is very unlikely to develop the inherited form of the condition (but may have a residual risk due to the incidence of the condition in the population generally, e.g., cancer). In contrast, when testing is being performed to either attempt to identify a causative mutation (mutation detection) or for mutations commonly found in a population, then the absence of a mutation is less than definitive. There are several reasons for this uncertainty: for some genetic conditions, there may be hundreds of mutations identified in a single gene, and it may not be feasible to test for all these; technical limitations may have prevented the identification of a mutation(s); or the condition may be caused by mutation(s) in an as-yet-unknown gene. In this context, failure to find a mutation is considered "uninformative," as it does not completely exclude the possibility that a mutation exists. For carrier screening, in which a defined panel of mutations is tested, there remains a residual risk of being a carrier as only the most common mutations are tested. Thus, it remains possible that, while the person has been shown not to carry a common mutation, he or she could carry one of the rarer mutations that has not been tested. For example, there are 1600 gene mutations known to cause CF, while screening for carriers is performed by testing for only a small number of the most common of these.

A final complication of interpretation is the *variant of uncertain significance* or *unclassified variant*. While some mutations are clearly disease causing, the impact of others on health are unclear. There may be insufficient information to determine whether the gene change is disease causing or part of the natural variation between individuals.

OPTIONS

Individuals can be motivated to share genetic information by a sense of responsibility to their relatives and a desire to provide them with options [24–27], which they can choose to pursue or ignore. Broadly speaking, these options relate to reproduction or to personal health, though these are not mutually exclusive. For example, a woman who experiences early menopause might be found to be a carrier of fragile X syndrome. This information has implications for her sisters—who are also at risk of being carriers—as carriers have an increased risk of developing early menopause, as well as a risk of having a child affected with fragile X syndrome.

Reproductive Choices

The range of reproductive choices available to couples now is shown in Table 2.3. Prior to prenatal diagnosis, couples had the options of choosing to avoid having biological children, to adopt, or to "take their chances." The introduction of testing for genetic conditions on fetal cells (chorionic villi or aminocytes) has meant that couples have an additional choice: to learn whether their pregnancy is affected by the specific condition of concern. This has been something of a double-edged sword, with people also required to face difficult choices about termination of affected pregnancies and dealing with the emotional impact of these choices on their experience of pregnancy. Despite lay beliefs that prenatal diagnosis is readily available for any condition of concern, in fact for most inherited genetic conditions it is necessary to know three pieces of information: *(1)* the precise condition in the family, *(2)* the mutation(s) causing the condition, and *(3)* that the parents seeking prenatal diagnosis are in fact carriers of these mutations.

A more recent alternative to prenatal diagnosis is preimplantation genetic diagnosis (PGD). Performed as part of artificial reproductive

Table 2.3 Reproductive Options

Prenatal screening for aneuploidies
Prenatal diagnosis for chromosome anomalies and/or specific genetic condition
Pre-implantation diagnosis for specific genetic condition
Donor gametes
Adoption
No (further) children

technologies (i.e., in vitro fertilization [IVF]), preimplantation genetic diagnosis ensures that only embryos shown not to have the condition are implanted. Preimplantation genetic diagnosis is generally only available if the couple is known to have a high risk of having an affected child and an accurate genetic test for the condition is possible. In some jurisdictions, it is necessary to obtain consent of a statutory government body before PGD can be performed. The issues inherent in PGD are discussed further in greater depth elsewhere [28]. Of course, an increasing array of options does not mean that they must be utilized, and some people choose not to undergo any of these procedures.

Personal Health Choices

Decisions relating to personal health are arguably more common for conditions with an onset in the adolescent or adult years. If the mutation(s) causing an adult-onset condition is known, then apparently healthy at-risk family members can have predictive or presymptomatic testing to determine if they will, or are more likely to, develop the condition at some point in the future. Predictive testing is well established for many hereditary cancer, cardiac, and neurodegenerative conditions. When there are management options available for risk reduction or early treatment, predictive testing can provide medical benefit by identifying those that carry the mutation and should consider these options and also those that have not inherited the mutation and do not therefore require medical intervention. However, treatment or preventative options are not always available and choices then relate purely to life planning, relief of uncertainty, and clarification of children's risks.

CONCLUSION

This chapter has provided only a simple introduction to the complexities of inheritance, genetic conditions, their psychosocial impact, and the genetic services that provide genetic counseling for families with or at risk of these conditions. The state of knowledge about genetic mechanisms that cause disease and the interaction between these mechanisms and environmental factors is growing rapidly. Skilled health practitioners will increasingly be needed to help family members integrate medical and scientific knowledge with their personal experiences of the condition, be aware of the implications for their relatives, as well as assist them to consider informing the relevant family members.

REFERENCES

1. Richards M. Families, kinship and genetics. In: Marteau TRM, ed. *The Troubled Helix: Social and Psychological Implications of the New Human Genetics.* Cambridge, England: Cambridge University Press; 1996:249–273.

2. Lander ES, Linton LM, Birren B, Nusbaum C, Zody MC, Baldwin J, et al. Initial sequencing and analysis of the human genome. *Nature* 2001 Feb 15;409(6822):860–921.

3. Venter JC, Adams MD, Myers EW, Li PW, Mural RJ, Sutton GG, et al. The sequence of the human genome. *Science* 2001 Feb 16;291(5507):1304–1351.

4. Gene Clinics. Growth of laboratory directory. 2008. Available at: http://www.ncbi.nlm.nih.gov/projects/GeneTests/static/whatsnew/labdirgrowth.shtml. Accessed December 20, 2009.

5. Rolland JS, Williams JK. Toward a psychosocial model for the new era of genetics. In: Miller SM, McDaniel SH, Rolland JS, Feetham SL, eds. *Individuals, Families and the New Era of Genetics*. New York: WW Norton & Company; 2006:36–75.

6. Jarvinen H, Aarnio M, Mustonen H, Aktan-Collan K, Aaltonen L, Peltomaki P, et al. Controlled 15-year trial on screening for colorectal cancer in families with hereditary nonpolyposis colorectal cancer. *Gastroenterology* 2000;118(5):829–834.

7. McAllister M, Davies L, Payne K, Nicholls S, Donnai D, MacLeod R. The emotional effects of genetic diseases: implications for clinical genetics. *American Journal of Medical Genetics Part A* 2007 Nov 15;143(22):2651–2661.

8. Walker AP. The practice of genetic counseling. In: Baker DL, Scheuette JL, Uhlmann WR, eds. *A Guide to Genetic Counseling*. New York: Wiley-Liss; 1998:1–26.

9. Resta R, Biesecker BB, Bennett RL, Blum S, Hahn SE, Strecker MN, et al. A new definition of genetic counseling: National Society of Genetic Counselors' Task Force report. *Journal of Genetic Counseling* 2006 Apr;15(2):77–83.

10. McAllister M, Payne K, Macleod R, Nicholls S, Donnai D, Davies L. What process attributes of clinical genetics services could maximise patient benefits? *European Journal of Human Genetics* 2008 Dec;16(12):1467–1476.

11. Wang C, Gonzalez R, Merajver SD. Assessment of genetic testing and related counseling services: Current research and future directions. *Social Science and Medicine (1982)* 2004 Apr;58(7):1427–1442.

12. Wang VO. What is and is not telephone counseling? *Journal of Genetic Counseling* 2000;9(1):73–82.

13. McCarthy Veach P, Le Roy BS, Bartels DM. *Facilitating the Genetic Counselling Process: A Practice Manual*. NewYork: Springer; 2003.

14. Ellington L, Baty BJ, McDonald J, Venne V, Musters A, Roter D, et al. Exploring genetic counseling communication patterns: The role of teaching and counseling approaches. *Journal of Genetic Counseling* 2006 Jun;15(3):179–189.

15. Kessler S. Psychological aspects of genetic counseling. IX. Teaching and counseling. *Journal of Genetic Counseling* 1997;6(3):287–295.

16. Veach PM, Bartels DM, Leroy BS. Coming full circle: a reciprocal-engagement model of genetic counseling practice. *Journal of Genetic Counseling* 2007 Dec;16(6):713–728.

17. Adelsward V, Sachs L. The messenger's dilemmas - giving and getting information in genealogical mapping for hereditary cancer. *Health, Risk and Society* 2003;5(2):125–138.

18. Forrest LE, Delatycki MB, Skene L, Aitken M. An international online survey of genetic health professionals' practice involving family communication. *European Journal of Human Genetics* 2008;18(S A-1035 EMPAG).

19. Parker M, Lucassen A. Concern for families and individuals in clinical genetics. *Journal of Medical Ethics* 2003;29:70–73.

20. McAllister M, Payne K, Macleod R, Nicholls S, Dian D, Davies L. Patient empowerment in clinical genetics services. *Jounral of Health Psychology* 2008 Oct;13(7):895–905.

21. Nisselle A, Forbes R, Bankier A, Hughes E, Aitken M. Consumer contribution to the delivery of genetic health services. *American Journal of Medical Genetics Part A* 2008 Sep 1;146A(17):2266–2274.

22. van Zuuren FJ, van Schie EC, van Baaren NK. Uncertainty in the information provided during genetic counseling. *Patient Education and Counseling.* 1997 Sep-Oct;32(1–2):129–139.

23. Navigenics. Genetics and health: powerful steps towards prevention. 2009. Available at: http://www.navigenics.com/visitor/genetics_and_health/. Accessed July 14, 2009

24. Gaff CL, Collins V, Symes T, Halliday J. Facilitating family communication about predictive genetic testing: Probands' perceptions. *Journal of Genetic Counseling* 2005 Apr;14(2):133–140.

25. McGivern B, Everett J, Yager GG, Baumiller RC, Hafertepen A, Saal HM. Family communication about positive BRCA1 and BRCA2 genetic test results. *Genetics in Medcine* 2004 Nov-Dec;6(6):503–509.

26. Forrest K, Simpson SA, Wilson BJ, van Teijlingen ER, McKee L, Haites N, et al. To tell or not to tell: Barriers and facilitators in family communication about genetic risk. *Clinical Genetics* 2003 Oct;64(4):317–326.

27. Ormond KE, Mills PL, Lester LA, Ross LF. Effect of family history on disclosure patterns of cystic fibrosis carrier status. *American Journal of Medical Genetics* 2003 May 15;119(1):70–77.

28. Knoppers BM, Bordet S, Isasi RM. Preimplantation genetic diagnosis: An overview of socio-ethical and legal considerations. *Annual Review of Genomics and Human Genetics* 2006;7:201–221.

29. McAllister M, Payne K, Nicholls S, MacLeod R, Donnai D, Davies LM. Improving service evaluation in clinical genetics: Identifying effects of genetic diseases on individuals and families. *Journal of Genetic Counseling* 2007 Feb;16(1):71–83.

3

SOCIETAL, EXPERT, AND LAY INFLUENCES

Roxanne Parrott, Michelle Miller-Day, Kathryn Peters, & James Dillard

Families are influenced by many messages about genetics and health, which then affect communication with health-care practitioners and communication within the family. Using a discourse approach, this chapter identifies the various sources of these messages and explains the influences they might exert.

At the start of the twenty-first century, publication of a working draft of the human genome sequence appeared in special issues of the journals *Science* (February 16, 2001) and *Nature* (February 15, 2001). Most families, of course, did not read these articles, but the news coverage and fanfare with which the research was received reached anyone watching televised reports or reading newspaper or online headlines. The stories suggest promise for revolutionizing medical care and preventing disease. In reality, the results of this research are far from therapeutic. Rather, this research was only a beginning, motivating patients and their families to ask questions about the role of genetics in health, while leaving clinical and public health professionals to answer those questions. As a result, our current era of "genomic health care" includes efforts to educate and train a wide range of health-care practitioners to guide the understanding of families with genetic concerns. The time and expertise that various health-care practitioners have to bring to conversations with families vary, as does the knowledge families bring into these interactions, affecting the outcomes arising from these consultations. Thus, how will families decide whether to be tested for these genes linked to health, nutrition, and even aging? How will family members explain to one another that they need more or less of a medication than some other families because a genetic test says their make-up enables their bodies to more readily metabolize important drugs? How will they understand the validity of needing to supplement with some vitamins in excessive amounts based on having inherited mutations linked to deficits in uptake and use? Why will families even be motivated to seek testing when possible employment or insurance discrimination looms at the end of results? In this chapter, we examine the influences that are often implicitly (and only sometimes explicitly) considered as families communicate about genetics and health. We apply a multiple discourse approach [1, 2] to this analysis of communication with families about genetics and health.

What is a discourse approach? At the broadest level, the term *discourse* encompasses conversations we have, talk we overhear others having, and dialogues in decision-making bodies (e.g., government), as well as a whole spectrum of verbal, visual, and nonverbal messages coming from different sources and through different modalities. A discourse approach emphasizes that, despite this vast array of sources and content, patterns appear across texts, messages, talk, dialogue, or conversation and reflect the context in which they occur [3]. As suggested by Figure 3.1, family communication about genetics and health simultaneously reflects three discourse fields: societal, expert, and lay domains. While only one arena may be the explicit focus, acknowledging the implicit influence of all spheres may enhance understanding about what takes place when families talk about genetics among themselves and with health-care providers. Contemplating communication about genetics in families from a discourse perspective enables one to consider the bigger picture by challenging one to step back from the individual theories and research. The ability to sort through a maze of sometimes confusing, contentious, and conflicting content can be enhanced from this more macro view.

Considering the bigger picture can enhance genetic counselors' and other health-care practitioners' communication with patients in several ways. First, it can lead to a more refined understanding of a patient's perspective, an important prerequisite to patient-centered care. For instance, understanding the religious discourse of a particular faith may help the practitioner to understand why a patient is reluctant to tell her sister about a diagnosis that could lead to suggesting the use of invasive fetal therapies such as blood or stem cell transfusion, gene therapy, or surgery which would rarely be approved within their religious doctrine. Second, awareness of these discourses may assist the counselor in helping a patient to plan how she will talk to her family. For example, being aware of images related to genetic mutations presented in movies or other entertainment venues suggests a starting place to discuss the meaning and implications of inheriting a mutation. Third, awareness of discourse about insurance or employment discrimination may contribute to practitioners' efforts to explain how information about a patient's genetic

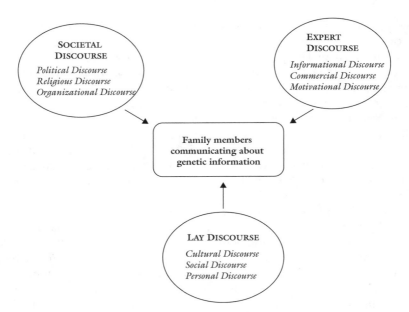

Figure 3.1   Types of discourse.

health will be safeguarded. For these and a myriad of other issues that contribute to the ways that interactions unfold for families when discussing genetics and health with counselors and other practitioners, a macro framework relating to the multiple discourses about health warrants consideration.

SOCIETAL DISCOURSE ABOUT GENETICS AND HEALTH

Societal discourse is the talk representing nations, rather than individuals, that we hear expressed in the news, that we talk about at the dinner table, and that we read about in Internet headlines. This discourse sometimes focuses on health and health care, addressing the allocation and use of a nation's resources, such as dollars for research and monies for health-care delivery. Societal discourse about health and health care is shaped by political, religious, and organizational agendas that guide decisions that lead to health knowledge and services [4]. This communication may not have anything explicitly to do with health education and everything to do with what is known about health and how this knowledge will be used to make diagnoses. Debates about what research to fund and who gets how much care at what expense is based on evidence that comes from many disciplines, including epidemiology, which provides support to determine how many people may be affected by a condition and its consequences [5]. Societal decisions about the allocation of scarce resources are frequently guided by the numbers of persons affected by a condition or its severity. Knowledge and comprehension of the patterns of health and disease are used in formal ways to encourage decision makers (such as law makers) to manage limited health resources and deliver health services in particular ways.

For families, their own communication about genetics and health, and the communication that they encounter in public health and clinical messages, reflects research completed and research yet to be done. Thus, prior to the identification of a link between thrombosis and the Factor V Leiden mutation, health-care practitioners could not talk with accuracy to families about possible genetic predispositions to risk of forming blood clots. With research dollars allocated to understanding the role of genetics in health and the findings linking mutations in the Factor V gene to thrombosis, clinical communication can reflect this new knowledge. Public health messages may follow, as in the case of the U.S. acting Surgeon General's "call to action to prevent deep vein thrombosis and pulmonary embolism" [6]. The press release emphasized the numbers of Americans affected, "350,000 to 600,000 each year," with "at least 100,000 deaths each year," and a role for "an inherited blood clotting disorder." Families thus reflect the politics associated with genetics and health when communicating about these issues, including ethical, legal, and social effects.

Political Discourse: Government and More

If an employer, or educator, or insurer can make the case that the "predicted" future status of their client matters, then discrimination—denial of opportunity for medical care, work, or education—can occur with impunity. Indeed, predictive genetic typing may create an underclass of individuals whose genes seem to have marked them for the nowhere track. [7] (p. 167)

Macro-level decisions linked to politics and government in society affect micro-level interactions about health, including not just what we talk about in a general way, but what we have to talk about in the first place. While doctors seek information that promotes the ability to diagnose conditions and prescribe suitable treatments, these conversations are guided by the existing state of knowledge. The knowledge base that is used to guide communication about genetic health depends fundamentally upon the origins and outcomes of debate by policy makers and funders about the status of knowledge and the need for research. That is because in the United States, France, Canada, and many other nations, political debates about whether to support some research compared to other research ultimately determines what research is funded and, thus, what knowledge will be generated and amplified.

The course of medical research toward the achievement of mapping the human genome included Mendel's discovery of the laws of heredity, identifying DNA as hereditary material, determining the structure of DNA, understanding the genetic code, developing recombinant DNA technologies, and discovering automated methods for DNA sequencing [8]. The research necessary to understand how genes and environments interact requires families to participate. Families are solicited to cooperate in giving lifestyle information, family health histories, personal medical information, *and* biological specimens [9]. Why? So that genetic databanks might be assembled with linkages to the multiple determinants of health, promoting better research and presumably the development of better treatments for many common diseases. This is largely the promise associated with an era of genomic health care in which genes have assumed a prominent role. But to achieve it, families will have to disclose information in ways like they never have before, and doing so will demand that they can trust that their participation will not be used to disadvantage them.

The study of political discourse highlights its strategic nature with links to coercion, information control, opposition and protest, as well as legitimization [10]. The implications of this reality make consideration of the role of political discourse on families' communication about genetic concerns critical. Such an analysis should address whether families feel coerced to give genetic samples, regard results linking their genetics to health status to be protected from disclosure and abuse, or feel inclined to protest the use of genetic information in some situations while supporting it in other cases. Barriers to families communicating about genetics and health often form around worries about discrimination, an arena in which government actions and policies may reduce or increase these concerns [11].

Concerns about discrimination are multifaceted [12], encompassing worries about employment and insurance, fears about reproductive rights and social standing, and anxiety that genetics will be inappropriately used in criminal investigations. Concerns that genetic testing will lead to insurance discrimination and lack of coverage pose a formidable barrier to the efficacy of the counseling process. These concerns must be addressed by societal policies, as individuals, families, and even healthcare practitioners can only do as the rules prescribe that they do [13]. Insurance companies in the United Kingdom have negotiated with government to reach an agreement not to use information from genetic tests that predict disease risk when setting insurance premiums until 2011 [14]. This illustrates a core concern around this issue as genetic testing becomes more important to diagnosis and treatment. It also emphasizes the reality that these debates are linked to lobbying by health insurers and others, widening the gap between families and their ability to control or even predict how personal genetic health information may be used.

A role for government in issues linked to health broadly is often justified by reference to "safety" and "quality." These terms form core constructs in efforts to expand and contract a role for government, and therefore awareness of their use should be promoted. Personal and professional reflection on the validity of invoking these terms to justify a role for government in genetic health and health care should be fostered. While current use of these terms commonly relates to quality of services and safety of the population, any changes in the definition of these terms should be recognized and care taken to avoid an approach that veers towards eugenics where questions are raised such as: What constitutes "quality" in terms of genes? Who decides how to enforce quality control when it comes to genes? What about the safety of genetic testing? Preimplantation genetic diagnosis? Age limits? Do effects on mental health count when "safety" is being discussed?

Families may have relatively little understanding about the specifics of sociopolitical matters relating to genetics and a rather short memory relating to issues such as eugenics boards, but they still have doubts that link back to these events. Daar and Singer [15] suggest that increased understanding of human genomic variation points to a greater need to look at interpopulation differences rather than interindividual differences. In part, this focus on difference is motivated by linkages between ethnic groups and vulnerability to certain diseases. A movement toward focusing on interpopulation differences, however, when juxtaposed with historical abuses of minorities in health care and contemporary health disparities, is being resisted by many for fear that it may exacerbate discrimination of minority groups [16].

The persistent belief that genetic testing needs to have value above existing tests for such diseases as heart disease has generated efforts to categorize genetic testing [17]. This is a partial response to the reality that there is a range of genetic testing "safety" and "quality" factors that can be operationalized. For example, some tests appear to have little to no harm and much benefit aligned with them. A child's test to determine if she has a rare allele of the thiopurinemethyltransferase (TMPT) gene can predict impaired ability to metabolize mercaptopurine, a chemotherapy agent commonly used in treating acute childhood leukemia. Children who are homozygous for this gene version may benefit by having other therapies and appear to suffer little or no societal harm. On the other hand, some genetic tests, such as APOE testing in the context of dementia, have lower accuracy in predicting a phenotype and may also be of less value at a societal level [17]. Policies are needed that represent efforts to acknowledge that not all genetic testing has the same promise to yield benefits for society and families. Policies are needed that reflect the reality that some genetic testing has more threats for the violations of individual rights which, in turn, cause families anxiety and worry.

Individuals, families, and health-care practitioners can advocate on behalf of such policies. Advocacy efforts among lay members of society who have been diagnosed with a genetic condition are too few. This is evident when science reporters seek lay quotes relating to genetics and behavior. Reporters have found activists and advocates among homosexuals who are willing to speak on the record about genetics and sexual orientation but have been unable to find advocates experiencing mental illness or diagnosed with alcoholism to speak on the record about possible genetic links to these behaviors [18]. Societal discourse framing these behaviors in ways that blame individuals or make reference to religion and God may also contribute to such reticence.

Religious Discourse: God and More

A second type of societal discourse that functions as a vital backdrop to families' reactions to communicating about genetics is religious discourse. Religious discourse relies on faith-based resources and perspectives to guide discussions and decisions about the derivation and delivery of health information and services. Faith-based positions do not have the authority associated with making laws and upholding policies relating to health. They do, however, have the power associated with invoking our conscience, our spiritual compass, and our morality. Religious discourse about health and health care may originate from personal faith, religious dogma, and spiritual beliefs and practices—partially illustrating the connectedness of religious freedom to fundamental values and decision making associated with health and health care in the U.S. [1]. Rabbis, pastors, Imams, and other religious leaders often counsel members regarding what political candidates' positions to support and how best to conserve and demonstrate regard for the sanctity of human life. These official positions may be spoken to individuals, couples, or families in religious counseling sessions, as well as from podiums, and also be posted as "rules for living" on Web sites.

Members of faith communities may perceive that the goal of promoting the sanctity of life limits interventions in which the individual appears to be "playing God." Thus, while there may be no direct awareness of doctrines denying the value of genetic testing and therapies, there may be a more broadly held doctrine that appears to deny the appropriateness of these activities. This may contribute to families' reticence to ask their faith leaders for guidance about such matters, as it may just seem so integral that asking itself is inappropriate. Faith discourse may be perceived to define defective genes as punishment for sins committed *or* as a life lesson. The former may contribute to an individual's resistance to disclose the need for care, while the latter may promote conversations with others who have similar views. Religious discourse may guide some to seek genetic testing to support the sanctity of life.

The dominant religion in the United States, Christianity, influences political discourse and decision making about health and health care at many levels. In 2001, the Evangelical Lutheran Church in America published a booklet called "Genetics!: Where Do We Stand as Christians?" It was designed to be an adult study group guide. As such, it begins with a chapter that is a primer in genetics. The second chapter advances a deterministic view of the role of genes for health and the age of genomics. It is called "Theology for the Age of Biological Control." The chapter reflects on the historical events linked to the eugenics movement. Included is a case study of a couple that has maternal serum testing and learns that there is a possible abnormality. Amniocentesis confirms that the fetus has an extra chromosome 18, which indicates Edwards syndrome. The guide includes chapters discussing genes and human behavior, gene patenting, and genetically modified organisms as well. As such, the guide serves as a concrete example of the role of religious discourse in communicating about genetics, as it will disseminate into the families who participate in discussions using the guide.

One review compiling the survey results of responses from representatives identified to speak on behalf of 31 major religious denominations in the United States revealed much consistency in the doctrines and practices relating to prenatal genetic issues linked to prenatal diagnosis and treatment [19]. Most representatives indicated that their members were free to elect or decline ultrasound or maternal serum screening, with the latter usually being conducted in the second trimester to identify certain birth defects, including Down syndrome. For both procedures, exceptions included the Mormon Church, which indicated that the decision should be made in consultation with Church leaders, while Conservative Judaism and Reform Judaism both specify it to be approved in order to make appropriate treatment decisions. The Eckankar Church was explicit in its statement that the Church has *no* position statement about any prenatal diagnosis or treatment decision as it is viewed as an individual decision. The Evangelical Free Church of America regards both choices to be individual ones so long as they are not performed with the intent to pursue an abortion. The Orthodox Church in America's position was that members are free to choose but often reject these procedures, as they are viewed as encouraging abortion—which is not allowed. Orthodox Judaism deems that the intent of having the procedures must be considered in deciding. The Unity School of Christianity asserts that the decision to elect or decline these procedures should be based on prayer and communion with God.

The positions of the churches surveyed on invasive prenatal testing [19], which requires entry of an instrument such as a needle into the womb (e.g., CVS, amniocentesis) and carries a risk for infection, fetal damage, or miscarriage, was similar to views on ultrasound and maternal serum screening with few exceptions. An emphasis on use to save the life of the fetus was emphasized by the Evangelical Lutheran Church in America. The General Association of Regular Baptist Churches emphasized the importance of having a corrective therapy to improve the "outcome of the fetus" if testing is performed. We do not have surveys or interviews of the various church members to assess how their personal views about what their church doctrine states align with published church dogma. Both statements reflect what may often frame a family's decision in these situations—do it if it will save the life of a fetus. There is less agreement among the doctrines relating to the use of such invasive fetal therapies as stem cell transfusion.

Faith-based doctrines influence the pursuit of medical science by taking positions on such issues as cloning or stem cell research. Religious discourse is often recorded in opposition with respect to genes and health, raising questions and challenging the science. Unfortunately, there is a tendency to pit science against religion in discourse associated with frontiers of discovery. The implicit assumption is that belief in God's role for humans denies belief in science and scientific explanations. Such simplistic conceptions have been and continue to be challenged and debated, with families sometimes caught in the middle of these debates and efforts to advance health and health care.

Organizational Discourse: Clinical and More

During the 19th and early 20th century, public health and genetics shared common ground through similar approaches to health promotion in the population. By the mid-20th century there was a division between public health and genetics, with eugenicists estranged and clinical genetics focused on single gene disorders, usually only relevant to small numbers of people. Now through a common interest in the aetiology of complex diseases such as heart disease and cancer, there is a need for people working in public health and genetics to collaborate. This is not a comfortable convergence for many, particularly those in public health. [20] (p. 894)

A third type of societal discourse in societies that affects what we know about health and our access to care occurs in and around organizations, specifically those that address the allocation and use of resources to provide clinical and public health care and services. Here, too, what health-care practitioners and patients do in relation to communicating about genetics and health is constrained by their access not only to valid tests with value added but also the availability of knowledgeable medical technicians to draw and prepare the blood for new genetic tests and skilled laboratory professionals to read and interpret the results. Payment policies also come into play. Thus, organizational discourse spans a broad array of content with consequences for families and genomic health care. These consequences often illuminate the tension between availability and affordability in promoting access to genetic health and health care. Interestingly, organizations often adopt broad practices linked to communicating about health, such as public health and clinical organizations' increasing tendency to promote the importance of knowing our "family health history." As family history "represents the contributions and interactions of unique genomic and ecologic factors that affect the metabolic profile and life course of a family and its members" [21] (p. 143), it has been progressively promoted as a tool to identify individuals with increased susceptibility to disease [22].

When it comes to the structural resources allocated to genetics and health care, the largest genetic screening program in the United States is the newborn screening program [23]. The Institute of Medicine of the National Academies of Sciences in the United States convened a study about "Educating Public Health Professionals for the 21st Century," and genomics emerged as a new area for training. The goals of training were defined as learning to apply public health science to genomics and identifying both ethical and medical issues associated with genetic testing as part of public health programs [24]. The strategic aims aligned with these goals include being able to use genomics to attain public health goals. This implicitly means communicating about genes and health with families who will be the targets of new science and products and businesses that emerge around genomics. The latter includes an array of genetic testing services, some already being offered online and through a myriad of other direct-to-consumer (DTC) advertisements in the United States, as we discuss later in this chapter.

Newborn screening programs have in many cases been the only experience individuals have with genetic screening. In the past, parents have not given newborn testing much thought because they were seldom asked whether they wanted to participate, but instead participated through "implied consent." This sets an unfortunate precedent when it comes to communicating in families about genetics and genetic testing. In the case of parents responding to a positive newborn screen for cystic fibrosis (CF) for their infant, there is documented evidence of organizational units failing to provide promised information, then offering conflicting instructions regarding where to obtain care [25]. None of the stakeholders were acting with malice, but the overall effect of completely decentralized communication was to increase the stress on parents at an already stressful time in their lives. As suggested by the newborn screening programs, organizational practice guides public policies and vice versa. Newborn screening policies worldwide challenge families and health-care practitioners to keep up with current standards in order to give informed consent and make informed choices [26].

In the mix of standards of care relating to whom to test, and for what, as well as why and when, organizational discourse reveals decisions about practices relating to counseling relatives of significant genetic test results. This often does not occur, raising debate about the need for genetic services to assure that relatives are informed [27]. Sometimes it does not occur because a patient has died before receiving test results and so is unaware of genetic status [28]. It can also fail to occur due to a lack of understanding about genetics. Health-care practitioners may be able to predict those most in need of genetic counseling services based on identifying and assessing family communication norms. However, practitioners can face further barriers *within* families, where risk *should be* communicated to other family members but doing so is difficult and lost in the translation of not understanding inherited risk information [29]. At a public health level, interventions related to genetics and health may need to emphasize the important role to be played by unaffected family members in conveying the relevance of hereditary disease information inside the immediate family and beyond [30].

EXPERT DISCOURSE ABOUT GENETICS AND HEALTH

Expert discourse (Fig. 3.1) consists of communication based on the derived or expert information and knowledge about health and health care collected through societal resources devoted to medical research and public health evidence. Expert discourse also often reflects knowledge not yet available or accessible, and multiple ways of conveying findings from the same research [4]. The knowledge gained about health and health care, and the services designed to support these insights form a foundation for expert discourse in health communication. This discourse impacts *both* health-care practitioners' and individuals' decision making about behavior with health implications. Expert discourse is comprised of conflicting content at times. This may happen because different expert sources look at the same evidence but reach different conclusions. It also happens because new knowledge may make old knowledge outdated, but we may still talk about and act on the old knowledge. Sometimes when new evidence about treating a disease is framed in terms of benefits for a patient with the disease, the message may suggest that benefits outnumber risks. When the same evidence is framed in terms of the financial costs related to treatment, the message may suggest that costs outweigh benefits. When discussions focus on our personal autonomy, the evidence may be mixed, as we may differ as individuals or in comparison to the expert source in views about the importance of making our own decisions or giving informed consent. Experts in varied topic domains or with training in a range of methods may also reach different conclusions about the meaning of research findings. They may emphasize different aspects of new knowledge in ways that seem contradictory at times. Expert discourse about health and health care is associated with informing, motivating, and profit making, all of which guide individuals' "informed" decision making about health.

Informational Discourse: Educating and More

> Rigid recommendations about how much information to provide to patients and about how much to involve patients in decision making are likely to be inappropriate. [31] (p. 597)

Informational discourse represents efforts to communicate about health based on disseminating the evidence of medical and public health science, sometimes with dramatic intent to draw attention to what is not known

[4]. In the midst of media fanfare and strategic clinical and public health communication conveying the promise of genomics, accurate translations of how new medical research findings affect families are needed. As illustrated above when considering newborn screening programs, societies organize to deliver these services to citizens based on the belief that the epidemiological database supports doing so, but in many settings communicating to inform parents about these tests usually only happens in the wake of test results that suggest something is wrong with the newborn's condition [32]. This truly is a worrisome and anxiety-provoking situation, not the best time to teach someone about complex science [25].

The United Kingdom's "informed consent" program to screen for phenylketonuria (PKU) is a model for strategic communication about genetics and health. If left untreated, this condition can retard brain development [33]. Per the established U.K. newborn screening protocol, a mother receives a prescreening leaflet in the third trimester of pregnancy to be discussed at least 24 hours before the baby's screening, which is prescribed to take place between 5 and 8 days after birth. The leaflet is to be used by the mother to make a decision about whether to consent. The benefits are clearly outlined in the leaflet. These include an emphasis on obtaining care at the earliest moment for any child diagnosed with PKU. Mothers are nearly unanimous in consenting, and they know what and why the test is being done. This is one path for health-care practitioners to advocate for and to assist with advancing both societies' and families' readiness to seek and be recipients of genomic health care.

News media sources of health and science information are often how individuals, including scientists and doctors, keep abreast of new knowledge [34]. Genetics and health is no exception. A number of researchers have examined the media coverage associated with genetics and health, finding that reports often accurately attribute partial causation for illness and disease to genes. For example, the headline "Obsessive Compulsive Disorder Is Partially Genetically Transmitted" [7] (p. 93) quite accurately reflects the scientific status of understanding and knowledge. Media stories about genetics and alcoholism include the following examples of such coverage: *(a)* "the susceptibility to alcoholism is inherited" (p. 11); and *(b)* "a specific gene that appears to greatly increase the risk for alcoholism" [35]. Once more, the reports do not assign total causation to inherited genes. The media do, however, tend to use shorthand phrases and terms, such as "the breast cancer gene," which may lead to misunderstanding among the general public [36]. Others find that a "narrative enlightened geneticization" characterizes the informational discourse, with factors other than genes being considered in discussions of disease causation but with genetic explanations ultimately being prioritized [37].

Beyond the news as a source of information about genetics and health, entertainment media are influential. One study that asked nearly 500 participants to indicate what was the first media message that came to their mind when they read the phrase "genes and health" generated the name of a movie as the most frequent response [2]. Participants named 33 specific movie titles with *Gattaca, Jurassic Park*, and *Multiplicity* comprising the top three. The latter focuses on cloning to solve the competing demands associated with work and family lives. Little research has been conducted to examine the accuracy of information about genetics presented in entertainment media.

From episodes of *The Twilight Zone* in the 1950s to *Heroes* in 2006, science-fiction media have integrated genetics into storylines. With the incursion of biotechnology research in the 1970s, several fictional plotlines emerged in popular culture with a focus on genetics, and since the 1980s there has been a substantial number of major Hollywood and other English-language fiction films in which genetic themes figured prominently [38]. These included *Jurassic Park* (1993) and television series such as *The X-Files* (1993–2002), which popularized genetics and how genes can alter lives. Then in the 2000s, crime dramas steeped in the science of DNA evidence such as *CSI: Crime Scene Investigation* (2000) popularized knowledge of DNA testing. Yet for every *CSI* effort to include accurate, science-based depictions of genetic information, there is a depiction of genetics gone awry such as in *Repo! The Genetic Opera!* a 2008 film with Paris Hilton whose plot synopsis reads, "A worldwide epidemic encourages a biotech company to launch an organ-financing program similar in nature to a standard car loan. The repossession clause is a killer, however" [39].

News and entertainment media are not the only source of information about genetics and health, of course. The mapping of the human genome and discoveries relating health conditions such as blood clotting risk to multiple genes and their variants has changed clinical communication about health. While we have always been asked about family history at medical appointments, a greater emphasis has begun to be placed on these questions and our answers. As described in the previous section, sometimes this emphasis is prescribed within organizations and has become important for public health initiatives such as the U.S. Surgeon General's campaign, urging people to "know your family health history" [40].

The rapidly changing landscape aligned with genomic health care challenges health-care practitioners' abilities to maintain competence in this arena. For example, a survey of 1054 practitioners revealed that just 52% were aware that *BRCA1/2* mutations can be inherited from either parent, while 46% knew that a woman with a sister with a known *BRCA1* mutation has a 50% risk for inheriting the same mutation [41]. Most patients know that changes in genes can be inherited, that changes can lead to disease, and that changes can be caused by radiation. Yet only 42% of more than 800 adults surveyed in community settings realized that the sun can cause changes in genes, 63% knew that changes in genes can occur over a lifetime, and 70% that every gene is able to mutate or change [42].

Research that examines health-care practitioners' communication with patients about genetics reveals that doctors tend to rely on objective and scientific facts about test results and do not address more subjective personal information needs [43]. Genetic counselors focus on informing clients about why something has happened and what might happen in the future as a result, using language to communicate probability [44]. Most families lack knowledge about genetics and inheritance [45]. When an individual has had a family experience with a genetic condition, what is most likely to be remembered are the effects of the disorder [46]. What is seldom understood, even with personal experience in the family, is how it affects individual risk for inheriting the condition [47]. A survey of parents showed that where one parent was a carrier and the other parent was not found to have a common mutation, the parent did not appreciate that there is a residual risk of having a child with CF [48].

In the genetic counseling clinic, it is not uncommon for people to demonstrate an understanding that a condition can be inherited, while at the same time they also show that they have a limited understanding of how a spontaneous mutation could occur [49]. In reality, all of us carry mutations, but research reveals that the use of the word *mutation* to describe variation in genes is linked to negative thoughts and feelings based on media images. In a study with 243 lay participants, rankings for the terms *mutation, alteration, variation*, and *change* in perceptions of good/bad, healthy/unhealthy, normal/not normal, desirable/undesirable, changing/unchanging, and intended/unintended, *mutation* was judged to be a more negative term when compared to all the other terms with regard to goodness, healthiness, normality, or desirability [50]. Interestingly, an alteration was perceived to be intended when compared to any of the other terms. The notion that a mutation could be a variation promoting human adaptation and survival does not appear to fit within these mindsets.

A proliferation of online sites with content about genetics and health demonstrates both the public's interest and need for information to enhance understanding. One survey of 780 Internet users found that perceiving a personal risk related to genes and health increases searches for online information about genetics [51]. In the end, these informational exchanges may actually help produce a more educated patient and family. While a diagnosis affects most directly the person being diagnosed, its implications for family members when it comes to inherited risk for a condition broaden the scope for an audience in relation to communicating about the diagnosis [29].

As the epigraph for this section makes clear, inflexible rules about how much or what kind of information to provide patients with are unlikely to be successful. In the case of genetic risk information, health-care recipients may vary widely in terms of their prior knowledge and preference for dealing with uncertainty. Those who are knowledgeable to begin with also acquire and retain new information more readily [52]. And where some individuals actively seek out genetic risk information from multiple sources, others are more passive [53], perhaps because they wish to wait for information from a medical professional or because they prefer not to deal with the possibility of genetic disease. The obvious solution would seem to be for the health-care practitioner to adapt the information to the knowledge level and preferences of the recipient. But often, in the case of genetic counseling following newborn screening, legal and/or organizational policies require standardized treatment of information recipients. In this way, informational discourse that should benefit patients is constrained by countervailing institutional concerns.

Commercial Discourse: Making a Profit

> Product placements expose us as viewers to health information, services, and products—options we may have no awareness of until viewing them in these entertainment outlets...We mostly frame medications as something to benefit our health, so we may more mindlessly respond to communication about them. We're not on our mental guard when health services and products come into scenes and settings for entertainment the same way we may have learned to be when alcohol use is being portrayed. [54]

Another very different path for the dissemination of expert knowledge derived about health is commercial discourse, which focuses on communicating to make a profit from providing products and services to support disease prevention and detection. Failure to address the profit motive of health and health care ignores the reality that where there is profit to be made from selling health and health care, a profiteer will not be far behind. The profit motive associated with health and health care occurs at many levels, as the pharmaceutical industry promotes an increasing number of products for consumers to use to treat all kinds of conditions. In this age of genomic health care, the messages families may be exposed to in relation to their health go beyond pharmaceuticals, nutriceuticals, and cosmeceuticals into the realms of pharmacogenomics, nutrigenomics, and cosmegenomics [55].

Traditional commercial appeals, such as cost comparisons, accessibility, and convenience, comprise core issues in efforts to promote products, activities, and other consumer goods related to health and health care. While published research in health communication often examines expert discourse and provides insights about both informational and motivational strategies and outcomes, far less study has systematically examined discourse in the commercial realm, especially in terms of positive effects on health and health care. Marketers aim to understand ways to sell products to consumers, and some of those products are health related or have potential health benefits. The field of advertising uses the desires of individuals to be healthy as a way to frame appeals as well. In the process of communicating to sell products and services, information may be included about how genes contribute to the likelihood of disease but only in service of profit. In the study previously mentioned which examined the first message that came to participants' minds in response to the phrase "genes and health," 19 commercials were identified [2]. These included a commercial about stem cell research to provide a cure for cancer, commercials about women and the fight for breast cancer, commercials about cloning, commercials about how the risk of heart attacks run in families, commercials about alcoholism running in the family, and commercials about genetics labs and curing illnesses [2]. Only the United States and New Zealand allow these direct-to-consumer (DTC) ads for medications and testing services.

There are three general types of DTC ads that have emerged. *Help-seeking ads* aim to educate us as consumers about a disease while also encouraging us to consult with doctors and discuss treatment options connected to prescriptions drugs based on our health status. If the ad makes no claims, no disclosure of risk in taking a drug is required. *Reminder ads* also contain drug names and offer very limited information about a drug's safety or efficacy. *Product-specific ads* promote particular prescription drugs and must provide information about the drug's safety and efficacy. These ads are supposed to pass strict Food and Drug Administration (FDA) guidelines. Direct-to-consumer ads do not necessarily enhance the accuracy of information for consumers and may lessen a sense of choice. A survey of hundreds of general practitioners and pharmacists in New Zealand revealed that doctors view the ads as contributing to participative decision making but also view them as often being *unreliable* sources of information [56]. The ads have increased individual awareness of products connected to genes and health, as some advertisements make reference to our family health histories.

Some have expressed concerns about DTC ads' references to race and possible stereotyping and racism [57]. Although health-care practitioners are encouraged to address racial issues associated with genes and health in working with clients [58, 59], existing data seem to provide evidence that linking genetics, race, and health in messages to the public can increase racism [16, 60]. This poses a barrier to communicating with families about genetics and health. Traditionally racial groups have been treated as if they were unified types defined by characteristics such as skin color, hair texture, and head shape and size [60]. However, as Kittles and Weiss pointed out [60], the arrival of genetic data revealed that within-group differences substantially exceed between-group racial differences. Yet despite the fact that all human beings share 99.9% of their DNA with each other and most of the 0.1% of difference is interindividual rather than intergroup [61], there is a growing movement in medical genetics to promote a model of race-based medicine—using race as a criterion for diagnosis, screening, and prescribing drugs [62].

The book *The Genius Factory* by David Plotz [63] tells the true story of a millionaire who created a sperm bank for Nobel Laureate sperm. Known as the genius sperm bank or the Nobel Prize Sperm Bank, the

Repository for Germinal Choice, not surprisingly, raised tremendous controversy. Between 1980 and 1999, 215 children were conceived from sperm out of the Repository and women who met the criterion of qualifying for Mensa, the high-IQ society. Even in the absence of awareness of this reality, societies express disdain for the elitist, racist, and sexist images aligned with thoughts of choosing the characteristics of not yet conceived children—and making money doing it. This may motivate some consumers to go online in search of anonymity when seeking genetic testing and products. Genetic testing services are increasingly offered online, including parentage confirmation, identity testing, and DNA banking, as well as health-related testing for such standard tests as CF and hereditary hemochromatosis as well as unconventional tests related to behavior, nutrition, and aging [64].

Other ethical issues emerge as well, including placement of such ads. For example, a biotechnology company advertised its commercial test for *BRCA1/2* genetic mutations in playbills for a theatre presentation about a woman's painful death from ovarian cancer [65]. A lack of understandable information, complicated social contexts surrounding genetic testing, and lack of consensus about utility of some tests limit their efficacy [66]. Do-it-yourself testing is particularly problematic [67] with online sources multiplying the effect [68]. Despite the reality that only the United States and New Zealand allow such commercialism, the public's confusion and autonomy form core arguments used in the United States to continue the practice of DTC ads [69, 70].

Motivational Discourse: Activating Thoughts and Action

Many of these women will not have a family history that suggests the presence of a highly penetrant breast cancer susceptibility gene. However, a small subset of such women will come from families with a striking incidence of breast and other cancers often associated with inherited mutations. [71] (p. 577)

The motivational discourse element of expert discourse reflects efforts to influence attitudes or behavior relating to health and health care, implicitly relying on a presumed level of knowledge or understanding. One of the most fascinating and at the same time frustrating areas of study within the strategic realm of health communication focuses on how to communicate in ways that motivate people to behave in healthy ways. Motivation often depends upon our awareness of information associating a practice with a desired or undesired outcome. Information can lead to motivation to seek genetic testing, for example, as suggested in this section's opening quotation. Women have increased their efforts to seek information regarding their individual breast cancer risk in the wake of media reports about a breast cancer gene [72]. Women who come from families with inherited mutations associated with breast and other cancers may benefit greatly from awareness of links between genetics and breast cancer to support their decision to seek testing. Women who do not have a family history, however, may impose undue emotional and financial burdens on themselves and their families. This case may also be associated with shaping public perceptions that inherited genes determine health and disease outcomes, and that genetically related technologies can save human beings from imperfect and unpleasant disease experiences. Research has shown that 60% of smokers surveyed anticipate they would be motivated to quit smoking if they had a gene linked to smoking-related disease, while 40% say they would feel demotivated [73].

Research that supports the impact of genetics on the expression of diseases such as cancer and neurological conditions, together with communication about these advances in knowledge, may also shape individual perceptions of the ability to act on genetic testing results to limit disease onset. Exposure to movies with content about human genetics has been found to be positively related to perceptions of one's ability to act on genetic information to benefit one's health and genetic self-efficacy [74] but not to affect belief in the efficacy of genetic therapies. Exposure to prime-time medical and crime television shows was, however, directly related to belief in the efficacy of genetic therapies but had no relationship to self-efficacy [74]. Unfortunately, genetics are often appropriated in media to inflame stereotypes and provoke rather than to resolve dilemmas [75]. This is a missed opportunity, especially considering that fictional media guide the public's understanding of genetics and are influential in making uses of genetic technology acceptable or unacceptable [76].

Smith [77] pointed out that as television dramas continue to include references to genetics, awareness of genetic testing and therapies will increase, prompting individuals to form attitudes and behaviors linked to these options. She reported Nielsen ratings in 2005 of an estimated 19,737,000 viewers who watched a *Grey's Anatomy* episode focusing on a character's decision to obtain genetic testing for ovarian cancer. Smith suggested that communicating about genetics and health on TV in conjunction with new technologies—such as pairing the episode with an ABC television network Web site to address viewer questions—provides an opportunity for shaping people's self-efficacy and control over gaining access to resources to make informed choices. Messages to motivate individuals in relation to genes and health are not limited, of course, to fictional media. Other research suggests that all media can play a critical role in shaping responses. Studies such as Weiner, Silk, and Parrott [62] report that media information can be particularly salient for individuals who have had personal experience with genetics (e.g., genetic testing). In this study, news shows and other media content relating to genetics and health were most valuable for individuals with at least a small amount of genetic knowledge.

Media frequently offer contradictory and contested messages about the role genes play in health. Parrott and colleagues [74] argue that uncertainty in the medical community about genetic and modifiable cofactors of disease leads to confusing messages in health promotion. Indeed, public messages about the role of genes in health are often overly deterministic and contribute to fundamental misinterpretations of how genetics research is done [78]. Many media messages increase fear and mistrust of genetic science [79], which, in turn, may reduce individual motivation to harness the understanding and resources necessary to benefit from testing and options linked to genetics and health. As an illustration of this point, Smith [77] reported that individuals consider one of the risks of genetic testing to be the threat of being labeled "a genetic mutant," along with the associated stigma, a further threat to the motivation to act on awareness. Smith pointed out that advertising campaigns using messages such as "Are you a carrier?" promote labeling and potential stigma. African Americans, in particular, have reported that the term *mutation* carries stigma related to race and ethnicity [80].

LAY DISCOURSE ABOUT GENETICS AND HEALTH

With the increasing reference to genes and genetic science in everyday life, it is important to understand what lay discourses influence understandings of genetics (Fig. 3.1). By "lay," we refer to people who are not trained and/or employed in genetics [81]. Cultural, social, and personal discourses guide how they think about genetics, behave in relation to genes and health, and importantly, what media they may use that will inform their understanding or when they seek clinical consultation for health. The ability to understand what health-care practitioners say and especially the value placed on medical interaction depends often on upbringing, combining family, cultural, and health experiences. A great deal of individual understanding and motivation relating to health and health care comes from indigenous knowledge conveyed through these discourses. Sometimes this information will be consistent with science and other times not. That does not mean that practices based on this knowledge will not produce good outcomes, nor does it mean that these insights and practices will not become a spark for funded research to build on the base of scientific understanding associated with health and health care. That is the reality. The channels responsible for disseminating this knowledge are the same ones that guide awareness of public health and clinical communication recommendations—interpersonal and media.

Cultural Discourse: Gendered and Racial Identities and More

> It's hard to talk about race in [the United States], but with a new medical enterprise focused on biological difference, we are forced to confront it. [82] (p. A11)

Some of what we know about health and health care comes from lay knowledge and practices associated with cultural membership and beliefs about health and health care. Cultural identities form around where one lives, ranging from the nation to the region of a country, and even whether one lives in rural or urban areas. Cultural identities also form around race, ethnicity, and gender. Given the importance of cultural identities and the recognition of the importance of non-Western medicine in the lives of a growing number of health-care recipients, a number of studies have sought to uncover and categorize common assumptions about genetic disease and genetic testing that are common among members of minority groups. For example, surveys and analysis of the disease causation beliefs of Latinos and African Americans [83, 84], Haitians [85], and Southeast Asians [86, 87] have been conducted. The outcomes of these studies may be academically interesting, as when Singer et al. [83] found that in their sample, Latinos and African Americans were more likely to express a preference for genetic and prenatal testing. Results should not be used to form rigid assumptions about a person's intentions or response to a genetic condition or genetic testing. Rather, health-care practitioners should view the research findings of ethnocultural differences as evidence that attention to cultural identities is vital for effective communication. Thus, the question changes from, What is this person's ethnocultural identity? to How best can I learn *from her* how her ethnocultural identity will affect communication regarding genetic health and her response to health-care recommendations/choices?

Culture contributes to cognitions and emotions about self and health, as well as the underlying motivations that may guide our actions or failures to act. As ethnographic research makes clear, many cultures construct different understandings of kinship, health, and illness and these differences are likely to affect the way that genetic risk is understood [88]. Since cultural discourse influences beliefs about genetics and health, this has implications for transcultural care. For example, consanguineous marriage, particularly between cousins, is common among some cultural groups. These marriages are seen to benefit family systems across generations due to shared family traditions and knowledge [89]. However, as this marital arrangement increases the chances of both parents being carriers for the same recessive condition, communicating about genetics and health within these families will clash with the cultural discourse.

Cultural beliefs and practices guide how one interprets clinical communication or whether one will even be exposed to strategic communication about health in clinical settings due to the standards for when one will seek expert care. Culture contributes to beliefs about such issues as whether one should be told about a terminal diagnosis and the appropriateness of having male physicians conduct exams of females. Patient participation norms also emerge from cultural discourse, contributing to commitment to medical decisions at times and other times, contributing to noncompliance with medical therapies. There is a reciprocal relationship, such that patients may comply more often and be more satisfied with formal systems of medical care because they accommodate to cultural practices when possible. Research has shown, for example, that some cultures believe that a cleft lip is caused by eating rabbit, hence the name "hare-lip" [86]. Nicolas, Desilva, Grey, and Gonzalez-Eastep's [85] discussion of Haitian beliefs reveal that Haitians often believe illnesses are supernaturally induced, rather than influenced by genetics. These cultural beliefs may present challenges for health-care practitioners who wish to respect cultural beliefs, while being reassuring about these concerns. Moreover, cultural practices may limit the likelihood that people will express uncertainty or doubt about a practitioner's diagnosis or explanation. Asian Americans, for example, are often silent partners in medical care, owing to cultural norms governing interaction [87].

In addition to the role of cultural identities aligned with ethnicity or race, gender is also a consideration when reviewing lay understandings of genetics and health. Women are the focus of much of the public discourse on genetics. Women are more often than not viewed as "kin-keepers," the center of the information network in terms of managing family health history information, and the primary client when a couple seeks genetic counseling [90, 91]. Moreover, research associated with reproductive processes and health tends to overemphasize the role of women, often excluding relevant findings pertaining to men [92]. Since women gestate and bear children, genetics information is often directed to them. Tuana [93] pointed out that lay understandings of genetics often give in to mother-blaming—holding mothers responsible for undesired traits in offspring. Consequently, women may be more inherently interested in genetic information than men.

Research that has examined whether differences exist between males and females in their actual understandings of genetic contributions to health finds few differences. Within gendered identities, race may affect beliefs. In a study that examined the lay public's perceptions of the influence of inherited genes, environment, social factors, and personal behaviors on human health, differences based on gender and race were considered [90]. For breast cancer, European American women assigned twice the emphasis to the physical environment as an influence than did African American women, and African American women perceived genes to have a greater influence on breast cancer than did European American women. The authors of this study draw attention to the need for more research in this area so that gendered understandings of genetics and health are improved.

Social Discourse: Families and More

A myriad of health habits have to be worked out through a second aspect of lay discourse, social discourse within families, which combines varied cultural backgrounds. Custodianship of genetic information faces barriers to telling linked to the reality that families vary in their communication norms and patterns of behavior. When families broach the topic of genetic health, in particular, the literal "blood ties" that link family members together may perpetuate blame, a psychological component related to disease causation

[94]. In theory, no single family member owns family health history information, because every member could potentially share certain genetic traits, links, or diseases. As a result, boundaries around disclosure of this information can be difficult to negotiate, though timeliness of the information may affect how individuals manage their well-being. Women considering oral contraception, for example, would likely prefer to be told about blood-clotting experiences and genetic risk factors within the family before making a decision to use this form of contraception. Couples planning their families would likely prefer to be informed of any clotting family history prior to the onset of pregnancy; and so on across contexts associated with increased risk for thrombosis linked to genetics [95]. Thus, health information becomes blurred when family medical history is comprised of information that may affect the health of *all* family members.

While some research suggests that media exposure to information about human genetics is related to more frequent family discussions of genetics research, there is little evidence that individuals are talking with friends or family members about their family health history [62]. This lack of exchange is concerning given the role of family communication in the formation of beliefs and behaviors of individual members. Moreover, as Phelan [96] notes, the most harmful effects of geneticization are for family members "tainted and rejected" via association with a genetically deviant relative (p. 319). Miller [97] reported a case study of one family whose members never shared information with one another about the legacy of depression and suicide among women in their family. This silence was striking because over the course of four generations there had been five suicide attempts—at least one female suicide attempt within *each* generation. It was not until a young woman in the fourth generation of this family was hospitalized for her suicide attempt that the spiral of silence regarding depression in this family was broken. The silence served to isolate individuals suffering from depression in this family and prevented each successive generation from getting necessary treatment.

Certain illnesses—or even illness itself—may be constructed as weakness in certain family cultures. As a result, discussion of the illness may be considered taboo. Moreover, actual discussions of genetic illness and history may be fraught with blame and guilt around responsibility for contributing faulty genes [98]. This situation offers unique challenges to the medical community because existing research suggests that more people with genetic disorders learn about their disorder from family members than from health-care practitioners [99, 100]. Indeed, family members are perceived to have a moral imperative to communicate genetic information to other family members [101, 102]. But do they?

While research literature in the area of family communication about genetics and health suggests that parents are responsible for disseminating information to their children, there is little evidence to suggest that they actually perform such a function and even less that uncovers the process of the information dissemination (see [103]). Studies that track the communication of parents to children [104] do so most often through self-report and give a post facto glimpse of behavior. Because of Gregory et al.'s [105] finding that participants drew a marked contrast between the nature of communication within the clinic and within the home, more studies like that conducted by Keenen, Arden-Jones, and Eeles [106], which occur outside of the clinical context and address communication patterns and interaction within family social networks, would be instructive.

Gaff et al.'s [103] systematic analysis of 26 studies of family communication and genetics revealed a variety of considerations that warrant additional examination, including considering the effects of disclosure, what information to disclose, timing of the disclosure, and the communication strategies employed in the disclosure. This study uncovered an interesting strategy of utilizing intermediaries to disclose information, especially across generations. This analysis revealed a "cascading of responsibility" wherein responsibility for informing others in the family is handed down along with the actual information [103] (p. 4). In addition to examining active disclosure, it may also be necessary to explore how patterns of information omission and the use of strategic ambiguity function in family communication about genetic health. Gaff et al. [103] call attention to the fact that, in some families, those managing genetic information may make the decision to withhold information altogether or deliberately present the information in an ambiguous fashion. A focus on communication is central to education in the area of genetic health since beliefs about disease inheritance are an integral part of family culture in the United States and other cultures [107].

Although, as noted above, intergenerational communication of genetic information appears to be rare, the same does not apparently hold true among siblings and partners. For example, in a study of the Wisconsin newborn screening program, after a positive screening result of cystic fibrosis (CF) for their infant, 88% of parents reportedly informed other family members that they might also be carriers [108]. Similarly, 80% of Belgian parents of a child with CF informed their brothers and sisters about the genetic aspects of CF [109]. In addition, women shown to be carriers of CF actively shared that information with members of their social network. In a study of 122 Danish women, 100% reportedly informed their partner, 89% informed their parents, 80% informed their siblings, and 57% shared the result with nonrelatives other than their doctor; transferal of this information was the presumed cause of partners and siblings obtaining a carrier test –100% and 26%, respectively [110]. The latter results suggest that knowledge of the carrier status of one individual has the potential to motivate carrier testing in others, perhaps because of the implications for family planning. However, from the data available, we cannot rule out the possibility that their communication was prompted by the false belief that testing could be followed up by some action that would remedy the genetic problem.

Personal Discourse: Experience and More

No matter what scientific or indigenous knowledge disseminates to individuals about genetics and health, in the final analysis, personal experiences in this arena will sometimes take precedence. This forms the final element of lay discourse. Beyond the communication about health and health care shared or avoided within cultural and social groups, one's particular life experiences with illness and health, and with health care, vary widely, deriving lay knowledge to guide future behavior. Once more, strategic health communicators must reckon with this reality in their efforts to intervene with information and motivation to guide decision making and action. Strategic health communicators give time and effort to understanding personal experiences individuals have with trying behaviors promoted to prevent or detect disease. If the practice is unpleasant, causing embarrassment or pain, will these be barriers to participation? Genetic tests have predominantly been blood tests. Fear of needles or personal beliefs about blood and blood tests may erect barriers to testing. Alternatively, the fact that genetic testing is viewed as a simple blood test may actually encourage uptake of genetic testing. Beyond our own personal experiences with specific health behaviors that are within our personal sphere of control, many health practices depend upon the cooperation or collaboration of others.

In the face of the seemingly inexplicable, such as the role of genes in health, some people rely on religious faith to guide their knowledge and outcome expectancies. Religious faith refers to the predisposition to think, feel, or act based on his or her belief in a spiritual power greater than humans to affect the course of nature and the role of humans within that realm. Religious faith is often guided by the prescriptions associated with the dictums and practices of different religions, as expressed in religious discourse. At the personal level, extrinsic religiosity, the outward and visible signs and practices associated with religious faith that include prayer and worship, provides solace, distraction, sociability, and even self-justification [111]. Intrinsic religiosity, the internalized expressions and integrated experiences of religious faith sometimes referred to as spirituality, has been found to be used by the sick and disabled for coping [111]. Prayer may be used by some of us as a strategy to seek peace with heritage linked to genetic mutations and disease. For others, prayer may reflect that the faithful depend upon belief in God's power for healing, for being saved from the health harms linked to a condition [112]. Religiosity has been found to affect the likelihood that individuals will be exposed to media with genetic health content [12]. Extrinsic religiosity relates to a greater likelihood of watching talk shows that contain information about genes and health. Intrinsic religiosity was negatively associated with exposure to newspaper content about genes and health.

Individual beliefs about a disease and its cause can inform treatment, especially since lay understanding of disease inheritance can be at odds with medical models [113]. Clinicians need to be aware of these personal "understandings, because they can influence patients' perceptions of their disease risk and its management" [114] (p. 584). While there are a multitude of beliefs relevant to specific genetic disorders, research by Parrott et al. [4] reveals a useful model for understanding meta-belief orientations—general frameworks people use for understanding genetics and health. This study developed a Genetic Relativism Instrument that identifies four lay frameworks for understanding the role of genes in health. Each of these frameworks includes beliefs about the role of personal behaviors, social environments, and religiosity on genetic expression. An *uncertain relativist* is an individual who is uncertain about the roles that personal behavior, faith, and environment play on genes and health. An *integrated relativist* believes that personal behavior, faith, and environment all contribute to how genes express themselves in health. A *personal control relativist* believes that personal behavior plays the most important role in the expression of genes on health—but doubts the role of faith and support. And, finally, a *genetic determinist* believes that none of these factors contributes much to how genes express themselves in health—the bottom line for these individuals is that you are born with your genetic blueprint and there is nothing that can be done. This study highlights the utility of considering the contributions of spiritual life on perceptions of genes on health.

Illness causation frameworks may be useful for health-care practitioners as a guide when assisting people in their efforts to integrate messages about health. For example, a practitioner can discuss how to combine and make sense of scientific genetic information about heart disease while presenting messages about personal lifestyle changes. This approach might help individuals integrate disparate messages about health and dispel beliefs that he or she has no control over the outcome of a genetically based disease. By applying these frameworks to better comprehend lay orientations to understanding genetics and health, practitioners may not only serve to educate patients and families, but empower them and increase personal efficacy to take control over their personal health. Lay attitudes about health care have been found to be shaped by media use, with greater overall consumption relating to pessimism about health care in the United States [115].

One vitally significant experiential and personal discourse that frames understanding and response to genetic diagnoses and testing, particularly prenatal testing, relates to disabilities. Pregnancy can be a stressful, worrisome time for virtually all couples. Even if a couple does not innately have their own worries, one trip to the obstetrician's office exposes the couple to a multitude of risk messages related to the developing fetus. Despite the strides individuals with disabilities have made in the past decades, such as the passage of IDEA (Individuals with Disabilities Education Act) and ADA (Americans with Disabilities Act), the birth of a child with a disability is often still viewed and discussed publicly, privately, and clinically as a tragedy—something that should have been avoided.

Disability and illness are grounded in real or imagined *experiences* with disability and illness. Like expert discourse (discussed earlier), discourse about disability experiences is often comprised of conflicting content and impacts both health-care practitioners and individuals making decisions in light of genetic information. Traditionally, the loudest voices of disability discourse forward the stigma [116, 117], hardships, and heartbreak associated with disability and dismiss as "denial" any attempt by others to proffer an alternative perspective on disability [118, 119]. The pharmaceutical and genetic testing companies profit from this view of disability, as negative views are related to genetic testing uptake and, in turn, growing market sales. Moreover, the media industry profits from negative messages about disabilities, as the images and stories draw viewers and readers [120].

Messages about disability presented by health-care practitioners also generally further a pessimistic view of disability in the context of genetic health [121–123]. Many practitioners have been criticized for presenting information about disability that is biomedical in nature, without sufficient context [124]. Further, some argue these same messages perpetuate discrimination against individuals themselves, not just their disabling trait. There is a plurality toward disability traits and genetic testing for disabling conditions [118]. There are significant differences in what counts as a serious trait, and many individuals with disabilities argue that negative views of disability are based on misinformation and fear. Many individuals and families with disabilities find value in the disability experience [118], even to the point of viewing the disability as an advantage [116]. As disability is a social construct, practitioners may play a role in the promotion of an improved view of disability. As clinical caregivers and advocates for individuals with disabilities, health-care practitioners can have a key voice in the promotion of improvements in society's concepts and infrastructure for individuals with disabilities.

CONCLUSION

As this chapter has illustrated, multiple discourses influence family communication about genetic information. These discourses are inherently linked. When talking to patients and families about genetic health, health-care practitioners are constrained by the state of knowledge about particular symptoms, which relates to the medical research that has been conducted. The state of such knowledge generally depends upon the funding of research associated with particular symptoms. The funding of medical research often depends upon the outcomes of political debate that shapes health policy. The arguments used in such debate depend upon social norms about what is important. These norms vary according to cultural beliefs and practices. To treat any of these events in isolation from the others limits understanding of communication about genetics in families. Efforts to communicate about genes and race must also carefully consider effects of these messages on both perceived threat relating to susceptibility and severity, and perceptions of biological essentialism. The former may enhance motivation to act in health protective ways, while the latter may contribute to genetically based racism and genetic discrimination, outcomes associated with health disparities.

While family intergenerational communication about health histories may function to meet needs related to emotion and action, it may also be complex, difficult, and result in misunderstandings or reinforce generational stereotypes. By the same token, perceived benefits relating to concealment include the possible benefit of allowing individuals to interact "normally" with others, without the stigma associated with the disease. In view of the vital role that promoting awareness of family health history will likely play in health care for the foreseeable future, consideration of conditions likely to motivate disclosure versus concealment is warranted. When families talk about health history, one motivation is likely to be the belief that awareness will promote attention to signs of the disease for which there is a history. Such communication may also relate to belief that therapies are available to prevent or detect the disease for which one has a family history, and/or that one's own behavior can prevent the disease. That was the promise underpinning funding to complete the mapping of the human genome. Prevention and detection, however, are frequently not possibilities, making necessary conversation about this reality in clinical and public health communication about genetics and health.

REFERENCES

1. Parrott R. Collective amnesia: The absence of religious faith and spirituality in health communication research and practice. *Health Communication* 2004;16(1):1–5.
2. Parrott R. A multiple discourse approach to health communication: Translational research and ethical practice. *Journal of Applied Communication Research* 2008;36:1–7.
3. Lupton D. Discourse analysis: A new methodology for understanding the ideologies of health and illness. *Australian Journal of Public Health* 1992 Jun;16(2):145–150.
4. Parrott R. Emphasizing "communication" in health communication. *Journal of Communication* 2004 Dec;54(4):751–787.
5. Miller DF, Price JH. Epidemiology: Assessing the health status of a population. In: *Dimensions of Community Health*. 5th ed. New York: McGraw Hill Company, Inc.; 1998.
6. Surgeon General. Acting surgeon general issues call to action to prevent deep vein thrombosis and pulmonary embolism. September 15, 2008. Available at: http://www.surgeongeneral.gov.news/pressreleases/pr20080915.html. Accessed September 17, 2008.
7. Nelkin D, Lindee S. *The DNA Mystique: The Gene as Cultural Icon*. New York: W.H. Freeman; 1995.
8. Collins FS, Green ED, Guttmacher AE, Guyer MS. A vision for the future of genomics research. *Nature* 2003 Apr 24;422(6934):835–847.

9. Friedrich MJ. Public education critical to population-wide genomics research. *Journal of the National Cancer Institute* 2004 Aug 18;96(16):1196–1197.
10. Chilton P, Schaffner C. *Discourse and Politics in Discourse as Social Interaction.* London: Sage; 1997.
11. Achter P, Parrott R, Silk K. African Americans' opinions about human-genetics research. *Politics and the Life Sciences* 2004 Mar;23(1):60–66.
12. Parrott RL, Silk KJ, Dillow MR, Krieger JL, Harris TM, Condit CM. Development and validation of tools to assess genetic discrimination and genetically based racism. *Journal of the National Medical Association* 2005 Jul;97(7):980–990.
13. Kausmeyer DT, Lengerich EJ, Kluhsman BC, Morrone D, Harper GR, Baker MJ. A survey of patients' experiences with the cancer genetic counseling process: Recommendations for cancer genetics programs. *Journal of Genetic Counseling* 2006 Dec;15(6):409–431.
14. Mayor S. UK insurers postpone using predictive genetic testing until 2011. *British Medical Journal* 2005 Mar 19;330(7492):617.
15. Daar AS, Singer PA. Pharmacogenetics and geographical ancestry: Implications for drug development and global health. *Nature Reviews Genetics* 2005 Mar;6(3):241–246.
16. Condit CM, Bates B. How lay people respond to messages about genetics, health, and race. *Clinical Genetics* 2005 Aug;68(2):97–105.
17. Burke W, Pinsky LE, Press NA. Categorizing genetic tests to identify their ethical, legal, and social implications. *American Journal of Medical Genetics* 2001 Fall;106(3):233–240.
18. Conrad P. Uses of expertise: Sources, quotes, and voice in the reporting of genetics in the news. *Public Understanding of Science* 1999 Oct;8(4):285–302.
19. Anderson RR. *Religious Traditions and Prenatal Genetic Counseling.* Lincoln, NE: Munroe-Meyer Institute; 2002.
20. Halliday JL, Collins VR, Aitken MA, Richards MPM, Olsson CA. Genetics and public health - evolution, or revolution? *Journal of Epidemiology and Community Health* 2004 Nov;58(11):894–899.
21. Kardia SL, Modell SM, Peyser PA. Family-centered approaches to understanding and preventing coronary heart disease. *American Journal of Preventive Medicine* 2003 Feb;24(2):143–151.
22. Yoon PW, Scheuner MT, Peterson-Oehlke KL, Gwinn M, Faucett A, Khoury MJ. Can family history be used as a tool for public health and preventive medicine? *Genetics in Medicine* 2002 Jul-Aug;4(4):304–310.
23. Holtzman NA. What role for public health in genetics and vice versa? *Community Genetics* 2006;9:8–20.
24. Gebbie KM, Rosenstock L, Hernandez LM, Institute of Medicine (U.S.). *Committee on Educating Public Health Professionals for the 21st Century. Who Will Keep the Public Healthy? Educating Public Health Professionals for the 21st Century.* Washington, D.C.: National Academy Press; 2003.
25. Dillard JP, Shen L, Laxova A, Farrell P. Potential threats to the effective communication of genetic risk information: The case of cystic fibrosis. *Health Communication.* 2008 May-Jun;23(3):234–244.
26. Kunk RM. Expanding the newborn screen: Terrific or troubling? *MCN: The American Journal of Maternal/Child Nursing* 1998 Sep-Oct;23(5):266–271.

27. Ormondroyd E, Moynihan C, Ardern-Jones A, Eeles R, Foster C, Davolls S, et al. Communicating genetics research results to families: Problems arising when the patient participant is deceased. *Psycho-Oncology* 2008 Aug;17(8):804–811.

28. Patterson AR, Robinson LD, Naftalis EZ, Haley BB, Tomlinson GE. Custodianship of genetic information: clinical challenges and professional responsibility. *Journal of Clinical Oncology* 2005 Mar 20;23(9):2100–2104.

29. Mellon S, Berry-Bobovski L, Gold R, Levin N, Tainsky MA. Concerns and recommendations regarding inherited cancer risk: The perspectives of survivors and female relatives. *Journal of Cancer Education* 2007 Fall;22(3):168–173.

30. Peterson SK, Watts BG, Koehly LM, Vernon SW, Baile WF, Kohlmann WK, et al. How families communicate about HNPCC genetic testing: Findings from a qualitative study. *American Journal of Medical Genetics* 2003 May 15;119C(1):78–86.

31. Nease RF, Brooks WB. Patient desire for information and decision making in health care decisions. *Journal of General Internal Medicine* 2007;10:593–600.

32. Dillard JP, Carson CL, Bernard CJ, Laxova A, Farrell PM. An analysis of communication following newborn screening for cystic fibrosis. *Health Communication* 2004;16(2):195–205.

33. UK Newborn Screening Programme Centre 2008. Available at: http://newbornbloodspot.screening.nhs.uk/. Accessed July 9, 2008.

34. Geller G, Bernhardt BA, Holtzman NA. The media and public reaction to genetic research. *Journal of the American Medical Association.* 2002 Feb 13;287(6):773.

35. Conrad P, Weinberg D. Has the gene for alcoholism been discovered three times since 1980? A news media analysis. *Perspectives on Social Problems* 1996;8:3–25.

36. Condit CM, Williams M. Audience responses to the discourse of medical genetics: Evidence against the critique of medicalization. *Health Communication* 1997;9(3):219–235.

37. Hedgecoe A. Schizophrenia and the narrative of enlightened geneticization. *Social Studies of Science* 2001 Dec;31(6):875–911.

38. Genetics and film: A short history [database online]. *The Human Genome.* December 3, 2006. Available at: http://genome.wellcome.ac.uk/doc_WTD023540.html. Accessed September 25, 2007.

39. Repo! The Genetic Opera! [database online] September 10, 2007. Available at: http://www.imdb.com/title/tt0963194/. Accessed September 25, 2007.

40. Surgeon General's Family Health History Initiative. U.S. Department of Health & Human Services; 2009. Available at: http://www.hhs.gov/family-history/. Accessed June 4, 2009.

41. Jacobellis J, Martin L, Engle J, VanEenwyk J, Bradley LA, Kassim S, et al. Genetic testing for breast and ovarian cancer susceptibility: Evaluating direct-to-consumer marketing-Atlanta, Denver, Raleigh-Durham, and Seattle 2003. *Journal of the American Medical Association* 2004;292:796–798.

42. Condit CM, Dubriwny T, Lynch J, Parrott R. Lay people's understanding of and preference against the word "mutation". *American Journal of Medical Genetics* 2004 Oct 15;130A(3):245–250.

43. Condit C, Parrott R, O'Grady B. Principles and practice of communication processes for genetics in public health. In: Khoury M, Burke W, & Thomson E, eds. *Genetics and Public Health: Translating Human Genetics into Public Health Action.* New York: Oxford University Press; 2000:549–567.

44. Sarangi S. The language of likelihood in genetic-counseling discourse. *Journal of Language and Social Psychology* 2002;21:7–31.

45. Chapple A, May C, Campion P. Lay understanding of genetic disease: A British study of families attending a genetic counseling service. *Journal of Genetic Counseling* 1995 Dec;4(4):281–300.

46. Royak-Schaler R, deVellis BM, Sorenson JR, Wilson KR, Lannin DR, Emerson JA. Breast cancer in African-American families. Risk perception, cancer worry, and screening practices of first-degree relatives. *Annals of the New York Academy of Sciences* 1995 Sep 30;768:281–285.

47. Lafayette D, Abuelo D, Passero MA, Tantravahi U. Attitudes toward cystic fibrosis carrier and prenatal testing and utilization of carrier testing among relatives of individuals with cystic fibrosis. *Journal of Genetic Counseling* 1999 Feb;8(1):17–36.

48. Mischler EH, Wilfond BS, Fost N, Laxova A, Reiser C, Sauer CM, et al. Cystic fibrosis newborn screening: Impact on reproductive behavior and implications for genetic counseling. *Pediatrics* 1998 Jul;102(1 Pt 1): 44–52.

49. Ponder M, Murton F, Hallowell N, Statham H, Green J, Richards M. Genetic counseling, reproductive behavior and future reproductive intentions of people with neurofibromatosis type I (NF1). *Journal of Genetic Counseling* 1998;7:331–344.

50. Condit C, Parrott R. Perceived levels of health risk associated with linguistic descriptors and type of disease. *Science Communication* 2004 Dec;26(2):152–161.

51. Bernhardt JM, McClain J, Parrott RL. Online health communication about human genetics: Perceptions and preferences of Internet users. *Cyberpsychology and Behavior* 2004 Dec;7(6):728–733.

52. Dillard JP, Shen L, Tluczek A, Modaff P, Farrell P. The effect of disruptions during counseling on recall of genetic risk information: The case of cystic fibrosis. *Journal of Genetic Counseling* 2007;16:179–190.

53. Dillard JP, Carson CL. Uncertainty management following a positive newborn screening for cystic fibrosis. *Journal of Health Communication* 2005 Jan-Feb;10(1):57–76.

54. Parrott R. *Talking About Health: Why Communication Matters.* Malden, MA: Wiley-Blackwell; 2009.

55. Yaktine AL, Pool R. *Nutrigenomics and Beyond: Informing the Future - Workshop Summary. Institute of Medicine Report.* Washington D.C.: National Academies Press; 2007.

56. Dens N, Eagle LC, De Pelsmacker P. Attitudes and self-reported behavior of patients, doctors, and pharmacists in New Zealand and Belgium toward direct-to-consumer advertising of medication. *Health Communication* 2008 Jan-Feb;23(1):45–61.

57. Bates BR, Poirot K, Harris TM, Condit CM, Achter PJ. Evaluating direct-to-consumer marketing of race-based pharmacogenomics: A focus group study of public understandings of applied genomic medication. *Journal of Health Communication* 2004 Nov-Dec;9(6):541–559.

58. Weil J. *Psychosocial Genetic Counseling*. Cambridge, England: Oxford University Press; 2000.
59. Weil J. *Multicultural education and genetic counseling*. *Clinical Genetics* 2001;59(3):143–149.
60. Kittles RA, Weiss KM. Race, ancestry, and genes: Implications for defining disease risk. *Annual Review of Genomics and Human Genetics* 2003;4:33–67.
61. Condit CM, Condit DM, Achter P. Human equality, affirmative action, and genetic models of human variation. *Rhetoric and Public Affairs* 2004;4:85–108.
62. Weiner JL, Silk KJ, Parrott RL. Family communication and genetic health: A research note. *Journal of Family Communication* 2005;4:313–324.
63. Plotz D. *The Genius Factory: The Curious History of the Nobel Prize Sperm Bank*. New York: Random House, Inc.; 2005.
64. Gollust SE, Wilfond BS, Hull SC. Direct-to-consumer sales of genetic services on the Internet. *Genetics in Medicine* 2003 Jul-Aug;5(4):332–337.
65. Hull SC, Prasad K. Reading between the lines: Direct-to-consumer advertising of genetic testing. *Hastings Center Report* 2001 May-Jun;31(3):33–35.
66. Gollust SE, Hull SC, Wilfond BS. Limitations of direct-to-consumer advertising for clinical genetic testing. *Journal of the American Medical Association* 2002 Oct;288(14):1762–1767.
67. Harding A. Do it yourself cancer gene testing raises concerns. *BMJ*. 2005 Mar 19;330(7492):617.
68. Williams-Jones B. Where there's a web, there's a way: Commercial genetic testing and the Internet. *Community Genetics* 2003;6(1):46–57.
69. Modra L. Prenatal genetic testing kits sold at your local pharmacy: Promoting autonomy or promoting confusion? *Bioethics* 2006 Sep;20(5):254–263.
70. Wasson K, Cook ED, Helzlsouer K. Direct-to-consumer online genetic testing and the four principles: An analysis of the ethical issues. *Ethics and Medicine* 2006;22:83–91.
71. Hoskins KF, Stopfer JE, Calzone KA, Merajver SD, Rebbeck TR, Garber JE, et al. Assessment and counseling for women with a family history of breast cancer. A guide for clinicians. *Journal of the American Medical Association* 1995 Feb 15;273(7):577–585.
72. Carter CL, Hailey BJ. Psychological issues in genetic testing for breast cancer. *Women's Health* 1999;28(4):73–91.
73. Sanderson SC, Wardle J. Will genetic testing for complex diseases increase motivation to quit smoking? Anticipated reactions in a survey of smokers. *Health Education and Behavior* 2005 Oct;32(5):640–653.
74. Parrott R, Silk K, Weiner J, Condit C, Harris T, Bernhardt J. Deriving lay models of uncertainty about genes' role in illness causation to guide communication about human genetics. *Journal of Communication* 2004 Mar;54(1):105–122.
75. Ness BD. *Encyclopedia of Genetics*. Pasadena, CA: Salem Press; 2004.
76. Bendle M. Teleportation, cyborgs, and the posthuman ideology. *Social Semiotics* 2002;12:45–62.
77. Smith RA. Picking a frame for communicating about genetics: stigmas or challenges. *Journal of Genetic Counseling* 2007 Jun;16(3):289–298.
78. Brookey RA. Bio-rhetoric, background beliefs and the biology of homosexuality. *Argumentation and Advocacy* 2001;37:171–183.

79. Turner SS. Jurassic Park technology in the bioinformatics economy: How cloning narratives negotiate the telos of DNA. *American Literature* 2002;74:887–909.

80. Baty BJ, Kinney AY, Ellis SM. Developing culturally sensitive cancer genetics communication aids for African Americans. *American Journal of Medical Genetics Part A* 2003 Apr 15;118A(2):146–155.

81. Goodnight GT. The personal, technical, and public spheres of argument: A speculative inquiry into the art of public deliberation. *Journal of the American Forensic Association* 1982;18:218–227.

82. Lehrman S. Race, genes, and illness. *Boston Globe*. April 19, 2007: Available at: http://www.boston.com/news.globe/editorial_opinion/oped/articles/2007/04/19/race_genes... Accessed December 9, 2009.

83. Singer E, Antonucci T, Van Hoewyk J. Racial and ethnic variations in knowledge and attitudes about genetic testing. *Genetic Testing* 2004 Spring;8(1):31–43.

84. Cohen LH, Fine BA, Pergament E. An assessment of ethnocultural beliefs regarding the causes of birth defects and genetic disorders. *Journal of Genetic Counseling* 1998;7:15–29.

85. Nicolas G, DeSilva AM, Grey KS, Gonzalez-Eastep D. Using a multicultural lens to understand illnesses among Haitians living in America. *Professional Psychology-Research and Practice* 2006 Dec;37(6):702–707.

86. Cheng LR. Asian-American cultural perspectives on birth defects: Focus on cleft palate. *The Cleft Palate Journal* 1990 Jul;27(3):294–300.

87. Young M, Klingle RS. Silent partners in medical care: A cross-cultural study of patient participation. *Health Communication* 1996;8(1):29–53.

88. Richards M. Lay and professional knowledge of genetics and inheritance. *Public Understanding of Science* 1996;5:217–230.

89. Bennett RL, Motulsky AG, Bittles A, Hudgins L, Uhrich S, Doyle DL, et al. Genetic counseling and screening of consanguineous couples and their offspring: Recommendations of the National Society of Healthcare Practitioners. *Journal of Genetic Counseling* 2002;11:97–119.

90. Parrott RL, Silk KJ, Condit C. Diversity in lay perceptions of the sources of human traits: Genes, environments, and personal behaviors. *Social Science and Medicine* 2003 Mar;56(5):1099–1109.

91. Rolland S. Genetics, family systems, and multicultural influences. *Families, Systems, and Health* 2006;24(4):425–441.

92. Parrott R, Condit CM. *Evaluating Women's Health Messages : A Resource Book*. Thousand Oaks, CA: Sage Publications; 1996.

93. Tuana N. *The Less Noble Sex: Scientific, Religious, and Philosophical Conceptions of Woman's Nature*. Indianapolis: Indiana University Press; 1993.

94. Finkler K. *Experiencing the New genetics: Family and Kinship on the Medical Frontier*. Philadelphia: University of Pennsylvania Press; 2000.

95. Buchanan GS, Rodgers GM, Ware Branch D. The inherited thrombophilias: Genetics, epidemiology, and laboratory evaluation. *Best Practice and Research Clinical Obstetrics Gynaecology* 2003 Jun;17(3):397–411.

96. Phelan JC. Geneticization of deviant behavior and consequences for stigma: the case of mental illness. *Journal of Health and Social Behavior* 2005 Dec;46(4):307–322.

97. Miller M. An intergenerational case study of suicidal tradition and mother-daughter communication. *The Journal of Applied Communication Research* 1995 Nov;23(4):247–270.

98. Mercer L, Creighton S, Holden JJ, Lewis ME. Parental perspectives on the causes of an autism spectrum disorder in their children. *Journal of Cancer Education* 2006 Feb;15(1):41–50.

99. Mellon S, Berry-Bobovski L, Gold R, Levin N, Tainsky MA. Communication and decision-making about seeking inherited cancer risk information: Findings from female survivor-relative focus groups. *Psycho-Oncology* 2006 Mar;15(3):193–208.

100. Wilson BJ, Forrest K, van Teijlingen ER, McKee L, Haites N, Matthews E, et al. Family communication about genetic risk: The little that is known. *Community Genetics* 2004;7(1):15–24.

101. Forrest LE, Delatycki MB, Skene L, Aitken M. Communicating genetic information in families - a review of guidelines and position papers. *European Journal of Human Genetics* 2007 Jun;15(6):612–618.

102. Godard B, Hurlimann T, Letendre M, Egalite N, BRCAs I. Guidelines for disclosing genetic information to family members: From development to use. *Familial Cancer* 2006 Mar;5(1):103–116.

103. Gaff CL, Clarke AJ, Atkinson P, Sivell S, Elwyn G, Iredale R, et al. Process and outcome in communication of genetic information within families: A systematic review. *European Journal of Human Genetics* 2007 Oct;15(10):999–1011.

104. Hallowell N, Ardern-Jones A, Eeles R, Foster C, Lucassen A, Moynihan C, et al. Communication about genetic testing in families of male BRCA1/2 carriers and non-carriers: patterns, priorities and problems. *Clinical Genetics* 2005 Jun;67(6):492–502.

105. Gregory M, Boddington P, Dimond R, Atkinson P, Clarke A, Collins P. Communicating about haemophilia within the family: the importance of context and of experience. *Haemophilia* 2007 Mar;13(2):189–198.

106. Keenan KF, Simpson SA, Wilson BJ, Van Teijlingen ER, McKee L, Haites N, et al. 'It's their blood not mine': Who's responsible for (not) telling relatives about genetic risk? *Health Risk and Society* 2005 Sep;7(3):209–226.

107. Davison C. Predictive genetics: the cultural implications of supplying probable futures. In: Marteau TM, Richards MPM, eds. *The Troubled Helix: Social and Psychological Implications of the New Human Genetics.* Cambridge, England: Cambridge University Press; 1996:317–330.

108. Ciske DJ, Haavisto A, Laxova A, Rock LZ, Farrell PM. Genetic counseling and neonatal screening for cystic fibrosis: An assessment of the communication process. *Pediatrics* 2001 Apr;107(4):699–705.

109. Denayer L, Evers-Kiebooms G, Van den Berghe H. A child with cystic fibrosis: I. Parental knowledge about the genetic transmission of CF and about DNA-diagnostic procedures. *Clinical Genetics* 1990 Mar;37(3):198–206.

110. Clausen H, Brandt NJ, Schwartz M, Skovby F. Psychological and social impact of carrier screening for cystic fibrosis among pregnant woman. A pilot study. *Clinical Genetics* 1996 Apr;49(4):200–205.

111. Genia V. A psychometric evaluation of the Allport-Ross I/E scales in a religiosity heterogeneous sample. *Journal for the Scientific Study of Religion* 1993;32:284.

112. Harris TM, Parrott R, Dorgan KA. Talking about human genetics within religious frameworks. *Health Communication* 2004;16(1):105–116.
113. Cox SM, McKellin W. 'There's this thing in our family': Predictive testing and the construction of risk for Huntington Disease. *Social Health and Illness* 1999;21:622–646.
114. Walter FM, Emery J, Braithwaite D, Marteau TM. Lay understanding of familial risk of common chronic diseases: a systematic review and synthesis of qualitative research. *Annals of Family Medicine* 2004 Nov-Dec;2(6):583–594.
115. Culbertson HM, Stempel GH. How media use and reliance affect knowledge level. *Communication Research* 1986 Oct;13(4):579–602.
116. Peters K, Apse K, Blackford A, McHugh B, Michalic D, Biesecker B. Living with Marfan syndrome: Coping with stigma. *Clinical Genetics* 2005 Jul;68(1):6–14.
117. Turner J, Biesecker B, Leib J, Biesecker L, Peters KF. Parenting children with Proteus syndrome: experiences with, and adaptation to, courtesy stigma. *American Journal of Medical Genetics Part A* 2007 Sep 15;143A(18):2089–2097.
118. Parens E, Asch A. Disability rights critique of prenatal genetic testing: Reflections and recommendations. *Mental Retardation and Developmental Disabilities Research Reviews* 2003;9(1):40–47.
119. Tyson JE, Broyles RS. Progress in assessing the long-term outcome of extremely low-birth-weight infants. *Journal of the American Medical Association* 1996 Aug 14;276(6):492–493.
120. National Center for the Dissemination of Disability Research. Disability Research and the Media 2009. Available at: http://198.214.141.98/products/researchexchange/v04n03/media.html. Accessed July 13, 2009.
121. Cooley WC, Graham ES, Moeschler JB, Graham JM. Reactions of mothers and medical professionals to a film about Down Syndrome. *American Journal of Diseases of Children* 1990;144:1112–1116.
122. Helm DT, Miranda S, Chedd NC. Prenatal diagnosis of Down Syndrome: Mother's reflections on supports needed from diagnosis to birth. *Mental Retardation* 1998;36:55–61.
123. Rapp R. Amniocentesis in Sociocultural Perspective. *Journal of Genetic Counseling* 1993;2(3):183–196.
124. Patterson A, Satz M. Genetic counseling and the disabled: Feminism examines the stance of those who stand at the gate. *Hypatia.* 2002 Summer;17(3):118–142.

4

FAMILY NARRATIVES

April R. Trees, Jody Koenig Kellas, & Myra I. Roche

'Family stories' can be used to make sense of a genetic diagnosis, construct an identity and communicate this to others. Families also are asked to provide a story in the form of a medical or family history by health-care practitioners. Narrative theories illuminate the way these stories are constructed and told, as well as the purpose they serve. By using the narrative process, practitioners can facilitate adjustment and thereby the capacity of the family to communicate with others.

Humans are storytellers, giving meaning to experience through narrative [1]. Narratives are communicative constructions organized by plot, character, and sequence and situated in social, historical, and familial contexts. Through telling stories, people construct and communicate identities and relationships and make sense of lived experiences. A variety of approaches to narrative guide research on family communication, although these are rarely referred to as "theories" in the formal sense [2]. These approaches focus on important processes of how narratives are constructed and used by both health-care practitioners and by the families with whom they work. The role of narratives in making sense of life experiences [3] has important implications for practitioners because it guides how information is elicited, conveyed, interpreted, and judged by both individuals and families in a clinical setting. Narrative theorizing can be especially relevant when considering the practitioner–patient interactions that revolve around the provision of genetic information. In this chapter, the use of narratives in shaping three components of this process will be emphasized: *(1)* the family history, *(2)* making sense of the diagnosis, and *(3)* coping with the implications of a genetic diagnosis.

GENERAL INTRODUCTION TO NARRATIVE THEORIZING

Narrative theorizing provides a frame for understanding how individuals make sense of their life experiences. Although much of narrative theorizing emphasizes the singularity of individual experience, noting that "narrators contending with life experiences struggle to formulate an account that both provides an interpretive frame and does justice to life's complexities" [4] (p. 24), families also use narratives to make sense of their shared life experiences and provide a way to understand and communicate their family history, values, and identities [5, 6]. During health consultations, narratives play a dominant role, from the ways families reveal their family and medical history to their later recounting of their experience in the clinic to relatives and friends and other health-care providers. Health-care practitioners can use these family stories to gain insight into family meaning and functioning in order to help facilitate effective family communication about the condition, its etiology, and implications and to promote coping with the diagnosis. The structure, content, and process of telling stories are highly relevant as the practitioner assesses the person(s)' history and counsels about the diagnosis.

Narratives provide a way for families to structure their shared experiences. The structural features of narratives include constructing a plot (what is the story about, who are the main characters and their relationship to one another, and from whose perspective is the story told), sequencing events (which events are included and which are omitted, which events are considered most important, and what order are they told in), and attributing motives (which characters or what events are assigned blame or credit). These structural elements both encourage and reveal sense making [3]. Three critical features of the narrative-building process are coherence, temporality, and perspective [7, 8].

Coherence refers to the degree to which the individual threads of the story are intertwined and hang together. Coherent stories show internal consistency, provide a logical sequence of events, and present the elements in an organized way [1, 9]. When multiple family members tell a story together, it can be completely incoherent or incoherent because there are conflicts between individually coherent but competing stories that together create a chaotic and inconsistent overall story [10]. Stories are the ways in which we explain ourselves intelligently in the social world [11, 12], and narrative theorizing typically assumes that a good story is a coherent story [1, 13]. Coherence helps individuals and families assign meaning to experiences and create consistency in relationship to their life stories. When family narratives seem chaotic, the health-care practitioner can attempt to identify the consistent parts of the story, ask for clarification about those parts that seem inconsistent, and/or add connections to help create coherence. One of the practitioner's tasks is to help families create a coherent story about their health experiences. The purpose of this coherence is twofold: the family can benefit from greater coherence by better making sense of their experiences, and medically coherent stories help the practitioner elicit critical pieces of information to create a version of the narrative that is communicated to other practitioners.

During a health consultation, an individual's structure of events and story content may not fit the medical model required to relate his or her history to other health-care practitioners. A second dimension of structure, temporality, is the way in which the storyteller establishes timeframes and chronologies within the narrative [14]. Narratives contain events that are ordered in particular ways; however, lay notions of narrative coherence, sequence, and plot often do not coincide with the structural features of a medical and family history that are required in the medical model (see Chapter 5). The family's story must often be reordered and restructured by the practitioner taking a family history in order to emphasize relevant aspects. Families typically have little understanding of which information is important to the medical historian and which is not. It is therefore important that the practitioner state the goals and needs for specific kinds of information early in the session to minimize the trial-and-error nature of gathering the family and medical history. In order to understand a story, listeners expect narratives to be sequential and coherent and adhere to what Labov and Waletsky [15] describe as a well-formed narrative—one that includes an abstract (preview), orientation (what led up to an event), complicating actions, resolution, coda (summary; moral of the story), and evaluation (the affective analysis of the story's meaning). Although families may not always create well-formed stories, this narrative structure should be recognizable to families and useful for practitioners working with families to develop a helpful narrative.

The complicating actions and the ordering of a sequence of events within the family's narrative may also hint at their search for the existence of a cause. Narrative sequencing intersects with a need to know why this particular sequence occurred as opposed to any number of alternative events and sequences. The need to ascribe causes is an important one in determining a genetic etiology for a condition, and determining the timing of the presumed causal events (prior to conception, during prenatal development, infancy, childhood, adolescence, or adulthood) is critical. For example, it is important to distinguish between growth delay that originates prenatally as opposed to postnatally.

The ways that a family orders the important events leading up to the diagnosis can reveal their assumptions about causality as well, providing insight into the family's beliefs about illness and/or genetics. For example, many women assume that their child's problems are due, at least in part, to something that occurred, or failed to occur, during the pregnancy. This misbelief, if uncorrected, can contribute to unnecessary feelings of guilt and shame. When a child has a new genetic change as the cause for his or her problems, mothers are often surprised and relieved to learn that they had no role in its development. Families' underlying beliefs revealed in their stories also have the potential to shape their behavior by influencing the way they communicate the possibility of risk to relatives and whether they share genetic test results with others. For example, misbeliefs about causality and transmission of genes through unaffected relatives may be a contributing factor as to why women with inherited forms of breast cancer are less likely to disclose risk information to their brothers than to their sisters [16].

The family's assumptions and viewpoints shape a third critical feature of the narrative sense-making process: perspective taking. Different members of a family may ascribe motives and describe experiences differently depending upon their perspective and their role in the story and their role in the family. In order to reveal this complexity, it is useful if multiple perspectives are used to construct the story. When stories have multiple narrators, there may still be one person who the family accepts as the "main" source of information. For example, the mother or other primary caregiver is typically the main narrator for a child and controls the structure and content of the narrative. Although others may add supporting information, they often defer to the primary narrator when their views conflict.

Perspective taking during storytelling recognizes that all family members may not experience the relevant events in the same way. Families may vary in the degree to which members attend to others' viewpoints, incorporate others' perspectives in the narrative being developed, and confirm or disconfirm these perspectives [9]. Attention to and confirmation of one another's perspectives during jointly told family identity stories and stressful experience stories predict the degree of family cohesion, adaptability, and family supportiveness [6, 17]. Families who engaged in more perspective taking during the joint telling of difficult experiences were more supportive than those who did not take each others' perspectives into account. Listening for the degree to which differing perspectives are allowed in the narrative can give the health-care practitioner valuable insight into family functioning, help identify who the family considers to be the main narrator, and determine the need for additional resources following the consultation. The family dynamics revealed in families' stories may also provide clues as to how likely it is that the genetic information, including the availability of genetic testing, will be communicated to relatives. When the practitioner senses strained relations in the family that may be a barrier to this communication [18, 19], it provides an opportunity to discuss specific strategies by which appropriate relatives can be informed.

The structure and process of storytelling provide insight into the meanings clients attach to their experiences and diagnoses as well as qualities of their family relationships. The health-care practitioner serves as a listener, interpreter, and facilitator in the context of these jointly told stories, and by drawing on key elements of narrative theorizing, he or she can help families arrive at a coherent, meaningful narrative. Practitioners may also facilitate the perspective-taking process that occurs during joint or multigenerational family interviews and help families arrive at a final, consensus story. This process can help the family by providing a more structured and coherent narrative to tell to future health-care providers or other family members. Narrative theory and family communication research provide insight to help practitioners engage in this process successfully, and this is discussed in more detail in the following section. The practitioner, however, also can guide families or family members to the benefits of narrative beyond the medical interview context. Thus, the latter two sections of the chapter focus on narrative theory and research relevant to the family's identity and coping processes following a diagnosis.

THE FAMILY HISTORY: HOW DO FAMILIES TELL THIS STORY?

Clinical genetics and especially genetic counseling rely heavily on the ability of individuals and families to provide coherent and accurate narratives about whatever problems have brought them to the clinic. The lost art of listening to what a patient says, recognizing how he or she says it, and translating the story into useful and recognizable patterns takes time, specialized training, and is poorly reimbursed in private health-care systems. Although historically, all of medicine was narrative based, the process of eliciting and translating detailed stories is being rapidly replaced in most specialties by technological methods that directly answer questions without needing to take into account the narrator's perspective. A body of research on the practice of narrative medicine [e.g., 20, 21] and on medical interviews [e.g., 22], however, argues for the value of approaching family history interviews as narrative processes.

The information sought in the genetic counseling evaluation process is distinct from most families' experiences with other health-care practitioners, and many families arrive in the clinic having little idea of what to expect or what is expected of them [23]. Some differences include the much greater depth and breadth of the family and medical information that is sought, unique components of the physical exam, and the large amount of time devoted to explanation and discussion of the potential genetic causes of the condition, genetic testing options, and resources for help and support. Additionally, families are usually ill prepared to furnish the amount of detail that is requested both in the questions asked of an individual relative and in recounting the number and type of relatives in the family. In the genetic counseling setting, counselors tend to spend more time eliciting family members' stories than typically occurs in other types of health contexts.

In health research, scholars have contrasted the "voice of medicine" with the "voice of the lifeworld" (14), suggesting that medical interviews can be a site at which the patient's situated experiences and individual meaning-making emerge and become accessible to the health-care practitioner. For this to happen, practitioners "need the ability to listen to the narratives of the patient, grasp and honor their meanings, and be moved to act on the patient's behalf" [24] (p. 1897). Narrative theorizing, then, highlights the value of narrative competence, for inviting and hearing families' stories as well as for restructuring and reinterpreting the narrative for other health practitioners.

The Value of Inviting a Story

Whereas the traditional medical history-taking interview tends to follow a question/answer pattern focusing on close-ended questions, *narrative expansion* [25] allows a person to introduce material of concern to him or her that may not directly answer the specific questions asked by health-care practitioners. In a structured, practitioner-dominated interview process, "the patient might not tell the whole story, might not ask the most frightening questions, and might not feel heard" [24] (p. 1899). Additionally, Charon [20] suggests that narrative processes require practitioners to seek their patients' point of view, helping them to develop empathy and create a whole picture of their experience. In the genetic counseling context, this whole picture can include the ability to gain insight into family experiences along with individual emotional and physical experiences. Narratives reveal information about families' shared understanding of their social environment, including the family's sense of mastery or beliefs about the value of taking action and seeking information in response to stress, solidarity or the degree to which the family defines problems as shared or individual, and closure or tolerance for ambiguity in the family [26]. These shared understandings shape family members' responses to stressful experiences such as being diagnosed with a genetic condition.

Genetic counseling's ethos of nondirectiveness depends on the ability of the practitioner to gain insight into clients' perspectives in order to help them weigh various options for diagnosis and treatment, to help them understand the genetic etiology of the condition, and to cope with its implications. Eliciting this information requires more time than a typical medical visit and is enhanced by creating a safe environment to encourage clients to share their lifeviews. The use of narratives also allows the counselor to gauge the client's level of education, cultural/religious background, and previous experiences that will then suggest optimal ways in which to tailor the educational aspect of the session. Finally, narratives can pinpoint specific emotional needs, such as the guilt of parents whose child has an inherited genetic condition, that require the counselor's ability to normalize this event by placing it in a broader context that everyone has some genetic changes. Other common themes that arise during these families' narratives include misconceptions about the genetic versus the

hereditary natures of conditions, the role of the family history in establishing (or not) the genetic etiology of a condition, and the mistaken association between the outward characteristics of someone with a genetic
condition and the altered gene. This latter assumption leads to the mistaken belief that an unaffected relative has the genetic alteration in the
family because of their physical resemblance or similar personality traits
to the affected family member.

Narratives can bridge differences between the health-care practitioner and the patient [20]. There are two underlying assumptions that can
impact the effectiveness of genetic counseling: beliefs about the cause of
a disease or disability and the contexts of illness. Charon [20] notes practitioners and patients may hold different understandings of the causes
of disease, something that may be encountered while trying to provide
information about a genetic etiology when a family has minimal understanding of biology and, therefore, has no experience in viewing causality
in a scientific way. Fisher [1] offers the concept of narrative rationality as
an alternative to technical, scientific rationality in part because narratives
are accessible to everyone, whereas technical rationality is restricted to
experts. Thus, narratives may enable an important bridge between practitioners and their clients. McAllister [27] argued that personal theories of
how conditions are inherited in families reflect ways that individuals make
sense of their family history and personal experiences and these sense-
making processes will also shape their beliefs about risks. Perceptions
of risk affect the responses to genetic testing results [28], and making
sense of risk is an important motivator, influencing whether an individual
chooses to disclose the results to family members [29] and governing how
much and who is told. The ways in which families explain the occurrence
of a condition can signal to the practitioner that the family's personal
beliefs may diverge in important ways from scientific explanations.

Secondly, health-care practitioners who focus on the medical consequences of the condition can benefit from hearing families' stories when
they encompass a multidimensional view of their life-world, including the
impact of the condition on family life. Families reveal important information about their identity and functioning in stories about their family
[e.g., 6, 30]. Both the stories individuals tell about their families, including story themes [30] and the use of "I versus we" in talking about experiences [6], and how family members tell stories together, including the
degree to which they attend to and confirm one another's perspectives
and the coherence of the story they construct together [17, 31], reveal
information about the quality of family relationships and how they have
coped with difficult situations in the past and how they are likely to cope
with them in the future. Practitioners who widen the topics of the interview to include family narratives create the opportunity for the various
contexts of illness to become a part of the story being developed.

Finally, narratives also provide moral frames, revealing the underlying values that motivate particular actions and grant the storyteller some

degree of control in constructing his or her story. Stories both recount the series of events and provide an accounting of how and why these events occurred [1]. Narratives allow clients to tell their story in the way that makes sense to them [21]. Adelsward and Sachs [32], for example, observed "narrative contests" between genetic practitioners and clients in family history interviews, with different meanings and values for what counted as newsworthy and where attention should be focused. They argue that "what you see when you look back influences your view of the future" (p. 131), and that understanding how an individual makes sense of family members' past health experiences can be important for developing insight into current and future behavior. To the extent possible, allowing families to tell their story in the order that makes sense to them can provide a richer view of the family experience.

Narrative Practices

Conducting the session as a narrative requires that the health-care practitioner have several key interpretive and behavioral competencies. Narratives are joint constructions, collaboratively created between teller and listener and requiring the coordinated activity of both participants [21, 33]. As an active listener and interpreter of the story, the practitioner's behaviors can facilitate the storytelling, eliciting a rich, insightful story that provides a window into the client's experience and understanding of the medical situation. Beginning with an open-ended question about a family's concerns, for example, is one strategy that provides space for families to begin to tell their story. Alternatively practitioners' responses and behaviors can shut down the narrative process and restrict the voice of the narrator. In a conversation analysis of medical interviews, for example, Clark and Mishler [22] found that remaining silent at critical junctures granted patients implicit permission to talk for an extended time, a component essential for telling a story. Practitioners who use engaged and attentive listening behaviors that acknowledge and legitimize the telling of the story encourage further narrative development. Charon [24] calls this kind of listening empathic engagement. In contrast, when the practitioner constantly controls the exchange, by conducting it in a predetermined order and by the pace of response to what the client says, this casts the patient rather than the practitioner as the attentive respondent. Although time limitations may make this difficult to achieve, particularly in one-time consultations, the creation of a coherent narrative is a joint effort that allows the themes and contexts important to both the patient and practitioner to be incorporated into the story being told.

In addition to collaborative construction of stories, Charon [20] argues that health-care practitioners need to develop narrative competence that increases their interpretive skills, helping them make sense of the stories that patients tell. Narrative competence includes the ability to closely listen to the story, focusing attention on features of the story such as the frame (e.g., what is included and what is left out, where is it set), the form or structure of the story, time (e.g., chronology of events, relationship of activities in time), plot (i.e., what happens in the story), and motivations. Additionally, practitioners can learn to listen for repeated elements that may occur in many families' stories. Charon advocates that practitioners create narratives about their patients, requiring that they attend closely to patients' experiences and think reflectively about their interpretation of those experiences.

DIAGNOSIS AND IDENTITY CONSTRUCTION: HOW DO FAMILIES SEE THEMSELVES AND UNDERSTAND THEIR EXPERIENCE?

Genetic testing and clinical genetic evaluations can reveal a broad range of diagnoses with differing implications for family functioning. On one end of the spectrum, discovering that one is a carrier of an autosomal recessive condition has implications for potentially adverse reproductive consequences but rarely has personal health consequences. At the other end of the spectrum is the presymptomatic discovery that an individual is at high risk for developing serious complications in addition to the significant chance that future generations will also be affected. The impact of a genetic diagnosis on the family can also vary by whether other relatives are at potentially substantial risk, the presence of stigmatizing physical differences as part of the phenotype, the degree to which the features of the condition affect daily living, and whether the condition can be confidently diagnosed. To varying degrees, depending upon the nature of the diagnosis, families may struggle with the identity implications of their diagnosis as both individuals and in their family roles. Specifically, families may struggle with both negative stereotypes or societal narratives as well as their own feelings of guilt, blame, and/or loss that disrupt their sense of identity. This is especially true for many rare genetic conditions that cannot be definitively diagnosed by laboratory testing [34] and that leave the family in doubt about the prognosis, implications, and even the name of the condition.

Following the confirmation that a condition is genetically determined, individuals and families may need to alter their views of the role of the affected individual in the family. For example, upon learning that their young son has fragile X syndrome (which causes developmental delay), a family must alter their goals and expectations of their child, cope with their anxiety about the child's future, and may dread having to tell relatives that they and their children may also be at risk, fearing both blame and stigmatization. Narrative theorizing can help health-care practitioners (*a*) better understand the societal discourse in which these stigmata are situated and, more importantly, (*b*) help individuals and families to reframe their narratives, thereby reshaping negative perceptions, potentially reducing psychological distress, and developing a story that they will be comfortable telling to members of their biological families and their extended social networks. Narrative theory and research can help practitioners understand the ways in which patients might frame the story of their diagnoses in light of potential societal or individual stigmatization as well as a need to cope with personal emotional distress.

Master Narratives

Narratives exist at multiple levels of abstraction [see 2, 12 for reviews]. Although individuals and families may tell stories of their diagnosis of a genetic condition to others, their initial reaction to a genetic diagnosis likely grows first out of their orientation to societal, historical, and contextual narrative ideologies about the diagnosis and about what it means that a condition is "genetic." Some narrative theorists refer to such societal level narratives as ideological forces or legitimacy narratives [35]. Others refer to them as master narratives or canonical stories "...that represent the generally accepted version in a particular culture" or the way things are supposed to be [36] (p. 120). For example, Harter et al. [35] illustrate the power of societal discourses in shaping perceptions of female reproductive health through the metaphor of the biological clock and the master narrative "age as decline." They suggest that these kinds of societal discourses support a negative preoccupation with aging and fertility.

Societal discourse about genetics includes the following types of master narratives: genetic determinism, the social view of a mutation as making a person "a mutant," that people with any genetic change should not have children, that all genetic changes are bad, that genetic changes are rare (it happens to somebody else), there is a parental responsibility for having healthy children, and that genetic conditions are both shameful yet also out of one's control. For example, when a child has a relatively common genetic condition, like Down syndrome, families are confronted with many harmful cultural assumptions about the prognosis and worth of their child. These assumptions exemplify master narratives of genetic determinism, genetic conditions as shameful, and that all genetic changes are bad. Furthermore, parents of children with genetic conditions that include physical differences as part of the phenotype (e.g., albinism, dwarfism) may experience more social stigma than those with less obvious differences (master narratives of parental responsibility and genetic conditions as shameful). Some conditions such as developmental disabilities are not usually recognized as being potentially genetically determined, while children with physical differences are usually assumed to have a genetic condition, regardless of their true cause. Alternatively, in some situations having a genetic cause for a child's problem may be viewed as preferable because it reduces blame. One example is the increasing number of children referred for genetic testing of osteogenesis imperfecta (OI), even though they have no features of it except a history of one or two fractures, in order to argue in court against the occurrence of nonaccidental trauma as the cause. Although little research has been conducted on master narratives of genetic diagnosis, narrative approaches have been applied to other contexts, such as therapy and illness, in ways that may also apply to helping individuals and families reframe the potentially negative stigmatization that accompanies diagnosis.

Narratively Reframing the Diagnosis

Stories help us make sense of life, but they also help us to construct identity [3, 37, 38]. A genetic diagnosis, particularly in light of societal stigmatization, has the power to upset an individual or family's sense of self and their view of the world. In the example cited above, the parents of a child newly diagnosed with fragile X syndrome may feel as if their identities as individuals, a couple, and as a family are drastically altered. Since the altered gene is inherited from only one side of the family, that parent may be blamed explicitly or implicitly. When others in the family are affected, parents may feel guilt at not having discovered that they were at increased risk before having their own children even when the pattern of inheritance is complex. In other cases, such as those with some forms of dwarfism or deafness, the condition or trait may be accepted in the family, especially if many other relatives share the same features. However, social stigma may still occur when the person moves outside his or her family and/or cultural group.

Arthur Frank's [39] work on illness narratives suggests that stories are essential in the face of unexpected diagnoses. Specifically, according to Frank:

> Becoming seriously ill is a call for stories in at least two senses....[First,] stories have to have to repair the damage that illness has done to the ill person's sense of where she is in life, and where she may be going. Stories are a way of redrawing maps and finding new destinations. The second complementary call for stories is literal and immediate: the phone rings and people want to know what is happening to the ill person. Stories of illness have to be told to medical workers, health bureaucrats, employers and work associates, family and friends. Whether ill people want to tell stories or not, illness calls for stories.

Although genetic diagnoses are not necessarily synonymous with illness, Frank's call for stories echoes the focus in narrative psychology [e.g., 38], narrative therapy [e.g., 40], and recent research in family communication [e.g., 6] on the importance of story framing and reframing in the construction of identity and managing problems. Ultimately, we fashion selves through narratives [3], compiling our experiences into an overall life story that enables a coherent sense of identity [38]. When we experience problems in life, however, we are apt to internalize those problems, considering them reflections of ourselves rather than the product of external forces. Parents of a child with a health problem or disability, for example, may feel personal guilt because they are not aware of the role chance events and new mutations can play in causing medical conditions. According to White [40], this can be problematic: "...People come to believe that their problems are internal to their self or the selves of others—that they or others are in fact, the problem. And this belief only sinks them further into the problems they are attempting to resolve" (p. 9). This seems especially true when children inherit a literal as well as an abstract part of the parent, thinking of genes as both physical entities and metaphorical symbols of our inner being. White, a founder of narrative approaches to individual and family therapy, traces this process of internalization back to Foucault's conceptualization of dominant discourses (i.e., master narratives), which divide individuals with "spoiled identities" from the rest of society, in part, through "normalizing judgment" (p. 25). Master narratives about spoiled identities, including some genetic diagnoses, often reify the internalization of responsibility. Based on these theoretical underpinnings, narrative therapists encourage practices such as externalizing conversations, which objectify the problem such that *it* becomes the problem as opposed to the person.

Thus, health-care practitioners can use narrative to deconstruct the individual's, or the family's, problem by challenging cultural assumptions about problems and helping the family to engage in a "reauthoring process" [41] (p. 20). This process entails restorying events or creating new plots that, in turn, allow people to identify positive aspects of their life experiences that may have been obscured by the problem. In other words, through reauthoring [40] or self-redefinition [41], people are encouraged to recall storylines of their lives that may have been neglected but that open up the possibility for constructing identities based on past triumphs, hopes, or experiences that counter the loss, frustration, worry, or sadness that have brought them to therapy. Additionally, Mishara [42] contended that telling the story of a problem allows a person to " 'transcend' one's past self through envisioning new possibilities," and it is this process that enables a significant change in attitude and outlook (p. 187). This restorying process can be especially important for families. Difficult or stressful experiences can have divisive effects on families, and narrative therapy focuses on externalizing and reauthoring the problem to avoid putting blame on one or more family members and to encourage family members to *work collectively against the problem* [40]. Ultimately, the process of restorying encourages a process of reframing problems and identities in productive ways.

Story framing is also important beyond the therapeutic context. In his research on life stories, McAdams [38] suggests that people create their own personal myths (i.e., life story, sense of identity) and that the ideal myth includes a number of characteristics, including coherence, openness, credibility, and generative integration, among others. Generativity is a concept that might be of particular importance to narratively reframing identities in the face of a genetic diagnosis. Specifically, generativity refers to a person's commitment to passing good things on to the next generation [38]. In the personal myths or stories we construct about our identities, "we seek endings that furnish new beginnings through which the self may live on. In our endings, we seek to defy the end, like the genes that replicate themselves from one generation to the next" (p. 224). Although genes in this context represent the particular problem, the metaphor of generativity and story framing are useful in the context of genetic diagnosis given its implications for future generations. Thus, the way in which an individual is able to frame the diagnosis in the larger identity story has potential implications across generations.

Empirical research supports the advantages of positive story framing and reframing. For example, McAdams, Reynolds, Lewis, Patten, and Bowman [43] researched the ways in which story framing reflected finding benefits (or faults) with adversity. They coded individuals' life stories for sequences of redemption (i.e., a potentially bad situation is reframed with a positive outcome) and sequences of contamination (i.e., a potentially good situation is reframed with a negative outcome). They found that individuals who told life stories with redemption sequences reported significantly higher levels of well-being and generativity than those with contamination sequences. The benefits of story framing are not limited to individuals, however. For example, Koenig Kellas [6] found that families who constructed jointly told stories framed in terms of accomplishment were much more satisfied and functional than families who framed their identity stories in terms of stress. According to Stone [44], "The facts of a family past can be selectively fashioned into a story that can mean almost anything, whatever they most need it to mean" (p. 294). Story framing and reframing, then, may be particularly important tools for health-care practitioners trying to help individuals and families come to terms with genetic diagnosis. Practices such as externalizing the problem, reauthoring or reframing the situation, and crafting redemption, rather than contamination, narratives might ease the potential burden that accompanies genetic diagnosis.

In the process of helping families construct productive narrative frames for their experiences, health-care practitioners also can assist families in creating a narrative about the genetic condition that can then be communicated to at-risk relatives. "By framing our experiences in the form of stories, we investigate what they mean to us, and we make what we understand about our experiences accessible to others by telling them our stories" [12] (p. 16). One barrier to communication with other family members is that concepts such as inheritance and genes are abstract and difficult to communicate for most families who have limited understandings of their meanings. Additionally, individuals are less likely to disclose test results with ambiguous meaning for them [18, 45], perhaps in part because they do not really understand their meaning and, therefore, find it more difficult to tell others, and in part because they are reluctant to disturb the family's normal functioning until they have to. Another barrier is the emotional risk families take when they confide in relatives that a genetic condition is present and that others could be at risk. In a survey of families with fragile X syndrome, parents encountered varying reaction from relatives [46]. Some were supportive and helpful but others disbelieved that *(1)* the child had a problem (assuring parents he would "grow out of it"), *(2)* that the problem was genetic (blaming poor parenting instead), and *(3)* that anyone else in the family was at risk. The narrative construction skills that practitioners can help individuals develop may facilitate the presentation of coherent complete narratives to other family members. This should, in turn, help the families to better understand and come to terms with the diagnosis. This narrative may include *(1)* the establishment of a goal state (e.g., "how I discovered my genetic condition and how we are going to cope with it"), *(2)* selection of events relevant to the goal state (e.g., the chronological steps and details relevant to the diagnosis), *(3)* an arrangement of events in chronological order, and *(4)* establishment of causal linkages [11]. This final step may be particularly important in helping to frame the story in a way that removes blame and defensiveness from family members to whom the story is being told.

BEYOND THE CLINICAL CONTEXT: HOW CAN STORYTELLING HELP FAMILIES COPE WITH STRESSFUL EXPERIENCES?

For families with a genetic diagnosis with significant and/or traumatic implications, narratives may be useful beyond the genetic counseling context. In particular, narrative theorizing suggests that telling the story of a stressful experience can be important for the health and well-being of family members, leading to adaptive coping [e.g., 47]. Telling the story of a problem helps us to "construct versions of reality that endow experience with meaning" [48] (p. 207). Specifically, research growing out of narrative psychology suggests that writing or telling stories about traumatic experiences can help individuals cognitively reframe, emotionally purge, and gain control over difficulty. In the case of genetic counseling, practitioners may be able to suggest narrative journaling practices to patients as a way to help them cope with a difficult diagnosis.

The *expressive writing paradigm* focuses on written narratives about a variety of traumatic experiences across a wide range of populations. A comprehensive meta-analysis of research in this area found that people who participated in at least three different writing sessions that were at least 15 minutes long demonstrated improved psychological and physical health as well as overall functioning [49]. The value of writing the story of a stressful experience has variously been explained using Inhibition Theory (i.e., failing to disclose stress requires inhibition which negatively impacts health), Cognitive Adaptation Theory (i.e., telling stories helps one create coherent meaning), Emotional Processing Theory (i.e., telling the story helps one process negative emotional responses), and Self-Regulation Theory (i.e., telling the story gives once a sense of mastery and control over their experiences). Meta-analyses of expressive writing studies suggest mixed support for each theory [50]; however, at some level each of these theories suggests that telling the story of a stressful experience is beneficial because it allows an individual to make sense of the trauma. "Language is a powerful way to organize complex emotional experiences" [51] (p. 216). Although studies have not specifically looked at expressive writing about genetic conditions, the wide empirical support for the health value of expressive writing suggests that families experiencing distress due to a genetic diagnosis may benefit from writing their story.

Specific features of narrative appear to be key predictors of well-being. Specifically narratives with more emotional language (both high levels of positive and moderate levels of negative emotion words) and cognitive language (both causal language such as *because* or *thus* as well as insight language such as *realize* or *understand*) that increased over the set of stories were related to better health outcomes [51]. These narrative qualities reflect the value of optimism and constructing a coherent storyline that helps to make sense of an experience. Health-care practitioners can utilize this research to suggest expressive writing to their patients following the medical interview. Practitioners may also demonstrate how to write about their experience, emphasizing the importance of writing about emotions and thinking about causes and insights as writing.

The benefits of writing may be different for different members of the family, however. In the context of family communication, it is important to note that these findings do not necessarily hold for children [52]. Fivush and Sales found that the expressive writing paradigm did not predict positive health outcomes for children. They point out that children have not yet fully developed their narrative skills, perhaps undermining the potential value of this practice. Parents, however, can help children develop effective narratives about difficult experiences. Children whose mothers helped them create a more coherent, explanatory, and emotionally expressive narrative of chronic stressors had higher levels of well-being [53].

Narratives are not only useful for collecting information from families and for understanding the ways in which families see themselves in the larger landscape of societal discourse about genetic diagnoses. The therapeutic function of narrative suggests health-care practitioners may also utilize narrative theorizing to suggest coping and communication strategies for their patients following a diagnosis.

CONCLUSION

Genetic counselors and other health-care practitioners who work with families provide an important resource helping them to make sense of their family history, their genetic diagnosis, and the implications this has for them as individuals and family members. Narratives are an important part of the sense-making process and can be a tool for health practitioners seeking to gain insight into families' lifeworlds. Additionally, this insight into families' meaning-making processes may reveal potential barriers to communication with other family members (e.g., beliefs about genetics, constructions of risk and experiences of ambiguity, perceptions of relevance to others, cohesiveness and distance in relationships) or aspects of the family culture that affect coping (e.g., family functioning and supportiveness, shared family understandings that shape responses to stress). Practitioners also can draw on narrative to help families cope with what may be a difficult and stressful health experience, working with them to develop the story of their experience, which they may then, in turn, share with their families.

REFERENCES

1. Fisher WR. *Human Communication as Narration: Toward a Philosophy of Reason, Value, and Action.* Columbia: University of South Carolina Press; 1987.
2. Koenig Kellas J. Narrative theories: Making sense of interpersonal communication. In: Baxter LA, Braithwaite DO, eds. *Engaging Theories in Interpersonal Communication: Multiple Perspectives.* Thousand Oaks, CA: Sage; 2008: 241–254.
3. Bruner J. *Acts of Meaning.* Cambridge, MA: Harvard University Press; 1990.
4. Ochs E, Capps L. *Living Narrative: Creating Lives in Everyday Storytelling.* Cambridge, MA: Harvard University Press; 2001.
5. Fiese BH, Sameroff W. The family narrative consortium: A multidimensional approach to narratives. *Monographs for the Society for Research in Child Development* 1999;64:1–36.
6. Koenig Kellas J. Family ties: Communicating family identity through jointly told family stories. *Communication Monographs* 2005;72:365–389.
7. Clark LF. Stress and the cognitive-conversational benefits of social interaction. *Journal of Social and Clinical Psychology* 1993;12:25–55.
8. Ochs E, Capps, L. Narrating the self. *Annual Review of Anthropology* 1996;25:19–43.
9. Koenig Kellas J, Trees AR. Finding meaning in difficult family experiences: Sense-making and interaction processes during joint family storytelling. *Journal of Family Communication* 2006;6:49–76.
10. Neimeyer RA, Levitt HM. What's narrative got to do with it? Construction and coherence in accounts of loss. In: Harvey JH, Miller ED, eds. Loss and Trauma: General and Close Relationship Perspectives. Philadelphia: Brunner-Routledge; 2000:401–412.
11. Gergen KJ, Gergen MM. Narratives of relationship. In: Burnett R, McGhee P, Clarke DC, eds. *Accounting for Relationships.* London: Methuen; 1988:269–315.
12. Bochner AP. Perspectives on inquiry III: The moral of stories. In: Knapp ML, Daly JA, eds. *Handbook of Interpersonal Communication.* 3rd ed. Thousand Oaks, CA: Sage; 2002:73–101.
13. Baerger DR, McAdams DP. Life story coherence and its relation to psychological well-being. *Narrative Inquiry.* 1999;9:69–96.

14. Sharf BF, Vanderford ML. Illness narratives and the social construction of health. In: Thompson TL, Dorsey AM, Miller K, Parrott R, eds. *Handbook of Health Communication*. Mahwah, NJ: Lawrence Erlbaum; 2003:9–34.

15. Labov, W, Waletsky, J. Narratives analysis: Oral versions of personal experience. In: Helm J, ed. *Essays on the Verbal and Visual Arts: Proceedings of the 1966 Annual Spring Meeting of the American Ethnological Society*. Seattle: University of Washington Press; 1967:12–44.

16. MacDonald DJ, Sarna L, vanServellen G, Bastani R, Giger JN, Weitzel JN. Selection of family members for communication of cancer risk and barriers to this communication before and after genetic cancer risk assessment. *Genetics in Medicine* 2007;9:275–282.

17. Trees AR, Koenig Kellas J. Telling tales: Enacting family relationships in joint storytelling about difficult family experiences. *Western Journal of Communication* 2009;31:91–111.

18. Stoffel EM, Ford B, Mercado RC, Punglia D, Kohlmann W, Conrad P, et al. Sharing genetic test results in Lynch syndrome: Communication with close and distant relatives. *Clinical Gastroenterology and Hepatology* 2008;6:333–338.

19. McGivern B, Everett J, Yager GG, Baumiller RC, Hafertepen A, Saal HM. Family communication about positive BRCA1 and BRCA2 genetic test results. *Genetics in Medicine* 2004 Nov-Dec;6(6):503–509.

20. Charon R. *Narrative Medicine: Honoring the Stories of Illness*. New York: Oxford University Press; 2006.

21. Frank AW. Enacting illness stories: When, what, and why. In: Nelson HL, ed. *Stories and Their Limit: Narrative Approaches to Bioethics*. New York: Routledge; 1997:31–49.

22. Clark JA, Mishler EG. Attending to patients' stories: Reframing the clinical task. *Sociology of Health and Illness* 1992;14:344–372.

23. Hallowell, N, Cooke, S, Crawford, G, Parker, M, Lucassen, A. Healthcare professionals' and researchers' understanding of cancer genetics activities: a qualitative interview study. *Journal of Medical Ethics* 2009;35:113–119.

24. Charon, R. Narrative medicine: A model for empathy, reflection, profession, and trust. *Journal of the American Medical Association* 2001;286:1897–1902.

25. Stivers, T, Heritage, J. Breaking the sequential mold: Answering "more than the question" during comprehensive history taking. *Text* 2001;21:151–186.

26. Reiss D, Oliveri, ME. Family paradigm and family coping: A proposal for linking the family's intrinsic adaptive capacities to its response to stress. *Family Relations* 1980;29:431–444.

27. McAllister, M. Personal theories of inheritance, coping strategies, risk perception, and engagement in hereditary non-polyposis colon cancer families offered genetic testing. *Clinical Genetics* 2003;64:179–189.

28. Ormondroyd E, Moynihan C, Watson M, Foster C, Davolls S, Ardern-Jones A, et al. Disclosure of genetics research results after the death of the patient participant: A qualitative study of the impact on relatives. *Journal of Genetic Counseling* 2007;16:527–538.

29. Forrest K, Simpson SA, Wilson BJ, van Teijlingen ER, McKee L, Haites N, et al. To tell or not to tell: Barriers and facilitators in family communication about genetic risk. *Clinical Genetics* 2003;64:317–326.

30. Vangelisti AL, Crumley LP, Baker JL. Family portraits: Stories as standards for family relationships. *Journal of Social and Personal Relationships* 1999;16(3):335–368.

31. Fiese BH, Wamboldt FS. Coherent accounts of coping with a chronic illness: Convergences and divergences in family measurement using narrative analysis. *Family Process* 2003;42:439–451.

32. Adelsward V, Sachs L. The messenger's dilemmas: Giving and getting information in genealogical mapping for hereditary cancer. *Health Risk and Society* 2003;5:125–138.

33. Eggly, S. Physician-patient co-construction of illness narratives in the medical interview. *Health Communication* 2002;14:339–360.

34. Roche M, Skinner D. How parents search, interpret, and evaluate genetic information obtained from the internet. *Journal of Genetic Counseling* 2009;18:119–129.

35. Harter LM, Kirby EL, Edwards A, McClanahan A. Time, technology, and meritocracy: The disciplining of women's bodies in narrative constructions of age-related infertility. In: Harter LM, Japp PM, Beck CS, eds. *Narratives, Health, and Healing: Communication Theory, Research and Practice.* Mahwah, NJ: Lawrence Erlbaum; 2005:83–105.

36. Bochner AP, Ellis C, Tillmann-Healy LM. Relationships as stories: Accounts, storied lives, evocative narratives. In: Dindia K, Duck S, eds. *Communication and Personal Relationships.* Chichester, England: John Wiley & Sons; 1997:12–29.

37. Kerby AP. *Narrative and the Self.* Bloomington: Indiana University Press; 1991.

38. McAdams DP. The Stories We Live By. New York: The Guilford Press; 1997.

39. Frank AW. *The Wounded Storyteller: Body, Illness, and Ethics.* Chicago: The University of Chicago Press; 1995.

40. White M. *Maps of Narrative Practice.* New York: W. W. Norton & Company; 2007.

41. Monk G. How narrative therapy works. In: Monk, G, Winslade, J, Crocket, K, Epston, D, eds. *Narrative Therapy in Practice: The Archaeology of Hope.* San Francisco: Jossey-Bass Publishers; 1997:3–31.

42. Mishara AL. Narrative and psychotherapy – The phenomenology of healing. *American Journal of Psychotherapy* 1995;49:180–195.

43. McAdams DP, Reynolds J, Lewis M, Patten AH, Bowman PJ. When bad things turn good and good things turn bad: Sequences of redemption and contamination in life narrative and their relation to psychosocial adaptation in midlife adults and in students. *Personality and Social Psychology Bulletin* 2001;27:474–485.

44. Stone E. *Black Sheep and Kissing Cousins: How Our Family Stories Shape Us.* New York: Times Books; 1988.

45. Claes E, Evers-Kiebooms G, Boogaerts A, Decruyenaere M, Denayer L, Legius E. Communication with close and distant relatives in the context of genetic testing for hereditary breast and ovarian cancer in cancer patients. *American Journal of Medical Genetics Part A* 2003;116A:11–19.

46. Bailey D, Skinner D, Sparkman KL. Discovering fragile X syndrome: Families experiences and perceptions. *Pediatrics* 2003;111:407–416.

47. Pennebaker JW. *Opening Up: The Healing Power of Expressing Emotions.* New York: Guilford; 1997.
48. Harvey JH. *Embracing Their Memory: Loss and the Social Psychology of Storytelling.* Needham Heights, MA: Allyn and Bacon; 1996.
49. Frattaroli J. Experimental disclosure and its moderators: A meta-analysis. *Psychological Bulletin* 2006;132:823–865.
50. Sloan DM, Marx BP. Taking pen to hand: Evaluating theories underlying the written disclosure paradigm. *Clinical Psychology: Science and Practice* 2004;11:121–137.
51. Ramirez-Esparza N, Pennebaker JW. Do good stories produce good health? Exploring words, language, and culture. *Narrative Inquiry* 2006;16:211–219.
52. Fivush R, Marin K, Crawford M, Reynolds M, Brewin CR. Children's narratives and well-being. *Cognition and Emotion* 2007;21:1414–1434.
53. Fivush R, Sales JM. Coping, attachment, and mother-child narratives of stressful events. *Merrill-Palmer Quarterly* 2006;52:125–150.

5

TIMESCAPES

Maggie Gregory, Anna Middleton, & Paul Atkinson

The implications of genetic information reverberate throughout a person's life cycle and over generations. A theoretical perspective on time offers a novel dimension for health-care practitioners to consider as they work with individuals or families adjusting to and communicating about a genetic condition.

Time pervades human life, but it is usually taken for granted. If you look around any of the main rooms in your home or workplace, it is almost certain that you will see some reminder of the importance of time in the organization of your life. Clocks, calendars, wall planners, and the small icon on your computer screen all map the hours of the day, week, or month. Time is central to the way that humans organize and plan the way that they live and work. It is also central to the concept of inheritance and families' experiences of and communication about genetics. In the course of this chapter, we use time as an organizing theme, drawing on theory that conceptualizes time within a social context. Consideration of relevant time theory offers a new dimension to understanding how genetic risk information is incorporated into the lives of individuals. It can also shed light on the process of disclosure of genetic risk information in a family.

Timescapes in our title derives from the work of the sociologist Barbara Adam [1–3]. She uses the term to encompass the multiple and complex forms of time that are involved in any given social organization. The term could be considered equivalent to a "landscape," although this obviously has the addition of spatial arrangements. In this chapter, we expand on the complexities of time and introduce some key ideas from Adam. We show how aspects of time pervade the genetic counseling process itself, drawing on examples of illustrative cases. We parallel our discussion of timescapes with a commentary on *genescapes*. By that we mean not just the biological distribution of genes among a family but also the social distribution of knowledge, beliefs, and actions relating to inheritance and genetics. Timescapes and genescapes together incorporate time, biology, and social perspectives simultaneously.

TIME AND SOCIOLOGICAL THEORY

Sociological theory distinguishes between four different aspects of time. *Time* itself measures the passage of time in seconds, hours, days, years, lifetimes, and eras; *temporality* is concerned with the process of change, of the irreversibility of what has taken place and the knowledge that life as we know it is impermanent; *timing* relates to the synchronization of events and actions (an important part of social interactions); and *tempo* relates to the speed and pace of activity. Further development of these elements includes time sequences (e.g., cause and effect); time extensions (duration of activity, continuity, time horizons, and the past, present, and future); and time patterns (rhythms, cycles, and periodicity) [1]. Thus, multiple facets of time intersect in daily life. An individual is able to hold several notions of time simultaneously in his or her mind—the present embracing the past and the future, the status quo being changed by new information, and so on. For instance, in consultations involving genetics, both the health-care practitioner and client are simultaneously required to consider past family health, present choices, and future outcomes, modifying these as additional information is provided.

One of the key messages of sociological theory is the way that the human conception of time has changed over the centuries. Capitalism and the industrial way of life wrought major changes on the human relationship with time. Our modern world places substantial emphasis on the measurement of time. Time is controlled, and the natural time patterns of life (e.g., the change of seasons, the rising and setting of the sun) have been evened out. Much of everyday life puts a value on the use of time, especially in the world of industry and institutions, where the "time is money" approach is evident. When time is understood and related to primarily as having a monetary value, the consequence is that the faster something happens, whether in an industrial or institutional setting, the better it is perceived to be [1, 3]. Both profitability (a primary concern of industry) and efficiency (a concern for institutions and industries alike) are tied to the pace (tempo) of the activity undertaken. Any underutilized time is regarded as wasted money.

Social time differs fundamentally from the "time is money" concept. Here, we may speak of "good times" and "bad times" and "the right time," of "quality time" with family, and of being "time poor" in our everyday life. People also perceive time passing more slowly or more quickly at different stages of their life. This has nothing to do with the linear, standardized time of the clock. Time might appear to accelerate as individuals consider what courses of action would be appropriate should a particular genetic test result be given; conversely, time might appear to slow down as a client waits "in limbo" to know his or her genetic status. In both cases the time of the calendar and the clock are fixed; it is the human perception of the passage of time that has changed as a result of the individual's specific circumstances.

Time is a fundamental part of human existence. However it is measured, whether by the natural order of the seasons or by the tick of the clock, it has a part to play in ordering daily life and social interactions. By using the sociological theory of time as an ordering tool, it is possible to see how what appears to be a straightforward human transaction—in this case, imparting knowledge to other family members—may be more difficult and thus protracted than might be assumed.

TIME AND THE GENETIC COUNSELING PROCESS

Time issues are fundamental to people's actions and thus have a bearing upon their relationship with the genetic counseling clinic. We consider some examples of clinical cases in order to examine how various aspects of time have an impact upon encounters with the health-care practitioner. We then explain the need to recognize, understand, and manage these aspects as part of the counseling process.

Case Study 1: An Uncertain Future

Amanda is 32 years old and has a family history of Huntington disease (HD), a neurological disorder involving loss of coordination, progressive physical disability, and a gradual loss of some mental functioning. Amanda's mother and maternal grandmother both had the disease, which started in their thirties, and Amanda has grown up knowing she is at risk of inheriting the HD disease gene. She has felt a "weight" on her mind about this since she was a little girl, and her future has always felt vague. In fact, she has not planned a future at all, having left school with few qualifications because she always felt uncertain about the careers that might be suitable for her if she developed the condition. Time is standing still. Amanda finds it hard to open her mind to a possible future because she is frightened that it may be taken away from her. It is easiest to live in the moment. Amanda comes for a routine genetic counseling session offered periodically to all clients at risk of having the HD gene fault; the genetics practitioner discusses the option of having a predictive genetic test. Amanda realizes that living with uncertainty is becoming intolerable, and she starts to wonder what the reality of a future might be like. The genetics practitioner spends a long time engaging with Amanda about her current coping mechanisms, and Amanda takes the lead on discussing the potential timing of a test and the plans that she could make on the basis of the results. A structure begins to emerge: Amanda begins to think about what she would do if she is found to have the family gene fault and what she would do if she does not. A future gradually materializes; the time ahead soon appears to have meaning.

Case Study 2: The Tempo of Action

Harry is in his fifties and has just learned that his sister, Mary, has terminal ovarian cancer. The diagnosis is quick, the prognosis is dreadful, and time is running out. Mary happened to take part in a research project at the time of her diagnosis and as part of this learns she carries a *BRCA1* mutation. This means that her ovarian cancer is likely to have a genetic cause, and her relatives are at risk of developing early-onset breast and ovarian cancer. Mary makes frenetic phone calls to her family with the news; she calls relatives she has not spoken to in years, urging them to seek genetic counseling and receive genetic testing quickly. Harry contacts his local genetic counseling department and demands an urgent appointment; he is frantic with worry, fuelled by Mary's anxiety. Harry has a 20-year-old daughter, and all he can think of is her risk of breast and ovarian cancer, imagining the worst, fearing he may lose her too. Time has sped up. Harry feels panicked and rushed. The genetics practitioner enables Harry to tell his story and gradually as she listens and he talks, the pace of the conversation begins to slow. At first he speaks in a manner that is fervent and without control, but then as he talks the pace of his language slows and in doing so the urgency dissipates. As the conversation develops, the genetics practitioner helps Harry to realize for himself that there is no urgency for genetic testing immediately. Harry begins to feel control again, and he visibly begins to relax in the consultation. Understanding his own grief reaction to Mary's news helps him to separate out Mary's need to do something for her family, to salvage useful information for her relatives, when she is helpless to do anything further for herself. Harry sees the genetics practitioner for several sessions and soon decides that genetic testing for himself and his own family can wait until another day, and he decides to focus on caring for Mary in the time he has left with her.

Case Study 3: Cycles of Events

Julie and David are referred to the genetics service because Julie has had seven successive, first-trimester miscarriages. After the first miscarriage, each subsequent pregnancy is embarked on with trepidation. Julie is frightened of the next miscarriage—the loss of a potential future, the loss of a dream, the loss of feeling normal. She is also frightened of the possibility that every future pregnancy will end in miscarriage—always the same conclusion with no prospect of anything different. Julie becomes obsessive about pregnancy; each time she sees a pregnant stranger on the street, she becomes jealous and wonders if she will ever have a normal pregnancy. Time appears to be repeating itself. Julie feels trapped in a nightmare that is always the same. Julie and David have their chromosomes tested in the genetics clinic and Julie is found to have a rearrangement of two chromosomes (translocation carrier), which means she has an increased risk of miscarriage as well a small risk of having a child with a serious disability. It also means that she has a good chance of having a successful pregnancy and a healthy child. The genetic counseling process helps Julie and David to reflect on their "living nightmare" and to wake up to their reality. Julie gradually begins to accept that a good outcome is possible if she can maintain a sense of patience. She continues to try for a new pregnancy, knowing that, in time, there is a chance that she will have a healthy baby.

Case Study 4: Wanting to Know the Future

Helen develops bowel cancer at the age of 20 and has most of her bowel removed. She copes well and feels reassured by the frequent screening she receives. She knows there is a 50/50 chance that her children may have inherited this condition, familial adenomatous polyposis (FAP), but feels optimistic that if they have inherited it that screening will pick up any cancers before they became life threatening. Helen's children are currently under the age of 5 and she knows that they are too young to be tested for the FAP gene fault at the moment. However, as they become older, Helen becomes more anxious to know. She begins to waiver from her calm state of mind, knowing the risks to her children and understanding the consequences. Helen begins to feel she cannot wait anymore for them to reach an age when they can be tested. Time is going too slowly; she needs it to speed up. She oscillates between wanting to relish the innocence they all have at the moment—not knowing either way—to needing certainty and clarity. On the one hand, Helen wants to plan, to construct their future, and wants time to speed up so she can know. Yet, on the other hand, she wants it to stand still, so that she never needs to know.

Case Study 5: Having to Face the Future

Valerie lives in an area where all newborn babies are tested for Duchenne muscular dystrophy, a progressive muscle wasting condition. Valerie does not remember that her new baby was tested for this, and so when the results show he is affected, she is shocked and cannot believe this new information. Ben is only 10 weeks old, is perfect in every way, and yet Valerie now knows that when he is around 4 years old he may begin to show signs of the condition that will gradually engulf him; the degenerative disease will take his life in his twenties and begin to take effect before he even starts school. Valerie feels cheated. The joy she felt initially when her new baby boy was born is soon tainted. She wrestles with this information; she feels her innocence has been stolen from her. She longs for an open future, she longs for a time when she does not know; she cannot look at Ben, even though he is now perfectly normal, without thinking how he will become in the future. The time that Ben is well seems so short; she can now count it in years on one hand. There is not enough time for him to be normal; there is not enough time for Valerie to have him before he becomes disabled. Time is slipping away, and she feels helpless to do anything about it.

Each of these cases illustrates a particular facet of time that is likely to be experienced in the clinical encounter. Pasts and futures are a dominant part of each account, interwoven with other aspects of social time. A sensitive health-care practitioner working regularly with clients grappling with issues relating to genetics, inheritance, and their family will be working with an awareness of *timescapes*, even if the practitioner is not consciously familiar with time theory. This is because the genetic counseling consultation naturally encompasses discussion about the past, present, and future, and the client will frequently change the tempo within a consultation as he or she incorporates new information. For example, it is quite common for a client to arrive at a consultation with a real sense of urgency about rushing through a quick predictive test; this is usually because the client has only just discovered that he or she is at risk of developing or passing on a dreadful genetic condition. This is demonstrated in the case study with Harry. The practitioner can use communication skills to help diffuse the urgency and panic. By focusing on the client, listening carefully, and using both verbal and nonverbal communication to show empathy, it is usually possible to slow the pace down and create an opportunity for a time extension. The genetic practitioner will often regulate the pace of his or her own speech and take care not to inadvertently match the pitch and panic of the client's voice. The genetic practitioner may also remain quite quiet and listen as the client tells his or her story naturally and eventually comes to a stop. This is a tactic that can help to restore a sense of balance. It is very important that the practitioner does not join the client in a state of alarm and stress (and thus ultimately helplessness); the practitioner can be of enormous benefit if he or she remains calm and on top of the situation because this helps the client to find this calmness too. In this way, the practitioner does not collude with the client's sense of panic and feel forced into ordering a fast-track predictive genetic test, which is usually unnecessary unless there are immediate diagnostic decisions to be made on the basis of the person's genetic status. Indeed, genetics services have predictive testing protocols that encourage clients to have at least two genetic counseling sessions first before blood is taken for testing [4]. This can allow time for reflection, further discussion with family, and careful and considered thought about what will be done with the results.

We turn now to a more detailed discussion of time in several relevant contexts: the family, health and illness, and, specifically, in genetic conditions. In concert, we explore some of the factors that impact upon family communication of genetic information.

THE FAMILY, BIOGRAPHIES, HEALTH, AND GENESCAPES

As the earlier sections of this chapter illustrate, time is a central part of human life and is integral to our way of being. This section seeks to show how time is implicated in family life, in general considerations of the experience of health and illness and in illnesses with a genetic underpinning. The temporal dimensions of these situations work together to produce interwoven cycles.

Family Timescapes: Generations and Life Courses

Temporal cycles are central to domestic relationships and family relations. Domestic groups have "developmental cycles" as generations progress, children are born and grow up, new marital alliances are entered into, members die, marriages are dissolved, and so on. These temporal cycles are part of the rhythms of domestic timescapes and are not based exclusively on the lapse of chronological time. They reflect the social and cultural marking of time. These include personal and calendar rituals (e.g., anniversaries, birthdays, and religious festivals) and celebrations of personal transformation (rites of passage, such as birth, marriage, and death). In these observances, social time and chronological time intersect.

Generations are among the ways in which the passage of time is recognized within kinship and domestic groups. They are simultaneously natural and social phenomena. Generation is linked directly to everyday, practical notions of growth and development. The life course and the cycle of generations shape, and are in turn shaped by, cultural assumptions and expectations. They include formal and informal ideas about childhood, the responsibilities of adulthood, and the limitations of older age. Transitions between such stages are dependent on status passages of various sorts; each stage of life carries with it responsibilities and presumptions of competence or incompetence, innocence and experience, and productive activities and leisure. Notions of temporal progression therefore underlie patterns and expectations concerning communication within kindred, including the management of genetic information. A new genetic diagnosis within a family can modify these transitions. For example, consider the case of an 18-year-old boy diagnosed with neurofibromatosis type 2 (NF2), a progressive, chronic condition involving tumors on the auditory nerve in the brain which cause hearing loss. Any 18 year old would usually be on the verge of a transition into adulthood, with plans to leave home and detach himself from his parents. However, an 18 year old with a new diagnosis of NF2 may need to put his plans for university on hold. The usual transition may become stalled because he now needs to stay at home with his parents as he and the family adapt to his sudden hearing loss; the 18 year old becomes a child again, relying on his parents to help him communicate and learn how to speak and understand without hearing.

Generational differences imply differential access to information. Age and generation affect what is kept private, what is divulged, and what is kept from family members [5]. The distribution of information and perceived competence are linked to social (and not merely chronological) age, and hence to membership of generation. Competence and coping are also linked to notions of maturity, "readiness," and other practical concepts of biographical development [6, 7]. The life course and generation shape patterns of disclosure, and of the distribution of information within a social network. For example, in the second case study, Harry may decide that his daughter does not yet have the maturity to participate in his conversations with Mary about hereditary breast ovarian cancer.

Generations and the succession of generations are ways of accounting for time, change, and succession. The importance of generations is evident in accounts of families with genetic conditions [8]. Families seek to make sense of change and continuity by looking to the past to account for the origin of a mutation or the route of its transmission. Past generations are inspected; everyday family pedigrees are invoked; and medical histories are located within that sense of the past [9]. All of this is part of the process of deciding which members of the family are at risk of the genetic condition and as a result need to be informed of the results of genetic testing and counseling.

Health and Genescapes

Health and illness always imply temporal dimensions. Acute illness can be a major turning point in people's unfolding lives, and chronic illness transforms the way a person's current and future life will be lived. Even when discovered genetic conditions have no immediate effect (e.g., discovering the presence of a *BRCA1* gene fault), this knowledge also changes the way a person thinks about his or her health and the choices the person makes. Thus, discovery of a genetic anomaly can lead to two different types of trajectories: the *trajectory of the illness* that the genetic anomaly gives rise to and the *trajectory of the gene* (over generations, across the boundaries of family and kin, and over the entire lifetime of the individual).

An *illness trajectory* is the path by which an individual progresses from the point of initial symptoms, through diagnosis into subsequent outcomes. Along similar lines, people affected by a condition have "patient careers." That is the stages through which they identify and evaluate symptoms, seek lay or professional advice, go through stages of treatment, and experience recovery, deterioration, or even death. Health and ill health always imply perspectives on the past as well as the present and the future [10–13]. The past is inspected for causes and origins of ill health, and future treatment or recovery is envisaged. Just as the past is inspected for causes and origins of ill health, similar narrative work is undertaken by those affected (directly or indirectly) by genetic illness. The search for origins includes not merely the work to understand and interpret the cause of the condition (the nature of genetic inheritance) but also the search for its origins in social relationships, the intersection of genetic constitution and lifestyle, and the routes of inheritance and risk transmission [9, 14].

There is a difference between a *genetic trajectory or career* and an *illness trajectory*. In contrast to illness, the disclosure of a predictive genetic test result to a healthy person provides a career or trajectory that is neither "acute" nor "chronic" in conventional terms. The master status [10] of being a carrier or being at risk is an emergent, but permanent one; it dominates a person's self-perception and interaction with others. It thus becomes different in form from a biographical "disruption" of illness diagnosis, being more akin to a biographical "translation" into a genetically defined past, present, and future.

Genetic trajectories are always socially shared and distributed among kin, and therefore they imply a somewhat different order of complexity from the individualized trajectories of acute or even chronic illness. *Genescapes* encompass the multiple constructions of the gene—biological and cultural—and inheritance. Beyond the temporal unfolding of an individual's genetic status and illness trajectory, for genetic conditions there are multiple family members' biographies to be constructed and reconstructed, and there may be multiple illness trajectories evident in the family [10, 12, 15]. As has been demonstrated from many disciplinary and theoretical perspectives, genescapes entail complex patterns of interpretation [16]. While we know that genetic understanding is not uniformly shared among kin, where there is sharing, narratives of past, present, and future may be jointly constructed and shared. As a consequence, the temporal dimensions of genetic knowledge are rendered potentially more complex than the narratives and interpretations of individual disease.

Biography and Health

There has been an emphasis on biographies and life histories in recent qualitative social research. Biographies are actively constructed by social actors, who make sense of their past and current lives, interpreting and evaluating experiences, events, and other people. They are, therefore, among the most significant ways in which the passage of time is understood in everyday social life. Biographies are not regulated solely by the passage of clock time or by the strict calendrical process of aging. Lives are constructed and understood in terms of *biographical time*. Key features include turning points, for example, the point of deciding to have a predictive test after years at risk (such as Amanda wanting to find out about Huntington disease, in the first case study); epiphanies (moments of revelation and identity transformation, such as Julie receiving a chromosome result identifying the cause of her miscarriages, in the third case study); and status passages such as transitions to adulthood, marriage, reaching the age when cancer screening must start, the birth of a child, or the death of a partner or parent. There are very general notions of time in the construction of a life: time to grow up, time to mature, time to "move on," time to start a family, time to settle down, and so on.

When thinking about genetic conditions, we need to recognize that there are different possible careers, biographies, and trajectories. First, there is the possible difference between a *genetic trajectory* (over generations, across the boundaries of family and kin, and over the entire lifetime of the individual) and a consequent *illness trajectory* mentioned above. So conditions like myotonic dystrophy or cystic fibrosis will follow a conventional illness trajectory (the symptoms and prognosis are recognized and fairly consistent), while the genetic trajectory may appear and disappear, seemingly at random, among relatives (i.e., some develop the condition and others do not). It also encompasses not merely the individual life but also that of previous and succeeding generations.

The future assumes a particular salience in the biographical work of individuals and families with genetic conditions. There is nothing unique in this: prognosis is always a feature of medical work, lay and professional, and all serious medical conditions carry possible implications for the future. Genetic conditions invite particular emphasis on future possibilities, however, in that they always, in principle, contain within them futures—for the individual, for their offspring, and for generations as yet unborn.

Turning Points

Rites of passage are among the classic, long-standing interests of social and cultural anthropology [17]. They mark the passage from one culturally defined stage of life to another or from one social category to another. The key events, and their social ceremonials, include birth, initiations, marriage, death, and bereavement. They are marked by collective celebrations. For instance, the birth of a child not only triggers the arrival of a new social person and redefines the status of the parents; it also reconfigures other members of the kindred (defining individuals as grandparents, aunts and uncles, cousins, etc.). These markers of social time and of biographical development thus have major implications for the patterns of social relations.

For families with genetic conditions, these junctures may precipitate major considerations of genetic information, the projection of genetic futures, and interpretations of genetic pasts. Relatives who are linked by the same genetic condition, such as women in a family who have all inherited the same family *BRCA1* mutation, share a common bond, both genetic and social in construction. This may unite the family within shared rites of passage, for example, a "coming of age" as younger women in the family reach an age where they can start breast/ovarian screening or make a decision to have a preventative mastectomy. These key turning points in the biographies of individuals and families are, therefore, key markers in the passage of time; they are also key moments at which genetic decision making may achieve enhanced salience.

TIME AND THE HEALTH-CARE PRACTITIONER

The intervention of the health-care practitioner is predicated on reconstructions of the past and projected futures, grounded in a present that is itself open to negotiation. As a number of authors have pointed out, the past is captured through a number of standardized procedures that make the past comprehensible, and that bring the past under the scrutiny of the professional gaze, for example, through the drawing of the pedigree [18, 19]. Alexias [20], for instance, argues that medical genetics reconstructs the past through its investigation and documentation of inheritance. It brings together the *social* past of the family and the *biological* past of inherited genetic material. The past history is not merely that of the individual attending the clinic. It is a shared past, defined by shared genetic inheritance between family members. The present always—potentially at least—implicates others beyond that person. The future extends well beyond the individual, as genetic risk and patterns of inheritance extend to offspring and to generations as yet unborn. The construction of the family tree or pedigree is one mechanism whereby the past is reconstructed and transformed into a clinical present and a potential future [21, 22].

The genetics clinic, therefore, is a point of surveillance of past, present, and future. Such surveillance is not, however, confined to the clinical setting. The same dimensions define the mutual gaze of "lay" family members. Featherstone et al. [9] show how mutual surveillance takes place across the generations within families. Previous generations may be inspected in order to construct etiological accounts of the origins and routes of inherited mutations. Equally, family members who have inherited a condition or a risk of developing a disease may inspect members of older generations in order to form an assessment of what might happen to them, the likely severity of their symptoms, and the trajectory of the condition. This is one practical way in which individuals may use the past and present to make assessments of their own future.

In the same way, surveillance and prediction operate from older generations to younger ones. Children and young people are inspected in order to predict whether they are developing a condition—whether the genetic cause is "coming out" in them. Resemblances to family members are used to try to make such assessments of future outcomes. Past and present appearances and health problems are used as a resource to predict the future by family members in the attempt to predict the outcomes of genetic predispositions.

THE RELEVANCE OF TIME TO FAMILY COMMUNICATION ABOUT RISK INFORMATION

We turn now to two specific examples relating to the temporal aspects of risk communication. At present there is no body of literature that deals specifically with time in this context, although previous studies of the communication of risk information have referred to some temporal issues. These include the belief that a family member is too young to be informed [23–29], that it is the responsibility of parents to inform their children [24, 30], and the timing of disclosure and finding the right time to tell [24, 26, 29, 30]. Further discussion on communicating genetic information with children can be found in Chapter 14.

The first of the examples relates to time processes following the genetic counseling appointment. It might be assumed that when a person leaves her appointment, armed with knowledge of her own risk of inheriting and passing on the condition and aware of the need to bring the risk to the attention of other family members, she has every intention of acting as a conduit for the passage of this knowledge to other members of her family. It is assumed that the person will feel a sense of obligation to other family members to protect them from harm. In the first instance, however, she may need to *take time* in order to come to an acceptance of the information that she has been given because it represents a shift in her understanding of her own future biography.

Thereafter, imparting this knowledge to other family members needs to take place in a way that is respectful of the *rhythms* of that family's communication patterns. Conversations with first-degree relatives are likely to be more regular than with those who are less close; attendance at genetic counseling will probably already have been raised as part and parcel of the usual interchange with close family members about how one's daily life proceeds. It is thus potentially easier for the person to communicate the results of the appointment as it affects him or her and, by extension, others who share a similar risk of inheriting the genetic defect.

However, even in these circumstances of close personal contact, there is a judgment to be made about whether it is the *right time* to impart information that may have serious implications for the *future* of another member of the family. It will take account of whether the age of the relative means that disclosure is appropriate. If that factor is not a stumbling block, a decision needs to be made about whether all should be revealed in one conversation or whether it is better to plant the seed by divulging results, following that up at a *later date* with a discussion of what the information obtained might mean for the relative.

In this process of disclosure, the right time has nothing to do with the time of the clock and the calendar. It is based on a judgment of whether at that particular time in the life of the relative it is appropriate to convey information that might provoke concern and anxiety. It takes account of other issues that the individual may be experiencing at that time that may make the disclosure inappropriate or unwelcome.

The second example deals with genetic information disclosure to more distant relatives. Many published studies of family communication have found that first-degree relatives are more likely to be informed about genetic risk than second- or third-degree relatives [28, 29, 31–33]. In the case of more distant relatives, it cannot be assumed that practical kinship involves close and intimate relations. The biomedical conceptualization of relationships does not map onto the emotional and social ties that are the reality of family life. For many families it is only at the times of rites of passage that more distant relatives are likely to meet face to face. Such occasions are likely to be celebratory (christenings, weddings, marking important birthdays or other anniversaries) or at more sombre occasions such as funeral or memorial services. Such occasions are not necessarily appropriate times for raising issues of genetic inheritance. So it is perhaps not surprising that clients tend not to communicate directly with their more distant relatives and that communication within the family is inclined to follow a more circuitous route.

CONCLUSION

From everything we have discussed so far, it is apparent that there are multiple trajectories and timeframes in play at any given time in relation to individuals and family members. Patterns of family communication are clearly shaped by such temporal (and spatial) constraints. We need, therefore, to recognize the extent to which *clinical* and *biographical* time-frames do not coincide.

The cycles of clinical intervention and consultation cannot be assumed to map onto the temporal cycles of families and domestic groups. Processes of information sharing and disclosure of genetic information are more complex than the organizational and professional imperatives of genetics clinics and professional personnel.

As Zerubavel [34] points out, organizations like hospitals and clinics are regulated by their own temporal imperatives. These rely heavily on the time of clocks and calendars, as described earlier. Appointments are scheduled within particular timeframes with regard to the efficiency of the organization. While they intersect with the biographical trajectories of clients and patients, such patients and clients are not constrained by organizational routines. While genetic counseling is not a one-off affair, and while families may be followed over long periods of time, the health-care practitioner cannot and should not assume that the timing of family processes matches the cycles of clinic encounters and counseling sessions. Genetic counseling, as with other medical encounters, is based on the efficient use of time. The disclosure and sharing of genetic information is—as numerous studies have shown—an event, or even a series of events, subject to uncertain timing, and grounded in the practical circumstances of everyday life.

Practitioners' counseling and expectations need to be sensitive, therefore, to the *timescapes* of family life described here as well as their *genescapes*.

REFERENCES

1. Adam B. *Time and Social Theory.* Cambridge, England: Polity; 1990.
2. Adam B. *Timewatch: The Social Analysis of Time.* Cambridge, England: Polity; 1995.
3. Adam B. *Timescapes of Modernity: The Environment and Invisible Hazards.* London: Routledge; 1998.
4. Craufurd D, Tyler A. Predictive testing for Huntington's disease: Protocol of the UK Huntington's Prediction Consortium. *Journal of Medical Genetics* December 1992; 29(12):915–918.
5. Petronio SS. *Boundaries of Privacy: Dialectics of Disclosure.* Albany: State University of New York Press; 2002.
6. Gregory M, Boddington P, Dimond R, Atkinson P, Clarke A, Collins, P. Communicating about haemophilia within the family: the importance of context and of experience. *Haemophilia* 2007;13(2)189–198.

7. Boddington P, Gregory M. Communicating genetic information in the family: enriching the debate through the notion of integrity. *Medicine, Healthcare and Philosophy* 2008;11(4):445–454.

8. Atkinson P, Gregory M. Idioms of generation and intergenerational information: The case of haemophilia. Paper presented at: Centre for Family Studies, Cambridge University; June 13, 2006; Cambridge, England.

9. Featherstone K, Atkinson P, Bharadwaj A, Clarke A. *Risky Relations: Family, Kinship and the New Genetics.* Oxford, England: Berg; 2006.

10. Bury M. The sociology of chronic illness: a review of research and prospects. *Sociology of Health and Illness* 1991;13(4):451–468.

11. Bury MR. Meanings at risk: The experience of arthritis. In: Anderson R, Bury M, eds. *Living with Chronic Illness: The Experience of Patients and Their Families.* London: Unwin Hyman; 1988:89–116.

12. Bury MR. Chronic illness as biographical disruption. *Sociology of Health and Illness* 1982;4:167–182.

13. Williams G. The genesis of chronic illness: Narrative re-construction. *Sociology of Health and Illness* 1984;6:175–200.

14. Featherstone K, Gregory M, Atkinson P. The moral and sentimental work of the clinic: the case of dysmorphology. In: Atkinson P, Glasner P, eds. *New Genetics, New Identities.* London: Routledge; 2006:101–119.

15. Corbin J, Strauss AL. Accompaniments of chronic illness: Changes in body, self, biography, and biographical time. In: Roth JA, Conrad P, eds. *Research in the Sociology of Health Care*, Vol. 6. Greenwich, CT: JAI Press; 1987:249–281.

16. Featherstone K, Atkinson P, Bharadwaj A. Inheritance in society. In: Cooper D, ed. *Nature Encyclopedia of the Human Genome*, Vol. 3. London: Nature Publishing Group; 2003:483–488.

17. van Gennep A. *The Rites of Passage.* Vizedom MB, Caffee GL, trans. London: Routledge; 1960[1909].

18. Bouquet M. Family trees and their affinities: The visual imperative of the genealogical diagram. *Journal of the Royal Anthropological Institute* 1996;2:43–66.

19. Pálsson G. The life of family trees and the "Book of Icelanders." *Medical Anthropology* 2002;21(3):337–367.

20. Alexias G. Medical discourse and time: Authoritative Reconstruction of present, future and past. *Social Theory and Health* 2008;6(1):167–183.

21. Nukaga Y, Cambrosio A. Medical pedigrees and the visual production of family disease in Canadian and Japanese genetic counselling practice. In: Elston MA, ed. *The Sociology of Medical Science and Technology.* Oxford, England: Blackwell; 1997:29–55.

22. Parsons E, Atkinson P, Featherstone K. Professional constructions of family and kinship in medical genetics. *New Genetics and Society* 2001;20(1):5–24.

23. Tercyak KP, Peshkin BN, DeMarco TA, Brogan BM, Lerman C. Parent-child factors and their effect on communicating BRCA1/2 test results to children. *Patient Education and Counseling* 2002;47:145–153.

24. Forrest K, Simpson SA, Wilson BJ, van Teiljlingen ER, McKee L, Haites N, Matthews E. To tell or not to tell: Barriers and facilitators in family communication about genetic risk. *Clinical Genetics* 2003;64:317–326.

25. Ormond KE, Mills PL, Lester LA, Ross LF. Effect of family history on disclosure patterns of cystic fibrosis carrier status. *American Journal of Medical Genetics Part C, Seminars in Medical Genetics* 2003;119(1):70–77.

26. Segal J, Esplen MJ, Toner B, Baedorf S, Narod S, Butler K. An investigation of the disclosure process and support needs of BRCA1 and BRCA2 carriers. *American Journal of Medical Genetics* 2004;125A:267–272.

27. Mesters I, Ausems M, Eichhorn S, Vasen H. Informing one's family about genetic testing for hereditary non-polyposis colorectal cancer (HNPCC): A retrospective exploratory study. *Familial Cancer* 2005;4(2):163–167(5).

28. Claes E, Evers-Kiebooms G, Boogaerts A, Decruyenaere M, Denayer L, Legius E. Communication with close and distant relatives in the context of hereditary breast and ovarian cancer in cancer patients. *American Journal of Medical Genetics Part A* 2003;116(1):11–19.

29. Gaff CL, Collins V, Symes T, Halliday J. Facilitating family communication about predictive genetic testing: Probands' perceptions. *Journal of Genetic Counselling* 2005;14(2):133–140.

30. Peterson SK, Watts BG, Koehly LM, Vernon SW, Baile WF, Kohlmann WK, Gritz ER. How families communicate about HNPCC genetic testing: Findings from a qualitative study. *American Journal of Medical Genetics Part C, Seminars in Medical Genetics* 2003;119(1):78–86.

31. d'Agincourt-Canning L. Experiences of genetic risk: Disclosure and the gendering of responsibility. *Bioethics* 2001;15(3):231–247.

32. Hamilton RJ, Bowers BJ, Williams JK. Disclosing genetic test results to family members. *Journal of Nursing Scholarship* 2005;37(1):18–24.

33. Blandy C, Chabal F, Stoppa-Lyonnet D, Julian-Reynier C. Testing participation in BRCA1/2-positive families: Iniator role of index cases. *Genetic Testing* 2003;7(3):225–233.

34. Zerubavel E. *Hidden Rhythms, Schedules and Calendars in Social Life.* Chicago: Chicago University Press; 1981.

6

FAMILY SYSTEMS
THEORY

Kathleen M. Galvin & Mary-Anne Young

The diagnosis of a genetic condition affects multiple family members, destabilizing the family system and resulting in new patterns of connection, disconnection, and communication. Family systems theory provides a lens for health-care practitioners to anticipate and consider the issues faced by families.

"**D**econtexted individuals do not exist." With these words family therapist Salvador Minuchin [1] captures the essence of a human systems perspective. A systems perspective assumes that an individual does not exist in a vacuum; individuals are parts of larger social systems, the most significant of which is the family. Familial interdependence is demonstrated clearly when one or more members confront health issues because, from a systems perspective, all members are affected by the health of other members. This is uniquely the case when a member is diagnosed with a genetic disorder.

A guiding principle for health-care practitioners discussing genetics is to consider the risk of a genetic condition not only for the individual attending the clinic but also for the individual's family. When a client enters the room, it is important not only to consider that individual and his or her family from the perspective of genetic risk but also from a family systems perspective. Guided by this perspective, health professionals ask themselves: Who else does this person bring into the room? What are the patterns of behavior and communication within this person's family? In what ways will the genetic information impact the established patterns of behavior and communication in this family?

From a systems perspective, a health-care practitioner considers the implications of a genetic diagnosis not only for the client but also that client's family due to the interdependence of family members. Communication in families about a genetic diagnosis and its resultant implications is viewed not as a single event or act, but rather as an ongoing, dynamic process that may occur over time. These ways of thinking and the information contained in this chapter may be novel for some practitioners who traditionally consider just the client as opposed to the client and his or her family. As well, they may expand on existing views for practitioners who are used to considering both the client and the client's family.

In this chapter we will examine the ways in which family systems theory can provide a useful lens through which to view families with genetic conditions and their communication, enabling health-care practitioners to consider additional and alternative ways to work with clients. This chapter will provide the following: *(1)* an overview of family systems theory and its ties to communication about family genetic issues, *(2)* a short case application of family systems theory and its relationship to counseling about genetic conditions, *(3)* a discussion of future directions, and *(4)* a review of strengths and weaknesses of using a systems perspective.

THE FAMILY AS A SYSTEM

The family may be viewed as "an example of an open, ongoing, goal-seeking, self-regulating, social system ..." [2]. When viewed as systems, families are dynamic, influenced by the ongoing development of family members and their relationships with each other. Ongoing fluctuations occur as every family member affects the others and is in turn affected by them. An example is parents who have previously come to a decision not to inform their children about the presence of an unbalanced chromosome translocation in the family. They review that decision as their children reach early adulthood as the information has greater implications and agree to provide the information to their children. Family systems foster the exchange of resources such as information and support. The family system influences action among family members and can change or evolve as a function of these actions [3, 4]. When two or more persons form a relational system, "the most important feature of such a relationship is communication" [5].

Family systems theory or family process theory [6] provides a framework for understanding the complexity of familial interactions. This theory describes the family as a complex and interactive social system, revealing the need for health-care practitioners to understand family structure, change, and development [7]. Health issues, such as a serious genetic disease, destabilize the family, creating new patterns of connection, disconnection, and resultant communication. To attend to the full impact of a diagnosis of a genetic disease, a person must be viewed within his or her family context. According to a family systems approach, all illness influences, and is influenced by, the family members who interpret the illness and manage interactions about the illness. This is evident in the way families respond and communicate with each other about illness. There may be open discussions of the implications of the illness, an attempt to avoid talking with the ill member about the health problem, or parents may keep the health information a secret from the children. The nature of genetic disease complicates the role of family members who are impacted on multiple levels by a diagnosis or a history of genetic disease. In cases of genetic illness, not only are family members concerned for the affected relative but become concerned for the implications of the diagnosis for their own health and the health of other family members. The diagnosis of a genetic disorder has unique systemic implications because "When one family member is tested, in a sense other family members are tested also" [8].

FAMILY SYSTEMS THEORY AND GENETIC ILLNESS

Viewing a family through the lens of family systems theory enables health-care practitioners to anticipate, explore, and understand the impact genetic information has on both individuals and families, as well as assess issues that individuals face when the diagnosis of a genetic illness occurs [9]. It may help practitioners to organize their conceptual approach when working with families faced with genetic illness. To fully understand an individual's needs, health professionals need to understand interactions and patterns in that individual's family, in particular patterns of communication, because these relationships are embedded in these patterns, consciously or unconsciously. Understanding patterns of communication in families is critical if individuals are to be supported in disseminating genetic information to their family. Finally, systems theory can inform the counseling approach utilized by practitioners when working with individuals and families.

Four basic assumptions underlie any systems perspective: "(a) systems elements are interconnected; (b) systems can only be understood as wholes; (c) all systems affect themselves through environmental feedback; and (d) systems are not reality" [6]. Although various authors emphasize different sets of family systems characteristics, eight characteristics are most commonly stressed for a social system such as the family [2, 6, 10, 11]. These are interdependence, wholeness, patterns/rules, calibration, interactive complexity, openness/boundaries, organization, and equifinality.

Interdependence

Interdependence implies that a change in one part of the system affects the entire system; accordingly, a health change in one family member impacts the entire family. Renowned family therapist Virginia Satir [12] vividly captured this concept through the metaphor of a mobile, a balanced hanging sculpture with parts that can be set in motion by air currents. She depicts family members on the mobile; as something affects one person, other family members reverberate with the impact. The genetics literature is filled with examples of the impact of one member's diagnosis on the entire family system's communication patterns [8, 13, 14]. In their study of women at risk for hereditary breast-ovarian cancer, Foster and colleagues [15] found that family communication could be hindered depending on the family members' test results; some of those who tested negative could not talk to those who tested positive or other relatives with the cancer due to feelings of guilt. In cases of asymptomatic carrier couples, Decruyenaere and colleagues [16] found predictive testing for the fatal neurodegenerative condition Huntington disease (HD) may result in an imbalanced partner system evidenced by the overprotectiveness of the unaffected partner.

Wholeness

This systems characteristic privileges the "whole" over the sum of its parts. Families have a history that is different from that of its individual members. Families exhibit characteristics reflecting both individual members and the relationships among them. Members' interaction patterns result in *emergent properties*, or characteristics that develop from members' synergistic interconnections [17]. Entire families may be characterized by emergent properties, such as humor, aggression, hopefulness, or skepticism that differentially represent each individual member. Distinctive communication patterns between and among family subgroups develop as a result of this wholeness; siblings may engage in incessant competition or parents may display predictable avoidance of certain topics. In some families, the experience of a genetic disease may emerge as a psychologically defining characteristic; in others, it may be one of many less specialized characteristics. Attitudes of hopefulness or hopelessness in the face of serious disease may characterize entire families, differentially affecting their response to ongoing diagnostic revelations. A dominant genetic illness, such as HD, may influence a family's self-definition, even for those unaffected members.

Patterns/Rules

Every family system develops communication patterns, often reflecting a multigenerational heritage. Over time such patterns may become communication rules or explicit or implicit relationship agreements that prescribe and limit a family members' behavior. Communication rules establish a sense of regularity and order while providing answers to questions, such as: What are you allowed to talk about? Who can you talk to about it?

How can you talk about it? How do you find answers when you do not understand? [10, 12]. These rules, which may be implicitly or explicitly learned, maintain stability in the system. Frequently rules differ by gender or generations. It is well recognized that implicit or explicit gendered rules influence dissemination of genetic information [18–21]. In many families implicit rules exclude males from discussions of members' genetic health, creating a powerful gendered pattern [13, 22]. Women tend to assume the primary role in communicating genetic information, even when the condition has health implications for both genders [23]. Gendered communication rules may play out as follows: only sisters are allowed to discuss the inheritance of a breast-cancer-predisposing mutation.

Faced with a member's genetic disease, many families enact rules regarding transmission of information to other relatives, such as the eldest female relative controls transmission of genetic health information. Aunts and uncles may be prevented from passing on information regarding hereditary hemochromatosis to their nieces or nephews by the rule that only parents may transmit information about serious medical information their children [13]. The nuclear family appears to be a boundary for discussion of genetic information. In a study of communication about Lynch syndrome genetic testing, Peterson and her colleagues [24] found that family members who were noncarriers and nonbiological relatives perceived discussion about genetic counseling and testing as less relevant to them and were subsequently less involved.

Two communication patterns—monitoring and blunting—may be enacted in families faced with the serious health issues of one or more members [25]. Monitoring occurs when family members are anxious; they tend to scan for and amplify threatening cues and engage in information seeking. Blunting involves minimizing and avoiding threatening cues. Blunters attempt to deny the risk and rarely seek genetic information. For example, by monitoring or blunting, family members may be following implicit or explicit communication rules regulating talk about HD.

A family script approach incorporates a range of patterns. A study of communication in families with a history of breast/ovarian cancer used a family script approach to identify five communication patterns: open and supportive, directly blocked, indirectly blocked, self-censored, and use of third parties [26]. Such patterns are likely to be highly regularized over time. Open communication about painful matters is considered to be desirable, or even necessary, for good relational adjustment [27, 28]. van Oostrom and colleagues [27] found family members who were less able to talk with their relatives about hereditary cancer reported more family difficulties and unwanted relationship changes.

Calibration

Ongoing family patterns are maintained through the process of calibration. Early systems theorists viewed the family system as committed to stability, reflecting a mechanistic perspective. This approach assumes families are "calibrated" or "set" through feedback mechanisms that regulate their behavior in accordance with the members' explicit or implicit rules. If one member breaks a rule, others are likely to provide feedback telling that individual to stick to the pattern; if the member is not pressured, it may be a sign that the calibrated pattern is open to change. Human systems, such as families, must change and develop in order to survive, although interaction patterns are constantly at work to maintain stability and prevent the family system from undergoing change that is too rapid or severe [29].

Knowledge that a family member has been diagnosed with a genetic disease, or is at risk of developing one, affects family interaction patterns. In a system calibrated to support observation and reject direct health-related comments, adult children avoid talking to their father about his increased stumbling; instead, they may develop an "observe-and-compare" pattern of surveillance, followed by sibling discussions, as they track their father's onset of HD. They live with the unwritten rule that the siblings do not talk directly with their father about what they see. If one sister mentions his increased stumbling to her father, that interaction breaks the calibrated pattern. Subsequently the other siblings will either try to bring her in line and maintain the status quo or they, too, will start to address signs of physical change with their father, enabling new communication patterns to develop.

Most families struggle to find a balance between forces maintaining stability and those enabling change. The calibration process has been problematized as theorists recognize the ongoing shifts in relationships that keep a human system in a state of flux, as well as the need for families to cope with developmental changes and unpredictable crises. For example, a systematic study assessing the quality of relationship with partners with predictive testing for HD found the impact of the test results varied after 5 years —some couples perceived no change in their relationship quality [16]. Noncarriers reported less distress and more communication. In either case, the marital systems had reached calibration over time, but there was great variability in each partnership system's initial adjustment to the news. In families undergoing cancer genetic testing, van Oostrom and colleagues [30] reported the impact of genetic testing on family relationships was more often perceived as positive as opposed to negative; some families reported improved communication and greater relational appreciation. These families recalibrated their interaction patterns. More recent thinking supports an evolutionary model of family change that incorporates the possibility of spontaneous or unpredictable change [31, 32].

Interactive Complexity

Interactive complexity suggests that, in ongoing, significant relationships, each individual's action is a response to a previous action and a trigger for a future action. Therefore, the ongoing nature of family interaction patterns renders meaningless any attempt to identify causality or "what action came first." Attempts to assign cause or blame to one member's behavior are considered useless; problems are viewed as the result of ongoing behavioral patterns, not as the fault of one member. This perspective creates an "illness-free" lens [5] through which to view relationships. This perspective holds that blaming one member for difficulties is senseless because all members play a part in creating the problematic patterns. And, even if a singular instigating event could be identified (X blamed Y for disclosing her health secret 5 years ago), the issue is so entwined in the family members' ongoing communication patterns that focusing on the isolated behavior is nonproductive.

A classic interactive pattern is the nag/withdraw cycle ("He withdraws because she nags; she nags because he withdraws"), demonstrating the pointlessness of identifying the "first cause." Focusing on current patterns serves to uncover ongoing complex issues. For example, after a diagnosis of a child's cystic fibrosis (CF), a fatal condition that affects the lungs, a husband and wife may develop a long-term demand–withdraw pattern. She may need to discuss the topic in order to talk about her anxieties and seek support; he may find enormous difficulty talking, or even thinking deeply, about the long-term implications of the genetic disease. Four years after the diagnosis he may tell a counselor that "Our marital issues started when Pat kept pushing me to talk constantly about Molly's future," while she may describe the problem saying, "Lee closes up anytime CF is mentioned and refuses to engage in any planning, leaving everything on my shoulders." From a systems perspective, even if a counselor could identify who "started" the pattern 4 years earlier, it would be a pointless finding. The therapeutic goal is to address the current problematic interactive pattern and how it could be modified.

Openness/Boundaries

Human systems are considered to be open systems, in contrast to closed systems such as mechanical ones, because they depend on interchange with the surrounding environments. Family members maintain constant interchanges, not only within the family boundary, but across the family boundary with the larger ecosystem that includes health, educational, legal, political, and economic institutions as well as friends and extended family. Boundaries can be likened to physical or psychological limits regulating access to people, places, ideas, and values. Internal boundaries guard family members' individuality and establish subsystems, such as generational subsystems [10]. Role confusion and conflict arise when boundaries are inappropriately constructed, such as when a child is co-opted into a parental role. Although boundaries vary, from strong to flexible to almost nonexistent, healthy families require some interchange with the environment to manage growth and change. Some families establish a closed boundary around a member's genetic disease, declining to tell extended family members, thereby denying these relatives knowledge of personal risk. Other families enact open boundaries, informing relatives of a member's diagnosis and, in some cases, burdening others with their need to talk [13]. Families with very loose and flexible boundaries as well as those who have rigid boundaries have been shown to be less able to cope with genetic testing and more prone to adverse changes in nuclear family relationships. van Oostrom and colleagues [27] described differentiation as an important family system characteristic for individuals adjusting to cancer genetic testing. Individuals more emotionally separated from their parents, particularly their mothers, while remaining connected reported less distress. A balance between rigidity and flexibility is important.

Complex Relationships

Families are organized into numerous interpersonal subsystems composed of two or more persons and the relationships and communication patterns among them. An example is a three-person subsystem that has three dyads (mother–son, brother–sister, and mother–daughter) with distinctive communication patterns for each dyad, as well as for the triad. Traditionally, the critical underlying concept of family organization was the generational hierarchy of power, such as the powerful parental subsystem with its secrets and emotional/sexual boundaries and the child's inability to control information or establish firm boundaries. Yet this varies across family forms; in a stepfamily, the mother and her three biological children may represent a more powerful subsystem than the couple subsystem.

Each family system reflects the members' cultural norms. For example, decision making regarding prenatal testing for genetic disease varies across cultures. Awwad and colleagues [33] found American couples to be less likely to involve extended relatives in the prenatal decision-making process than Native Palestinian couples.

Additional factors add to the complexity. Currently, more families are experiencing generational reversals due to immigration and technological change. Immigration may render a child as the language/culture broker for the older generations; technological sophistication may also place a child in the role of family expert. Such generational differences may also appear in attitudes and knowledge regarding genetic testing because younger generations may view testing as more acceptable. Lack of interest in learning about personal genetic risk for cancer has been shown to be associated with less education, minority status, and infrequent performance of other protective health behaviors [34].

As families cope with the long-term impacts of certain genetic diseases, subgroups may develop representing those who decide to be tested and those who resist testing. For example, Sobel and Cowan [14] found that, in families with a history of HD, subgroups emerged that included (1) those who chose to be tested and those who did not and (2) those who tested normal and those who did not. Such subgroups managed grief and losses in varying ways, as reflected in their communication patterns.

Coalitions, especially triangles consisting of two insiders and an outsider, may form as members align strongly, establishing highly stable interaction patterns. When a two-person relationship is stressful, members frequently draw in a third person to serve as the focal point of attention, relieving the stress on the original pair. Boundary problems may involve intergenerational coalitions (e.g., grandmother and grandson only speak of health as "God's will"), and parental or sibling alliances. In addition, boundary problems may arise due to member differences on the extent to which outsiders (friends and colleagues) are allowed to hear any genetic disease information.

Finally, illness may alter the roles played by family members. An 11 year old may become the "parentified child" who significantly assists an affected parent by assuming caretaking responsibilities; another may become the clown, desperate to bring laughter and distraction into the situation.

Equifinality

Family systems are considered goal-oriented entities. Equifinality implies that a particular final state or goal may be accomplished in different ways from different starting points and that there are many ways to reach the same end [10]. For example, the goals of "raising successful children" or "creating a happy family" may be achieved in various ways across diverse families. Romantic partners may face negotiating a marriage commitment involving biological children if one of them is a carrier for a mutation causing hereditary breast-ovarian cancer. In one case their discussions may lead to an even deeper tie between the couple and the agreement to use in vitro fertilization; in another case a decision to adopt may result. All these systems characteristics interact to create rather predictable patterns of response to family stressors, including responding to a member's diagnosis of a genetic disorder.

Genetic technologies continue to develop at a rapid rate, resulting in an increasing amount of complex information for individuals and their family members to understand. Future discussions about genetics and its relationship to disease, including options available to individuals and their families, will become increasingly complex. Systems theory may be applied explicitly to a particular family or partnership as the primary framework for analyzing members' interactions and is of particular relevance to health professionals to understand how families communicate and integrate genetic information into their lives. Conversely, a systems approach may serve as a general worldview, establishing a larger frame for responding to a family's issues. Systems theory may be paired with other more restricted theories such as Communication Privacy Management (see Chapter 7) or uncertainty theory (see Chapter 8).

ILLUSTRATION OF FAMILY SYSTEMS THEORY IN PRACTICE

In order to illustrate how these concepts may be evident or applied in a genetics consultation, we offer the case of the Wilmington family. Barbara Wilmington was an only child, her mother having died from bowel cancer when she was 8 years old. All her mother's relatives were deceased, many from cancer. Barbara was raised by her father, whom she described as a kind and caring man. Barbara and her husband were divorced and had three children, Damien, 28, Rebecca, 24, and Samantha, 22. Barbara spoke highly of her son, Damien, particularly in terms of the care and responsibility shown toward his mother following her own diagnosis of cancer and subsequent to the divorce. She also spoke of the role model he was for his sisters. Damien, a human resources manager, lived at home with his mother and sisters and managed many of the affairs of the household.

Recently Barbara was invited to return to the hereditary bowel cancer clinic for further discussion after an *hMSH2* mutation was found. Damien attended the appointment with his mother. The genetic findings were discussed with Barbara and Damien, including the availability of predictive testing for Damien and his sisters. After Damien expressed interest in predictive testing for himself, the genetic counselor suggested that he make another appointment to discuss such testing. The counselor also indicated that, if Damien had a partner, his partner would be welcome to attend the subsequent session. Damien explained he did not have a partner.

As part of the consultation, the counselor asked how the genetic findings would be discussed with Rebecca and Samantha. Damien responded, suggesting that this was information Rebecca and Samantha may not need to know at this stage. The genetic counselor asked what Barbara thought about Damien's comment. Barbara stated that, while she felt it was important for Rebecca and Samantha to be informed of the newly found *hMSH2* mutation, they would be upset by the information. She noted that the girls were very young when she developed bowel cancer and, coupled with the divorce, Barbara felt their lives had been difficult enough. She also reported feeling responsible for their current situation. Barbara suggested that she and Damien would talk further about when and how to tell them. The genetic counselor asked how Rebecca and Samantha might respond to the information if they were here today. Barbara replied that Rebecca would be upset, although interested in predictive testing, whereas Samantha would be very distressed and "run a mile."

Then the counselor asked Barbara how important or potentially distressing information was usually discussed in the family. Barbara replied that she would usually talk about the situation with Damien and they would devise a plan as to how to discuss it with the girls. When asked if she ever sought input from the girls' father or anyone else in her family if there was important or distressing news, Barbara indicated she did not. The genetic counselor agreed to telephone Barbara after she had time to consider the additional genetic information and the possibility of discussing the information with Rebecca and Samantha.

Adopting a systems approach enabled the genetic counselor to consider roles and communication patterns in the family, which informed the approach taken, specifically the questions asked by the genetic counselor of Barbara and Damien, as well as the suggestion to schedule future appointments. This case highlights a number of issues related to systems theory, including interdependence, openness/boundaries, patterns/rules, and calibration.

Because *interdependence* implies that a change in one part of the system affects the entire system, the additional genetic information and the availability of predictive testing represented a significant change for every member of this family. The genetic counselor was mindful of the reverberations that could occur as a result of finding the *hMSH2* mutation, which is consistent when viewing the family as a system.

Boundaries maintain family members' individuality and establish subsystems such as generational subsystems [10]. Generational subsystems separate parents (assumed to have an executive function or leadership role) from the child/sibling subsystem. Clear boundaries enable family members to develop a sense of autonomy and a sense of belonging. Role confusion and conflict arises when boundaries are inappropriately constructed. For example, when boundaries are diffuse, family members experience a sense of belonging but not a sense of independence; members may experience psychological problems due to overinvolvement. Children may be co-opted into the spousal role [3, 10]. The genetic counselor considered the relationship patterns in the family, in particular Damien's role. The genetic counselor wondered about Damien's differentiation from his mother, and therefore his ability to make autonomous decisions for himself, in particular about predictive testing. Family systems theory defines interpersonal differentiation as the extent to which an individual feels separated from emotional attachment to his or her parents without damaging the relationship and is necessary for healthy psychological adjustment [35]. Interpersonal differentiation is helpful to consider when thinking about parental influence and decision making. Barbara's prior description of her son and the experience of meeting Damien left the genetic counselor wondering whether Damien had assumed the role of his father following the divorce of his parents; therefore, he had a powerful role when it came to decision making. It was as though Damien and his mother were the parents and Rebecca and Samantha the children. The counselor also wondered whether Damien had been co-opted into co-parenting with his mother. Had Damien become the "parentified child," acting as an emotional sounding board and as "partner" for his mother? As such, this would have resulted in the separation of the sibling subsystem, with Damien acting as "father" to his sisters in this regard rather than brother. Was Damien the competent, protective adult and his sisters the incompetent/needy sisters? It is possible Damien and his mother made executive decisions about when and how to communicate the genetic information to Rebecca and Samantha, and even whether they should or should not have predictive testing.

While the genetic counselor was aware the family was not presenting for family therapy, adopting a family systems approach enabled the genetic counselor to make assessments of the roles and communication patterns within the family, which in turn informed the counseling approach adopted. The primary aim in understanding roles and communication patterns in the Wilmington family was to anticipate, explore, and understand the impact genetic information would have for their family. More specifically, the genetic counselor wished to know whether the genetic information would be communicated to others in the family, how this communication would occur, and identify whether this would be problematic. It also enabled the genetic counselor to consider strategies that might improve communication and support for the family.

Patterns and rules serve to make life predictable and manageable. Each family system develops and maintains communication patterns, usually based on agreements to follow a set of rules. This maintains stability, or *calibrates* the system. The genetic counselor determined that the communication rules in the Wilmington family sanctioned Barbara discussing the situation with Damien and the pair jointly devising a plan for communicating with the girls. She did not discuss the matter with their father or any other people. This led the genetic counselor to understand that Barbara identified Damien as her support when communicating with the girls and to anticipate challenges that may arise for this family as a result of their usual communication patterns (e.g., Barbara and Damien may choose not to tell Samantha and Rebecca, who were both approaching the age where they would be considered genetically at risk).

A family systems perspective enabled the counselor to appreciate the interactions and patterns in this family, including members of the family not present at the appointment (Samantha and Rebecca). Genetic counseling provided a platform for Barbara and Damien to consider whether the communication patterns in their family enabled the relational system to develop and change or if the communication patterns would remain the same, therefore maintaining the status quo.

IMPACTS OF GENETIC INFORMATION ON A FAMILY SYSTEM

Established family communication patterns and ways of behaving can be challenged and change as members address genetic health issues. Weak points in family interaction will be tested under the strain of confronting a genetic condition and the potential for genetic testing and, as a result, increased communication may occur in family members who are usually disengaged. Likewise, those who are comparatively involved may find themselves distancing from each another or even in conflict [36].

Even when a family member tests negative for a genetic disease, the process of getting tested and waiting for results impacts the family system. McDaniel [36] describes a couple in which the male's mother had been diagnosed with HD and he had not yet been tested. The couple's anxiety, and the wife's hypervigilance to every twitch or moment of forgetfulness, altered their marriage. Even after the husband tested negative for HD, it took several months for his wife to see her husband as "whole" and for the couple to enact communication patterns similar to those practiced before the mother's diagnosis. The tensions experienced by the marital subsystem would have affected any children or extended family members.

The impact of a mutation on the entire family system remains understudied. According to McDaniel [36], in addition to knowing who is affected genetically, there is a great need to know "who is 'affected' psychologically and interpersonally, who may benefit from family therapy consultation or treatment" (p. 27). Relatives who are noncarriers may feel a sense of responsibility for the future care of relatives with mutations or feel guilty about escaping a future with cancer [27]. For example, Tibben and colleagues [37] found that in cases of HD, partners respond with similar thoughts and feelings as tested individuals, such as carriers, and their partners show an increase of hopelessness over noncarriers at 1 week post testing.

Although members of married couples and committed adult partnerships have been addressed in the literature, certain key familial relationships have received far less attention. These include sibling ties and nonbiological kinship ties, related to adoption, in-law relationships, and fictive or social kinship ties. For example, in their examination of barriers to carrier testing for adult CF siblings, Fanos and Johnson [38] suggest the impact of one sibling's diagnosis on another's decision making. They provide eight reasons why siblings may wish to remain unaware of their carrier status including the following: "a) global sense of guilt, (b) guilt over the relationship with their sib, (c) survival guilt, (d) fears of an early death for themselves" [38].

Understandably the focus for health-care practitioners is often the biological family because their primary concern is related to genetic risk, although it is evident genetic information impacts the entire family system. A family systems perspective is concerned with all family members, biological and nonbiological, and the impact genetic information has for them all. Nonbiological ties are often overlooked in genetics research. Although there is minimal acknowledgment of adoptive kin or step-relationships in studies of disclosure [13], such relationships are seldom addressed.

In-law relationships remain seriously understudied in the family literature and particularly in genetic implications. But these ties can be powerfully affected as genetic issues surface. McDaniel (2005) describes the emotional cutoff between a mother-in-law and daughter-in-law after the son/husband underwent testing at his mother's urging and learned that he tested positive for both the *BRCA1* and *BRCA2* gene mutations. The outcome devastated his wife, who reported seeing death on the faces of her daughters and became estranged from her mother-in-law. Families formed through commitment, rather than blood or traditional legal means, create ties of "practical kinship" that may serve to separate members. Practicing with a family systems perspective, health-care practitioners can identify and provide support for those who are not only affected biologically but also those psychologically and interpersonally affected by genetic information. Most genetic counseling research investigates the initial impact of a genetic diagnosis and the psychosocial impact of genetic counseling and genetic testing on the individual. Few studies have investigated family system characteristics, family interactions, and the impact of genetics on family relationships [23, 27, 36].

HEALTH-CARE PRACTITIONER PRACTICE

As illustrated in the case study above, a family systems approach can enable health-care practitioners to encourage individuals, partners, and their family members to anticipate the impact genetic information may have, specifically on ways of communicating and relating to each other. Anticipating the impact of genetic information, particularly testing results, may have a number of positive benefits. As well as reducing tension, it may allow growth and development of the family as they come to understand ways they communicate and behave with each other. In addition, a family systems perspective enables practitioners to assist and support individuals and their family while they adjust.

Recently the profession of genetic counseling has acknowledged the need for research that identifies theoretical models that guide practice. Although there are many descriptions of the tasks of genetic counseling and what genetic counseling involves, there is limited discussion about what theoretical models underpin practice [39]. Genetics is concerned with families, including the impact of genetic technology on families. Therefore, it seems evident that a family systems approach is considered and articulated as one of the guiding theoretical approaches to inform the practice and profession of genetic counseling.

Adopting a family systems approach does not equate to practicing family therapy. When an individual/family presents for family therapy, the therapist focus is to develop specific interventions to improve/change family communication, usually as a result of a problem being identified (e.g., a child with behavioral problems). Usually in consultations, the genetic practitioner seeks to understand how the genetic information will impact on the family system so that they may develop strategies to assist families and support them in communicating about genetic information.

Health-care practitioners who wish to utilize a systemic approach in enacting specific counseling techniques and systemic interventions may benefit from additional training in counseling techniques specific to family therapy. As compared to other types of psychosocial therapy, family therapy focuses on improving family functioning. Family therapy focuses on concerns such as interaction patterns, coalitions, and roles [29]. These goals and focus are similar to the goals and focus of genetic counseling.

A systems perspective helps provide psychosocial meaning to families with members who are diagnosed with a genetic disease or with a genetically influenced condition. Given the evolving sophistication of medical treatments, dealing with genetic and genomic issues across the life span will become the "new normal" for countless family members. In adopting a systems theory approach, health-care practitioners can engage with a range of family members and assist them in learning how to face living with familial health challenges.

STRENGTHS AND LIMITATIONS

Systems theory has influenced research and practice in family communication, family therapy, and genetic counseling, serving to keep a focus on the familial interdependence of any individual. Systems theory reinforces the idea that families are constantly changing while calling attention to patterned interaction. Practitioners focus on family patterns that support or interfere with well-family functioning. The interdependence of members is emphasized. Yet there are limits to the theory. In addition to the claims that it is too abstract, systems theory has been criticized for denying gender inequalities between males and females. The marital pair "may be viewed as an equal unit whereas greater power may reside with the male" [40]. The systems theory may reify the family roles when, in some cases, families may need to function with fluid roles due to unique pressures. A final concern involves the possibility of losing sight of individual issues, such as alcoholism or depression, when attending to relational concerns [41].

CONCLUSION

Discussions of systems theory and genetic counseling must be embedded in the evolving ecosystem of therapeutic approaches because systems theory, family communication research, family therapy, and genetic counseling are inextricably linked. Systems theory remains a central element of family therapy training programs [42, 43], although advances in areas such as evolutionary theory and biopsychosocial systems theory are also informing therapeutic practice [44]. Health-care practitioners may incorporate a systems perspective when working with individuals or a set of family members. Recent work includes the development of colored eco-genetic relationship maps (CEGRMS) to depict the various system resources—informational, functional, and emotional—provided to clients through their social networks [45]. Given the stream of ongoing research emerging from the Human Genome Project, practitioners must prepare clients for the "new normal, " or the integration of a continuous stream of alternative treatments developed from the research findings.

Finally, family therapists must be prepared to incorporate genetic knowledge into their practices and to collaborate with health-care practitioners working in the realm of genetics.

Practical applications of a systems perspective accomplish the following:

- Allow health professionals to recognize the systemic implications for all family members following the diagnosis of a genetic condition, enabling them to anticipate and consider the issues family members face
- Provide valuable insights into the interactions and communication patterns in families, informing the therapeutic approach for both individuals and family subgroups
- Aid health professionals in developing counseling interventions as they attempt to determine family communication patterns to help identify barriers to communication and identify families who may require additional psychosocial support
- Support the professional collaboration of health professionals, family therapists, and family communication scholars, all of whom are committed to providing meaningful support to families with whom they work.

The need for understanding the family as a system is clear: "As more and more becomes known about the genetic components of disease, the family becomes a multifaceted crucible of biological and psychological connection" [46].

REFERENCES

1. Minuchin S. *Family Kaleidoscope: Images of Violence and Healing.* Boston: Harvard University Press; 1984.
2. Broderick, C. *Understanding Family Process: Basics of Family Systems of Theory.* Newbury Park: CA: Sage Publications; 1993.
3. Hayes, H. A re-introduction to family therapy: Clarification of three schools. *Australian and New Zealand Journal of Family Therapy* 1991;12:27–43.
4. Giddens, A. *The Constitution of Society: Outlines of Theory and Structuration.* Cambridge, England: Polity Press; 1984.
5. Duncan BL, Rock JW. Saving relationships: The power of the unpredictable. *Psychology Today* 1993;21:46–51.
6. White JM, Klein DM. *Family Theories.* 2nd ed. Thousand Oaks, CA: Sage; 2002.
7. Loukas A, Twitchekk GR, Piejack LA, Fitzgerald HE, Zucker RA. The family as a unit of interacting personalities. In: L'Abate L, ed. *Family Psychopathology: The Relational Roots of Dysfunctional Behavior.* New York: Guilford Press; 1998:35–59.
8. Sorenson JR, Jennings-Grant T, Newman J. Communication about carrier testing within Hemophilia A families. *American Journal of Medical Genetics Part C: Seminars in Medical Genetics* 2003;119C:3–10.

9. Kim K. Case report: A systems approach to genetic counseling for albinism. *Journal of Genetic Counseling* 1999;8:47–54.
10. Galvin KM, Bylund CL, Brommel BJ. *Family Communication: Cohesion and Changes*. 6th ed. Boston: Allyn & Bacon; 2008.
11. Littlejohn SW, Foss KA. *Theories of Human Communication*. 9th ed. Belmont, CA: Thomson Wadsworth; 2008.
12. Satir V. *The New Peoplemaking*. Mountainview, CA: Science and Behavior Books; 1998.
13. Forrest K, Simpson SA, Wilson BJ, van Teijlingen ER, McKee L, et al. *Clinical Genetics* 2003;64:317–326.
14. Sobel S, Cowan D. *Family Process* 2003;42:47–57.
15. Foster C, Eeles R, Ardern-Jones A, Moynihan C, Watson M. *Psychology and Health* 2004;19:439–455.
16. Decruyenaere M, Evers-Kiebooms G, Cloostermans T, Boogaerts A, Demyttenaere K, et al. Predictive testing for Huntington's disease: relationship with partners after testing. *Clinical Genetics* 2004;65:24–31.
17. Whitchurch GG, Constantine LL. Family communication. In: Sussman M, Steinmetz SK, Peterson GW, eds. *Handbook of Marriage and the Family*. New York: Plenum Press; 1999:687–704.
18. Green J, Richards M, Murton F, Statham H, Hallowell N. Family communication and genetic counseling: The case of hereditary breast and ovarian cancer. *Journal of Genetic Counseling* 1997;6:45–60.
19. Hallowell N. Doing the right thing: Genetic risk and responsibility. *Sociology of Health and Illness* 1999;21:597–621.
20. d'Agincourt-Canning L. Experiences of genetic risk: Disclosure and the gendering of responsibility. *Bioethics* 2001;15: 231–247.
21. d'Agincourt-Canning L, Baird P. Genetic testing for hereditary cancers: The impact of gender on interest, uptake and ethical considerations. *Oncology Hematology* 2006;58:114–123.
22. Gaff CL, Collins V, Symes T, Halliday J. Facilitating family communication about predictive *genetic* testing: Probands' perceptions. *Journal of Genetic Counseling* 2005;14:133–140.
23. Koehly LM, Peterson SK, Watts BG, Kempf KK, Vernon SW, et al. A social network analysis of communication about HNPCC genetic testing and family functioning. *Cancer Epidemiology, Biomarkers and Prevention* 2003;12:304–313.
24. Peterson SK, Watts BG, Koehly LM, Vernon SW, Baile WF, et al. How families communicate about HNPCC genetic testing. *American Journal of Human Genetics Part C: Seminars in Medical Genetics* 2003;119:78–86.
25. Miller SM. Monitoring versus blunting styles of coping with cancer influence the information patients want and need about their disease: Implications for cancer screening and management. *Cancer* 1995;76:167–177.
26. Kenen R, Ardern-Jones A, Eeles R. We are talking, but are they listening? Communication patterns in families with a history of breast/ovarian cancer (HBOC). *Psycho-Oncology* 2004;13:335–345.
27. van Oostrom I, Meijers-Heijboer H, Duivenvoorden HJ, Brocker-Vriends AH, van Asperen CJ, et al. Family system characteristics and psychological adjustment to cancer susceptibility genetic testing: A prospective study. *Clinical Genetics* 2007;71:35–42.

28. Watzlawick P, Beavin JH, Jackson DD. *Human Communication: Forms, Disturbances and Paradoxes.* Oxford, England: Hans Huber Publishers; 1969.
29. Glick I, Kessler D. *Marital and Family Therapy.* New York: Grune and Straton, Inc.; 1974.
30. van Oostrom I, Meijers-Heijboer H, Duivenvoorden HJ, Brocker-Vriends AH, van Asperen CJ, et al. A prospective study of the impact of genetic susceptibility testing for BRCA 1/2 or HNPCC on family relationships. *Psycho-Oncology* 2007;16:320–328.
31. Hoffman L. Constructing realities: An art of lenses. *Family Process* 1990;29:1–12.
32. Yerby J. Family systems *theory* reconsidered: Integrating social *construction theory* and dialectical process. *Communication Theory* 1995;5:339–365.
33. Awwad R, Veach PM, Bartels DM, LeRoy BS. Culture and acculturation influences on Palestinian perceptions of prenatal genetic counseling. *Journal of Genetic Counseling* 2008;17:101–116.
34. Andrykowski MA, Munn RK, Studts JL. Interest in learning of personal genetic risk for cancer: A general population survey. *Preventive Medicine* 1996;25:527–536.
35. Bowen M. *Family Therapy in Clinical Practice.* New York: Arenson; 1978.
36. McDaniel SH. Psychotherapy of genetics. *Family Process* 2005;44:24–44.
37. Tibben A, Timman R, Bannink EC, Duivenvoorden HJ. Three-year follow-up after presymptomatic testing for Huntington's disease in tested individuals and partners. *Health Psychology* 1997;16:20–35.
38. Fanos JH, Johnson JP. Barriers to carrier testing for adult cystic fibrosis sibs: the importance of not knowing. *American Journal of Medical Genetics* 1995;59:85–91.
39. Gaff, C.L., Clarke, A. J, Atkinson, P., Sivell, S. Elwyn, G. Iredale, R. et. al Process and outcome in communication of genetic information within families: A systematic review. *European Journal of Human Genetics* 2007, 1–13.
40. Galvin KM, Dickson FC, Marrow SR. Systems theory: Patterns and (w)holes in family communication. In: Braithwaite DO, Baxter LA, eds. *Engaging Theories in Family Communication: Multiple Perspectives.* Thousand Oaks, CA: Sage; 2006: 309–324.
41. Booth A, Carver K, Granger D. Biosocial perspectives on the family. *Journal of Marriage and Family Therapy* 2000;62:1018–1034.
42. Breunlin DC, Schwartz RC, Mac Kune-Karrer B. *Metaframeworks: Transcending the Models of Therapy.* San Francisco: Jossey-Bass; 2001.
43. Pinsof WM. *Integrative Problem-centered Therapy.* New York: Basic Books; 1995.
44. Pinsof WM, Lebow JL, eds. *Family Psychology: The Art of the Science.* New York: Oxford University Press; 2005.
45. Kenen R, Peters J. The Colored, Eco-Genetic Relationship Map (CEGRM): A conceptual approach and tool for genetic counseling research. *Journal of Genetic Counseling* 2001;10:289–309.
46. McDaniel SH, Rolland JS, Rubin LR, Miller SM. "It runs in the family." Family systems concepts and genetically linked disorders. In: Miller SM, et al., eds. *Individuals, Families and the New Era of Genetics: Biopsychosocial Perspective.* New York: W.W. Norton & Co.; 2006:118–318.

7

MANAGING PRIVACY OWNERSHIP AND DISCLOSURE

Sandra Petronio & Clara L. Gaff

Family members may be unwilling to share genetic information with one another, with reluctance often arising from concepts about ownership of the information. Communication Privacy Management Theory illuminates family and individual expectations about genetic information and assists health-care practitioners in identifying privacy problems that can face families, as well as strategies that may help them address these issues.

At the root of many concerns about genetic testing is the debate regarding ownership, as cogently pointed out by Barnoy and Tabok [1]: "If information about the medical state of one person is also information about the medical state of another, then all parties must confront the questions: Who owns the information? Is it only the person directly tested or also others implicated in the test findings? In addition, who has the right to decide the answer to this question? [A final problem] is that genetic testing can uncover information that people do not want to know" (p. 280).

As seems clear from this statement, ownership, privacy, and confidentiality are intrinsically linked. Because people believe they own the private information about their personal genetic makeup, they assume the right to control who knows, how much they know, how they know, and what is done with the information. When others appear to presume control by making decisions about a person's genetic information, that individual is likely to feel compromised [2]. Thus, the act of sharing genetic information with another person carries an expectation that the confidant will handle that information according to the confider's "privacy rules." In other words, the confidant will regulate access by revealing or concealing the information in the same way as the confider [3]. However, these rules may or may not be explicitly stated by the confider. Nevertheless, conflict can arise when information is not treated in ways either party expects. The concept of "ownership" is distinct in this chapter from the legal concepts discussed in Chapter 13. We consider privacy ownership in this discussion as defined within and arising out of a *personal and relational* context [2, 4].

For families, navigating privacy and confidentiality around genetic testing and results is fraught with dilemmas [5, 6]. An individual's desire to retain information defined as personal may compete with a concomitant ethical need to inform relatives. Additionally, concealing information about results may be further complicated by inconsistent assumptions about who the rightful owners are of genetic information [7]. Likewise, respecting a relative's confidentiality may compete with needs to share the information with other members impacted by the genetic findings. Privacy dilemmas occur when a person attempts to manage disclosures about genetic issues while also balancing the protection of family members from perceived harm such as stigmatization [8]. Clearly, the family is not alone in these struggles. Health-care practitioners also grapple with a dilemma between "duty to warn" and preserving the confidentiality of their patients [9].

The way people conduct themselves and the choices they make regarding disclosure have consequences for both loved ones and themselves [10]. Yet, we tend to find that making one "choice" produces a series of other obstacles in managing disclosure and confidentiality of private genetic information [3, 11]. For example, Hallowell and colleagues [12] found that some men in their study undergoing testing for breast cancer–predisposing mutations made a decision not to tell their daughters they were seeking testing, even though the testing was apparently motivated by a desire to protect their daughters. The fathers encountered difficulties with their daughters when they finally revealed the test results to them. Some daughters felt they should have been involved in the initial decision and were uncertain about the implications of the results for them personally. As this example illustrates, people face embedded dilemmas as they weigh decisions to reveal or conceal genetic information. Frequently, there is no clear way of knowing which decision is the "right" choice for whom, where, and how to tell the genetic information, or when it is best to kept the information secret [2]. Consequently, it is more productive to find a way to manage the situation rather than expect to find a clear solution to the dilemma. These difficult circumstances require an approach that serves to illuminate both the health-care practitioner's understanding and the client's grasp of the choices as well as the privacy rules that the client explicitly or unconsciously applies to these decisions. Likewise, practitioners often need to help clients avoid obstacles they are contemplating when deciding to reveal or conceal information about genetic testing and results. Thus, for practitioners, the best approach is to strive to develop "privacy management strategies" in collaboration *with* clients that determine the most productive set of decisions, given the circumstances, that effectively handle regulating private information about genetic testing, results, and overall decision making.

The evidenced-based theory of Communication Privacy Management (CPM) can facilitate understanding of the ways people "manage" revealing and concealing private information. As such, CPM serves as a viable framework for health-care practitioners to help client decision making of disclosure to and among family members about genetic testing results [2, 13]. Communication Privacy Management has been applied to a multitude of privacy situations across a number of contexts [e.g., 14–21]. The application of CPM has potential to assist the practitioner in understanding the how, when, and why decisions take place as family members communicate with each other about genetic information. The CPM road map works to provide practitioners with signals to recognize and address the critical issues facing people as they decide a course of action regarding genetic testing and results [2].

COMMUNICATION PRIVACY MANAGEMENT

Communication Privacy Management defines private information as something people believe they own and therefore have the right to control [2, 22]. Access to private information is controlled through the use of privacy rules that are developed and employed to regulate the privacy boundaries that house the information. When private information is shared (either through disclosure or granting access in some way), the act of doing so makes the recipient a co-owner or stakeholder of the information. In the context of family communication about genetics, the act of giving access or revealing the genetic information to a recipient family member transforms the privacy boundary surrounding that information from one that is personally owned and operated to a boundary collectively owned and operated with that relative. Families have two kinds of privacy boundaries they traverse—external and internal [2, 23, 24].

External family privacy boundaries reflect control of private information flow to those outside of the family (e.g., friends, work colleagues), while internal family privacy boundaries define information sharing between family members. These internal family "cells" do not necessarily include all family members. Thus, there are internal privacy cells that house private information co-owned by only certain members, not all. As the research indicates, families range in the level of permeability they grant to both insiders and outsiders [25, 26]. We know that families fall on a continuum from very open to very private, even extending to the point of being completely secretive with insiders and outsiders [17, 21]. They also manage the level of ownership and co-ownership rights of those inside and outside the family boundary to make independent decisions about the information [16].

Co-owners have responsibilities to treat the information according to the needs and desires of the original owner and learn these expectations by negotiating jointly agreed-upon privacy rules that are used to govern protection or access to the mutually controlled information. For instance, in disclosing to one family member, the original owner of the information may tell a new co-owner not to reveal the information to a particular relative. The outcome is best if there are negotiations that achieve a coordinated effort among the owner and co-owners agreeing on privacy rules that determine how they will regulate the ebb and flow of information surrounding genetic information. However, if no such negotiations take place or they break down because privacy rules are misunderstood, used incorrectly, or intentionally breached, CPM predicts that the breakdown causes a state of turbulence (i.e., privacy violations, privacy dilemmas, privacy intrusions, and/or privacy misunderstanding). To reduce turbulence, the root cause of the privacy rule disruption must be determined and mutually agreed-upon rules identified that can be used to control jointly owned and operated privacy boundaries [2].

As this discussion illustrates, CPM offers five fundamental principles that guide our understanding about privacy management:

1. Communication Privacy Management defines the nature of private information as something that people believe they own and therefore want to control. To better conceptualize this idea, CPM uses a boundary metaphor to illustrate information that is owned resides within a privacy boundary.
2. In order to control private information, people develop privacy rules that are based on decision criteria people use to reveal or conceal.
3. When private information is shared with others, the act of revealing creates co-owners of the information.
4. Because it is presumed that co-owners of the private information have a level of responsibility to care for the information, there is an expectation that privacy rules used to make decisions about third-party disclosures are negotiated and coordinated between the original owner and co-owner.
5. Although there are often expectations that the parties will coordinate the kind of rules that are used to manage the co-owned private information, at times there are intentional or unintentional breaches of that understanding resulting in boundary turbulence [2].

COMMUNICATION PRIVACY MANAGEMENT AND GENETIC DISCLOSURES

Communication Privacy Management offers guidance to deal with the knotty problems found in genetic testing. The best way to illustrate how CPM functions as a road map that directs us toward a better understanding is through analyzing genetic testing cases. We present four cases. Although they may not necessarily represent situations health professionals encounter frequently in their daily work, they do exemplify the ways in which genetic information may challenge existing family communication and lead to the identification of patterns that can be recognized and responded to by health-care practitioners.

Case Study 1: Renegotiating Privacy Rules

Mr. Andrews attended an appointment for a risk assessment with his adult children. He had been diagnosed with cancer 20 years earlier and reported that this affected his physical and mental health greatly. His personal and family history was consistent with a particular hereditary cancer condition, so Mr. Andrews was offered genetic testing to find the causative mutation. Mr. Andrews decided to proceed because he believed that this knowledge might help his children. Thus, if a mutation were found, they could have predictive testing to determine whether they had inherited the mutation and were therefore at high risk. His children agreed that he should proceed with testing.

When the genetic test results were available, Mr. Andrews attended an appointment to receive the results of his genetic testing with his wife but without their children. They were told that genetic testing had found a mutation responsible for causing a hereditary cancer condition. Mr. Andrews and the genetics practitioner assumed the next step was to tell his adult children about the test results. However, his wife insisted that they should *not* be informed. She thought that only she and her husband should know; she said that giving this information may adversely affect their children in the same way she perceived her husband was affected by his cancer diagnosis. She was also concerned that knowing the test results (if positive) may affect one of the daughter's forthcoming marriages. Hence, if the daughter's fiancé was to know, his family would also know, and he may not be willing to go through with the marriage because of his own reservations or his family's concerns. In addition, there was the potential (in Mrs. Andrews' mind) that the future in-laws might treat her child differently with this knowledge about genetic predisposition.

People typically negotiate three issues regarding management of a mutually held privacy boundary, according to CPM. These include who else can know (regulated by *linkage rules*); how much information is told (*permeability rules*); and the degree of control each party has over the particular information *(ownership rules)*. Married couples usually have a shared privacy boundary that houses private information belonging to both members of the couple (also called marital privacy boundaries) with commonly agreed-upon privacy rules about access to this information by others [2, 23, 25]. Because marital couples tend to talk about these privacy rules over time as they develop their relationship, in long-term marriages, as with Mr. and Mrs. Andrews, determining what information is jointly controlled and who has the right to make a choice about the way to manage this information is often more a matter of habit than discussion [25]. Clearly, Mrs. Andrews felt that the information about her husband's mutation was hers to dictate which privacy rules should be used for access/protection, even concerning access by her children. She saw herself as more than a co-equal owner of the information because she took control away from her husband and acted on the rights she believed she had to conceal the information from her children.

Although these privacy rules may become "taken for granted" where marital couples are concerned, there are situations when privacy rules need to be *renegotiated* because they are no longer useful and may create a feeling of turbulence—unease between the couple managing the private information. Particularly in cases where the issues are new or volatile, as we see in this case, and can arise with unexpected genetic information, there is the potential need for change in the privacy rules and the way they are coordinated. Mrs. Andrews' statement about concealing the genetic test result was inconsistent with the way Mr. Andrews defined ownership rights to the information. Mr. Andrews, in this case, considered genetic information to be within the *family privacy boundary*, rather than the marital one, and therefore belonging to all family members. Hence, Mrs. Andrews' claim that the children should not know likely disrupted long-standing marital privacy rules and functioned as a catalyst, or change agent, calling into question the utility of existing privacy rules. As happens in many cases, this kind of crisis is heightened when an explanation for regulating private information concerns the welfare of others. The mother believed that the threat inherent in disclosure justified restricting her children's access to information about the mutation and predictive testing.

Because Mr. and Mrs. Andrews were managing not only marital privacy boundaries but also family privacy boundaries, the issues were complicated. In family privacy boundaries, members expect to know the information because they see it as belonging to all, not just a few family members. Families develop rules for revealing and concealing that are a blend of privacy expectations the marital couple learned from their family of origin and the couple's own negotiations of rules [2, 14, 23, 24]. When marital couples have children, one of their parental jobs is to socialize them to learn how to regulate privacy according to the parent's expectations. In this way, children learn agreed-upon rules that the whole family deems important for managing access.

For the Andrews family, we can determine that there are potential dilemmas between what information belongs to the whole family, what information belongs to an internal privacy cell between the parents, and what information is defined as personally private belonging only to the individual [e.g., 14]. Further, we also know that the parameters for all of these boundary types in families are often defined differently for parents and children [27, 28]. In particular, adult children may assume that where parents hold information salient to them and where the information is directly relevant, as in this first case, they should have the right to know. In fact, it may be that the adult children define the genetic information as more personal than familial-owned information because it involves their well-being. At the very least, the adult children are likely to presume that they are rightful co-owners of the information with the ability to determine who knows, how much they know, and the capacity to control whether they are privy.

Case Study 2: Changes in Privacy Boundaries

Mr. Bryant had a hereditary heart condition that could cause fainting and sudden death. During genetic counseling, Mr. Bryant revealed that he also had a teenage child, Bill, by an earlier relationship; however, he was not a part of this child's life and did not have an amicable relationship with the child's mother, Brenda. Yet he felt a certain responsibility toward Bill regarding disclosure of this genetic finding and said that he attempted to inform the child's mother of the risk. When he contacted the mother and told her about the genetic possibility that Bill, their son, could contract this disease, she grew angry asking if he was trying to ruin their lives, hanging up the phone, and cutting off communication. Mr. Bryant was racked with guilt and felt uncomfortable, but he tried again to make contact. This time, she told him that she had no intention of having her child tested or informed about the information that Mr. Bryant had revealed.

Although Mr. Bryant was clearly taking responsibility for contacting his son's mother to alert her to his condition, one of the complications involved penetrating a family privacy boundary to which this man was no longer privy [14]. Once a former shareholder of information is no longer considered a member of a privacy boundary and privy to the information, all rights tend to be terminated. Only after a significant amount of trust is re-established can there be an attempt to reinstate access rights to private family information. In cases of divorce or estrangement, the circumstances that sever family ties and the relationships that members currently have with each other impact how opened or closed they are with private information belonging to the new family members [14]. When there is an unequivocal termination of any communication between a former family member and current members, seen in the case of Mr. Bryant, it is difficult to break back into a privacy boundary.

As Mr. Bryant experienced, even when circumstances seemed essential that a line of communication be opened and access to private information be restored, the severed membership in the family privacy boundary that Mr. Bryant had with his former wife and child was so damaged that he was not allowed access to Bill even when he had critical health information. In what appears to be a protective move, Brenda declared more ownership rights than her ex-husband or her child regarding regulating access to the child's privacy boundary. This mother likely considered it her prerogative to regulate the kind and amount of access to her child given the relationship she and Bill had with his estranged father. Becoming estranged, by definition, is often defined as cutting off privileges to private information because having those rights signals a level of intimacy that no longer exists. Likely, the thickness of the boundary walls that had been erected by Brenda, grew thicker the longer her ex-husband made no effort to maintain contact.

Yet as we see in this case, regardless of being estranged, the father wished to do the "right thing" by his child. Nevertheless, he paid the price for severing a relationship not only with his ex-wife Brenda but also with his son, Bill. Unfortunately, Bill also paid a hefty price when his mother confiscated his right to decide whether he was able to learn about possible genetic predispositions. By stopping the flow of information into Bill's privacy boundary, his mother denied access to critical health information. Obviously, she felt that making this judgment was within her rightful domain regarding her child. Yet doing so diminished the child's ability to voice his own privacy rules for personal information within his sphere of judgment. While his mother was likely to consider herself a legitimate co-owner of the information, Bill's perspective might be different. If he finds out, he may feel that she had exceeded appropriate levels of control over the private information.

Case Study 3: Being Outside a Privacy Boundary

Mrs. Carroll presented pregnant at 15 weeks. She had only recently found out that there was a family history of an inherited condition causing intellectual disability in boys and potentially intellectual impairment in girls. A cousin had an affected child. Although Mrs. Carroll knew the child had problems, she was only recently told (indirectly) by a family member in a passing conversation that the child in question had an inherited condition. She was angry that she was not told earlier so that she could have had carrier testing and considered the implications before her pregnancy.

In this case, Mrs. Carroll's anger stemmed from being kept outside the privacy boundary that held the information about a possible genetic condition. Mrs. Carroll clearly felt she had the right to know so she could make informed choices. Although Mrs. Carroll believed this information should be revealed (according to her privacy rules), the cousin appeared to have not defined Mrs. Carroll within the internal family privacy boundary. As a consequence, she was not privy to the information.

This case illustrates the difficulty of how family privacy boundaries are defined and the parameters of privilege given to extended members who are considered outside of their immediate family. Mrs. Carroll judged the privacy rules for knowing the child's condition as important to her own welfare, while it seemed evident that the child's close relatives did not have the same expectations regarding granting access to the child's condition. The child's family restricted disclosure of the information to protect the child and the immediate family members from negative reactions by others. On the other hand, Mrs. Carroll was focused on believing that knowing the information likely would have affected her choices. She was clearly functioning from a different set of privacy rules than the child's family.

Conversely, a person who perceives themselves as being outside a privacy boundary may elect not to seek information from those within that boundary. For instance, genetic services commonly ask their clients to obtain more information about other family members, but a client can feel uncomfortable potentially breaching boundaries by approaching relatives about this private information [29].

Case Study 4: Permeability Conflicts—Telling Too Much

Mrs. Duggan was a woman in her mid-fifties. Her father died of cancer and her brother was diagnosed 20 years ago with the same type of cancer. When he had a second cancer, he was referred to a genetic service for genetic testing because it was suspected that there was a hereditary cancer syndrome in the family. This was shown to be the case. Her brother, Greg, was found to have a mutation causing the cancers and several of his currently healthy children were also found to have inherited the mutation and therefore to be at higher risk themselves. Mrs. Duggan, Greg, and their other siblings appeared to be pragmatic about their situation and declared that it was best to know so that their health could be well managed medically. Each individual describes the family as close knit, supportive, and open about sharing genetic information and test results.

As Mrs. Duggan returned to receive her own test results, she commented that Greg's wife, Jo, was waiting to hear Mrs. Duggan's results as well. So far, only Greg, her brother, and his children had received a result that indicated a risk. All of the other siblings had normal results and therefore they and their children were not at increased risk. When Mrs. Duggan learned that she too had the mutation, her first comment was that Jo would be pleased. Mrs. Duggan stated that her sister-in-law tended to "go on" about how difficult it had been for her family, how much they had suffered, and Mrs. Duggan believed that her sister-in-law was resentful of the others' good fortune.

Mrs. Duggan was more distressed by her test results than she expected. Although this particular clinic had a policy of suggesting that a patient take some time to adjust to the results before telling others, it was different in Mrs. Duggan's case. Because of their family orientation toward high disclosure, the extended family was already aware of her appointment and expected her to reveal the results without delay. Unfortunately, Mrs. Duggan did not have the luxury of coming to grips with her risk before having to confront relaying the information to her family members. She anticipated that her sister-in-law would call her soon after the session to find out the results and dreaded the prospect of telling her mother and children.

This case illustrates the complexities of family privacy management that is particularly salient to issues in genetic testing and counseling. The perception of this family regarding privacy is noted when they indicate they are close and openly disclose to each other. As we mentioned earlier, the research using CPM indicates that families develop privacy orientations and regulate the ebb and flow of information according to whether they have a high or low degree of permeability (how much is told), who they link into their family privacy boundary (telling confidants), and how frequently this occurs, as well as the degree of ownership they accord others inside and outside the family [2, 25]. For this family, the statement appears to suggest that the members believe that they readily tell other inside family members, tell them as much as they know, and give them equal ownership rights to make judgments about who might have access to the information outside the family.

While this statement describes the family's assumptions about the way they define themselves, we see that there are several limits to the notion of openness indicated in the discussion with Mrs. Duggan. Through her information we begin to observe that even though the members consider themselves open, they actually have more complex sets of privacy rules, particularly when it comes to the genetic issues discussed in this case. We see some tensions between Mrs. Duggan and her sister-in-law, suggesting that the sister-in-law, Jo, may have disclosed too much information about how difficult she felt it was for her family and how much they had suffered. Mrs. Duggan clearly implies that she felt uncomfortable with receiving Jo's unsolicited disclosures about her family's medical challenges. In CPM terms, Mrs. Duggan's privacy rules are different than Jo's, in that Mrs. Duggan did not want Jo to be so open about her feelings.

COMMON PATTERNS

From a health-care practitioner's perspective, the conflicts over ownership, permeability of the privacy boundary, and granting access to information can seem enormous [30]. Communication privacy management provides a framework for practitioners to determine the lines of demarcation regarding level of ownership, determination of who may know (linking), and the rules for permeability.

As exemplars of family communication, these cases offer some signals about the processes that occur when genetic information is disclosed or concealed. From a CPM perspective, several patterns are predicted. These patterns revolve around privacy management of revealing and concealing; families find themselves in privacy dilemmas that emanate from turbulence surrounding ownership rights, disagreements about permeability, and inconsistencies concerning who can know and who cannot know the genetic information. Isolating these patterns helps us to predict and recognize recurring issues in cases like the ones in this chapter. The analysis of the patterns also provides a basis for the reasons these patterns seem to develop.

By examining these cases through the lens of CPM, we can identify some pathways that allow us to determine a better understanding of the choices clients and their families make. Thus, there are some clear directions for helping clients with privacy management about genetic testing results. These patterns assist health-care practitioners to recognize "warning signals" for privacy management that can be stumbling blocks for family interactions about genetic results. These warning signals alert counselors so they may be able to suggest different paths to alleviate possible negative outcomes where privacy management is a concern. Counseling strategies will be considered in more depth in Chapter 15.

Warning Signal 1: Blocking

With one exception (Case 4), we find that someone in the family *blocks* knowledge of the genetic results from other members. In Case 1, Mrs. Andrews actively prevented her children's access to information about her husband's genetic testing results that had health ramifications for these adult daughters. In Case 2, Mr. Bryant's ex-wife likewise *blocked* his attempts to tell his son about genetic results that might impact the son's life. In Case 3, Mrs. Carroll was not told about a cousin's affected child, and while this case has evidence of blocking the passage of information, it illustrates how a person who defines herself as a rightful recipient feels when access to genetic information is denied. When people indicate that they intend to or have blocked *access* to family members of genetic information, this signals the grounds for a potential problem. The health-care practitioner may be able to redirect clients to alternative strategies by working with them to gain insights into exploring the way they define the parameters of these boundaries (very restricted access versus more open access) and the rules they use to manage access (who is given permission to know, how much others are allow to know, and who has restricted access). The client may not have considered that other family members feel they justifiably deserve the information because they are legitimately a member of the privacy boundary guarding genetic results. These members may believe they should be privy because they have been granted access to similar kinds of information in the past or because they believe the information has direct implications for their own health or that of their children.

Warning Signal 2: Sudden Rule Change

We also find that there is a consistent pattern for all cases presented here regarding changing or redefining privacy rules for boundary access or protection. In Case 1, we see that Mrs. Andrews *redefined privacy rules* for permeability by limiting the sharing of information to the marital couple, whereas her husband believed the whole family should be privy to the genetic information. In Case 2, Mr. Bryant recognized that the *privacy rules for access* to disclose information to his son had *changed* by the nature of his estrangement with the son's mother. Unfortunately, Mr. Bryant's attempt to help his son by telling him about the genetic results illustrated the depth and breadth of the rule changes post divorce. In Case 3, Mrs. Carroll's experience again is somewhat different in that instead of a rule change, Mrs. Carroll learned from her encounter that her *relatives used different privacy rules* than she expected. In Case 4, Mrs. Duggan and her family maintained that they had a consistent set of family privacy rules, that is, they continued to remain open with each other. However, for Mrs. Duggan, there was a point at which she wished she could *change the privacy rules* regulating access and limit when people knew her result and how they learned about the information.

This second pattern of sudden rule change suggests that there are times when a person redefines the privacy rules, changes the rules, or has a very different set of rules than others involved with the genetic information in question. By recognizing that a change has occurred, the health-care practitioner can work with the client to explore the nature of that change and impact of that chance on his or her own expectations and those of other family members. Untangling the misconceptions held about privacy rules, particularly those relating to who may be told or how much may be said, and making explicit the nature of conflicting privacy rules held by each party, helps to determine where the privacy dilemmas are and the basis for these dilemmas. Identifying a root cause for privacy rule conflict that arises is likely to help identify a communicative path to follow for redirecting the flow of information.

Warning Signal 3: Appropriating Control

The third pattern found is a common theme, though presented some-what differently in each case. This pattern reflects the way that certain family members *appropriate ownership* of the information, thereby tak-ing over total *control* and treating the genetic result as though they had more rights than other seemingly rightful co-owners. In Case 1, Mrs. Andrews clearly defines her ownership rights as ones that limit or negate choices her husband wishes to make and restricts her children's knowledge about the tests results, thereby absolutely controlling how the information is managed. She closes off the privacy boundary holding the genetic results and actively works to make choices for her family without their input. Parents often do this with young children and, in many cases, rightfully so. However, with adult children, the rule structure changes dramatically and in most cases, actions that appropriate control are typ-ically deemed inappropriate, at best. Undoubtedly, this type of action has great potential for undermining the nature of the relationship for Mrs. Andrews and negatively impacting the other members [16]. In Case 2, Mr. Bryant's ex-wife took control over the information he shared with her about the possibility of their son's genetic predisposition. She manipulated the situation so that she could hold the information tightly within the privacy boundary. In Case 3, Mrs. Carroll's relatives had initial control of genetic information, deciding that only the immediate family should know. Given the indirect way that Mrs. Carroll leaned about the genetic information after she became pregnant, she felt that her extended family members took away options she wanted to have regarding her decision to become pregnant. Case 4 offers another view of ownership appropriation. Interestingly, because Mrs. Duggan's family ascribed to open boundaries where access to private information among family members was permissible, when Mrs. Duggan needed a level of privacy, the family's open privacy orientation did not allow her that option. Consequently, the privacy orientation and the effectiveness of it for the family essentially worked to appropriate ownership where Mrs. Duggan was concerned , thus limiting the choices she had to manage her own genetic results.

As these cases illustrate, a person sharing information tends to assume that the co-owner will treat the information in the same way as the original owner. Dilemmas arise when a co-owner takes over control in ways that limit other rightful co-owners' ability to manage the genetic information. In many of these cases, appropriating control has meant that the information is locked away (see warning sign 4 in the following section), but it may also mean that information is shared in ways that the original owner had not anticipated or did not intend. In our experience, health-care practitioners are very likely to respond to a person who states that he or she intends to retain complete control through not sharing information by exploring the consequences of this action with the person. However, the practitioner may be less likely to prepare those who intend to inform relatives by using different privacy rules than their relatives may hold. While not wishing to deter someone from sharing with others, some prudence might be exercised. From CPM we know that sharing or not sharing in ways that are inconsistent with the privacy rules people use and expectations they have about access impacts their reactions to receiving or being denied the information. There is benefit in helping people explore their understanding of how the family members in question actually treat privacy information. Do they believe in telling all and as soon as possible? Do they believe people should tell a little at a time? Do they believe that only a sketch of the facts should be told? Helping individuals consider family expectations of disclosure will help in the preparation of telling.

Warning Signal 4: Locking Information Away

As implied in the previous section, a final pattern is the *locking away of information*. We can only speculate about the effect on those who appropriated ownership and dictated the closed privacy boundaries surrounding genetic results. From CPM research, it is likely that they might ultimately find they have taken on a burden for which they did not understand the consequences [7]. Keeping control over highly emotional or charged information, such as genetic results, is often difficult. Research suggests that people have to sustain mindfulness about who is privy and who is not. The management of such restricted boundaries takes considerable energy and the person must remain proactive to protect any access [31]. This kind of management can be particularly difficult with genetic information where there is often an ongoing threat that the information will be "released" through the diagnosis of another family member. The toll may be high ultimately for the person who assumes the strategy of locking the information away and denying any access. Consequently, it is useful for the health-care practitioner to help the client face the reasons why this information seems so volatile and scary to talk about with others. Doing so may help reframe the issues and reduce the thick boundary core around the genetic information so that the person can come to terms with the results and prepare to talk with family members about the genetic ramifications.

CONCLUSION

Communication privacy management provides a predictive, conceptual framework for health-care practitioners to understand the privacy rules families and individuals have for sharing information. These rules are often implicit because they develop gradually over time; therefore, a person may assume that genetic information will be shared by family members according to the same expectations he or she holds. Where there is, in fact, a common and shared understanding, it is likely that genetic information will be communicated within a family with few negative consequences. However, as we have demonstrated here, it cannot be assumed that family members hold the same privacy rules, especially when they are adults who have established new rules that are often different than the family of origin. As a result, privacy rule violations and conflict can occur. Because genetic information carries a complex set of issues and is potentially volatile, sometimes existing privacy rules change because of the immediate needs a person has in coping with the results (see Case 4 as an example). Thus, practitioners are charged with helping people traverse the terrain of privacy rules that necessarily shift and change given the circumstances. Nevertheless, the one consistent issue that practitioners can depend on to help their clients is that even if there have been changes in privacy rules, there will be privacy rules to uncover. Doing so will give a window into the maze of privacy and disclosure management that can help the practitioner assist the individual to better understand choices that can be made and outcomes that can be expected. Thus, CPM can help practitioners chart a map toward a better understanding of privacy and disclosure of genetic information, particularly genetic test results, and of the scope of issues that families face as they deal with the new horizon of genetic issues and new technologies to test predispositions.

REFERENCES

1. Barnoy S, Tabok N. Israeli nurses and genetic information disclosure. *Nursing Ethics* 2007;14:280–294.
2. Petronio S. *Boundaries of Privacy.* Albany: State University of New York Press; 2002
3. Petronio S, Reierson J. Privacy of confidentiality: Grasping the complexities through CPM. In: Afifi TD, Afifi W, eds. *Uncertainty and Information Regulation in Interpersonal Contexts: Theories and Applications.* New York: Routledge; 2009:365–383.
4. Petronio S, Kovach S. Managing privacy boundaries: Health providers' perceptions of resident care in Scottish nursing homes. *Journal of Applied Communication Research* 1997;25:115–130.
5. Forrest LE, Delatycki MB, Skene L, Aitken M. Communicating genetic information in families: A review of guidelines and position papers. *European Journal of Human Genetics* 2007;15:612–618.
6. Rothstein MA, ed. *Genetic Secrets: Protecting Privacy and Confidentiality in the Genetic Era.* New Haven, CT: Yale University Press; 1997.
7. Petronio S, Durham W. Understanding and applying Communication Privacy Management theory. In: Baxter LA, Braithwaite DO, eds. *Engaging Theories in Interpersonal Communication.* Thousand Oaks, CA: Sage; 2008.
8. Greene K, Derlega V, Yep G, Petronio S. *Privacy and Disclosure of HIV/AIDS in Interpersonal Relationships: A Handbook for Researchers and Practitioners.* Mahwah, NJ: Erlbaum; 2003.
9. Offit K, Groeger E, Turner S, Wadsworth EA, Weiser MA. The "duty to warn" a patient's family member about hereditary disease risks. *Journal of the American Medical Association* 2004;292:1469–1473.
10. Orentlicher D. Genetic privacy in the patient-physician relationship. In: Rothstein MA, ed. *Genetic Secrets: Protecting Privacy and Confidentiality in the Genetic Era.* New Haven, CT: Yale University Press; 1997:77–91.
11. Pullman D, Hodgkinson K. Genetic knowledge and moral responsibility: Ambiguity at the interface of genetic research and clinical practice. *Clinical Genetics* 2006;69:199–203.
12. Hallowell N, Ardern-Jones A, Eeles R, Foster C, Lucassern A, Moynihan C, Watson M. Communication about genetic testing in families of male BRCA 1/2 carriers and non-carriers: Patterns, priorities, and problems. *Clinical Genetics* 2005;67:492–502.
13. Johnson S, Kass NE, Natowicz M. Disclosure of personal medical information: Differences among parents and affected adults for genetic and nongenetic conditions. *Genetic Testing* 2005;9:269–280.
14. Afifi TD. "Feeling caught" in stepfamilies: Managing boundary turbulence through appropriate communication privacy rules. *Journal of Social and Personal Relationships* 2003;20:729–755.
15. Afifi TD, Olson L. The chilling effect in families and the pressure to conceal secrets. *Communication Monographs* 2005;72:192–216.
16. Caughlin J, Petronio S. Privacy in families. In: Vangelisti A, ed. *Handbook of Family Communication.* Mahwah, NJ: Erlbaum; 2004:35–49.
17. Caughlin JP, Afifi TD. When is topic avoidance unsatisfying? Examining moderators of the association avoidance and dissatisfaction. *Human Communication Research* 2004;30:479–513.

18. Cochran PL, Tatikonda MV, Magid JM. Radio frequency identification and the ethics of privacy. *Organizational Dynamics* 2007;36:217–229.
19. Helft PR, Petronio S. Communication pitfalls with cancer patients: "Hit-and-run" deliveries of bad news. *Journal of the American College of Surgeons* 2007;205:807–811.
20. Petronio S, Jones SM. When 'friendly advice' becomes a privacy dilemma for pregnant couples: Applying CPM theory. In: West R, Turner L, eds. *Family Communication Sourcebook*. Thousand Oaks, CA: Sage; 2006:201–218.
21. Petronio S, Jones SM, Morr MC. Family privacy dilemmas: Managing communication boundaries within family groups. In: Frey L, ed. *Group Communication in Context: Studies of Bona Fide Groups*. Mahwah, NJ: Erlbaum; 2003:23–56.
22. Petronio S, Caughlin JP. Communication Privacy Management theory: Understanding families. In: Braithwaite DO, Baxter LA, eds. *Engaging Theories in Family Communication: Multiple Perspectives*. Thousand Oaks, CA: Sage; 2005:35–49.
23. Petronio S. Communication boundary perspective: A theoretical model of managing the disclosure of private information between marital couples. *Communication Theory* 1991;1:311–332.
24. Serewicz MCM, Dickson FC, Morrison JHTA, Poole LL. Family privacy orientation, relational maintenance, and family satisfaction in young adults' family relationships. *Journal of Family Communication* 2007;7:123–142.
25. Serewicz MCM, Canary DJ. Assessments of disclosure from the in-laws: Links among disclosure topics, family privacy orientations, and relational quality. *Journal of Social and Personal Relationships* 2008;25:333–357.
26. Petronio, S. Communication privacy management theory. What do we know about family privacy regulation? *Journal of Family Theory and Review* in press.
27. Hawk ST, Keijsers L, Hale WW, Meeus W. Mind your own business! Longitudinal relations between perceived privacy invasion and adolescent-parent conflict. *Journal of Family Psychology* 2009;23:511–520.
28. Petronio S. Privacy binds in family interactions: The case of parental privacy invasions. In: Cupach WR, Spitzberg B, eds. *The Dark Side of Interpersonal Communication*. Hillsdale, NJ: Lawrence Erlbaum Associates; 1994:241–258.
29. Adelsward V, Sachs L. The messenger's dilemmas—Giving and getting information in geneaological mapping for hereditary cancer. *Health Risk and Society* 2003;5: 125–138.
30. Biesecker LG. Strike three for GLI2. *Nature Genetics* 1997;17:259–260.
31. Lane JD, Wegner DM. The cognitive consequences of secrecy. *Journal of Personality and Social Psychology* 1995;69:269–280.

8

MANAGEMENT OF UNCERTAINTY

Heather Skirton & Carma L. Bylund

*The inherent uncertainties of life are often increased significantly in
light of a genetic diagnosis or genetic risk information. Uncertainty
management theory highlights types of uncertainty and different
ways in which individuals and families may choose to respond to
these. Strategies that health-care practitioners can use to help manage
uncertainty within families are discussed.*

Living with uncertainty is inherent to the human condition. At every
life stage, uncertainties about the past, present, and future are part
of the context of daily living. Members of a family known to be affected
by, or at risk of, a genetic condition face numerous uncertainties about
their own futures and the future of relatives, even those as yet unborn.
Consequently, uncertainty is central to conversations about genetic
information—whether these occur between family members or between
health-care practitioners and patients. Furthermore, family communication can be challenging in this environment of uncertainty.

In this chapter we provide an overview of the principles of uncertainty
management theory [1] within a context of communication about genetic
information. In contrast to many of the other theoretical perspectives presented in this book, uncertainty management theory has arisen from work
in interpersonal communication, rather than studies of families or family communication. Thus, its applicability to family communication has
not yet been fully explored. However, uncertainty management theory has
been shown to be relevant to communication about health conditions such

as HIV [2] and we believe that, given the uncertainty intrinsic to many genetic conditions and the difficulty in conveying uncertain information [3], further exploration of this theory in the context of genetic conditions is warranted.

We begin with an explanation of uncertainty and then move to a description of types of uncertainty. We then describe various appraisals of and emotional responses to uncertainty and how those affect multiple ways in which people manage uncertainty. We further describe how seeking or avoiding information relates to the management of uncertainty. We proceed to describe how clients' individual needs and approach can influence their decisions, and we conclude with some specific suggestions for health-care practitioners.

In the past, communication theorists viewed uncertainty as unidimensional, as something that needs to be reduced or eliminated in order to feel a sense of control [4]. However, current research paints a more complicated picture of uncertainty. Contemporary scholars emphasize three important points [2, 4, 5]. First, in attempting to reduce or eliminate uncertainty, more uncertainty may be created. For instance, in wanting to find out whether one may develop a condition in the future, a person may seek information through genetic testing, attempting to eliminate uncertainty about the presence of the predisposing mutation. However, finding out that one carries this mutation may actually lead to further uncertainty about whether the disease will actually manifest. Second, at times persons may want to maintain or even increase uncertainty. For example, a man with a history of the fatal neurodegenerative condition Huntington disease (HD) may prefer to maintain his uncertainty about whether he has the disease-causing gene expansion. He may feel that *not* knowing is better than knowing. Third, uncertainty cannot always be reduced. For example, there are still a number of genetic conditions for which gene testing is not definitive. In a family in which there is an extremely strong history of breast cancer but no *BRCA1/2* mutation is detected in affected women, an at-risk woman will be unable to further define her chance of developing breast cancer through genetic testing. In studying uncertainty, contemporary scholars use the term "managing uncertainty" to describe the process that people undertake in dealing with uncertainty. Communication plays a key role in managing uncertainty, as "uncertainty is created, sustained and transformed by both spontaneous and strategic interaction" [4] (p. 1813). Conversely, uncertainty may also play a role in the willingness to communicate with relatives, with mutation-positive results being communicated more often than uninformative and mutation-negative results. Definitive genetic testing results, such as the presence of a cancer-predisposing mutation, appear to be communicated more frequently than uninformative results that leave open the question of causation [6–8]. Brashers [1] delineates a theory of communication and uncertainty management that explains that how people manage uncertainty is determined by their appraisals of an experience and emotional response to the experience. We illustrate the tenets of this theory throughout the chapter.

TYPES OF UNCERTAINTY

There are a number of types of uncertainty that persons may experience [9, 10]. For those at risk of a genetic condition, these include uncertainty about illness complexity, uncertainty about the genetic information, uncertainty about the timescale, uncertainty about the likelihood of a particular outcome, and uncertainty that comes from a 'nondiagnosis'. We discuss each of these in the sections that follow.

Uncertainty about Illness Complexity

Uncertainty arising from the complexity of the illness is common with genetic conditions. Genetic conditions can be variable in expression: the same gene mutation can result in many different signs and symptoms of the disease in different individuals. Thus, it is difficult to predict how a condition may manifest. For example, the signs and symptoms of neurofibromatosis type 1 can vary from café-au-lait patches on the skin to sarcoma, even within the same family. A mildly affected parent may have a more severely affected child. A further complexity of genetic conditions that leads to uncertainty is variable penetrance. That is, *not* all those who have inherited the gene mutation will go on to develop the condition; it is not usually possible to distinguish between those mutation carriers who will develop it from those who will not. The inherited cardiac condition long QT syndrome is one such condition, in which a person with the inherited gene mutation may or may not develop the ECG abnormality or arrhythmia associated with this condition.

Uncertainty about the Genetic Information

Individuals may be uncertain about how reliable or valid the genetic information is or how sufficient it is for their particular purpose. In a genetic counseling service, it is not uncommon for people given bad news after genetic testing to question whether there could have been an error that resulted in inaccurate results.

Timescale

Uncertainty can also differ in terms of how long or short lived it is [5]. For example, in the short term, an individual may experience uncertainty while waiting a few weeks for a test result. Or an individual may wonder about how a relative will react to news of the diagnosis, as he prepares to pass this information on. In contrast, chronic uncertainty exists when a person who may have inherited a predisposition to an adult-onset condition learns of her risk years before the expected age of onset. Long-term uncertainty may also exist for an at-risk individual thinking about pregnancy, and not knowing if future children will inherit the condition.

The Likelihood of a Particular Outcome

Uncertainty is also present in the consideration of the outcome of a genetic test. An individual who thinks it is highly likely that he will be found to have the mutation causing a familial condition may experience uncertainty differently from a person who thinks this event is highly *un*likely. Others who have not considered their likelihood may experience it differently again. Each of these states is likely to influence how the person communicates with those around him.

Uncertainty That Comes from the Nondiagnosis

Cases of nondiagnosis also present uncertainty [11]. Despite the advances in genetic science, there are still situations in which a definitive diagnosis is not made. This may be due to the fact that the condition is so rare that few cases are seen, or there is no accurate test for the condition. It has been shown that parents who have a child with unexplained learning disabilities are strongly motivated to find a diagnosis through the genetic service [12]. However, in some cases it is not possible to make such a diagnosis, leaving them with uncertainty about the cause of their child's condition, the prognosis for the future, and risks of recurrence in future pregnancies.

LAY KNOWLEDGE, APPRAISALS AND EMOTIONAL RESPONSES

A key tenet of uncertainty management theory is that people judge the meaning of an event (in this case genetic risk) based on their appraisal of the event—or how they believe it will affect them. Their management of uncertainty arises, in part, from these appraisals. These appraisals, in turn, often result from a person's lay knowledge about genetics. For example, a person who enters a genetic counseling situation with a relatively sophisticated lay knowledge through reading and contact with a lay support group may be better able to manage uncertainty that arises from illness complexity. Similarly, a client with very little lay knowledge about genetic information may feel unable to make a judgment about the reliability or validity of the genetic information, increasing uncertainty. A client's lay knowledge may also directly affect her judgment about the likelihood of a particular outcome. The next section explains in more detail how lay knowledge influences the appraisals and emotional responses to uncertainty.

Lay Knowledge

Hallowell and Richards [13] have emphasized the importance of prior knowledge, beliefs, and values brought into the process by both the genetics practitioner and the client. According to the theory of lay epistemics [14], which concerns the way in which information is acquired, the client's interpretation of the information provided—and consequently the degree of the client's uncertainty about those results—will be based to some extent on the store of previously learned material in his or her mind, which may vary enormously in its relevance to genetics and genetic counseling. Therefore, a person's mind is not a blank canvas on which scientific information can be imposed, but that person will bring preconceptions about the genetic condition and his or her own susceptibility to it. For example, an individual may utilize her past experience of medical encounters to inform the way in which the genetic counseling session will run and become confused if not given direct advice about how to proceed. Lay knowledge may be conceived of as the basis of information the client brings to the genetic counseling encounter.

In order to think about any issue, the mind constructs a tangible representation of the relevant object or situation. Lau and Hartmann [15] devised a model describing the five disease domains that contribute to the construct of a condition created by the client: disease identity (i.e. symptoms, signs, name), timeline (i.e., duration), consequences, causes, and controllability. These attributes may be based upon acquired information, the client's experience of the condition personally or in affected family members, and/or inferences made by reference to other conditions deemed to be similar. When faced with a threat to health, the illness representation is used to help assess the threat and devise strategies to deal with it [16]. The representation of the condition is of special significance when it is to be used as a basis for important life decisions (such as reproductive plans) or influencing behavior (such as attending a cancer screening program). However, Leventhal et al. [16] have also identified a difficulty in persuading clients to attend for screening when it is the threat of disease occurring rather than the presence of signs and symptoms that is the only motivating factor. This is particularly relevant to genetics service provision, where risk of disease to the client or the client's offspring is frequently the focus of discussion. It may explain why in some families, people do not present for predictive genetic testing until a close relative or someone in their own generation is diagnosed with the condition. The threat may appear too nebulous, and the uncertainty created is not sufficient to warrant action. An extension of this argument is that people may not be motivated to communicate to relatives until their perception of the certainty of their own or relatives' risk is greater.

Many factors may influence a person's lay knowledge of a condition, including the following:

- *A basic understanding of genetics.* Marteau and Senior [17] draw attention to the fact that even dominantly inherited conditions such as the hereditary colorectal cancer condition familial adenomatous polyposis (FAP) may be considered multifactorial diseases by an affected family.
- *The social and support structure of families.* In a study of knowledge of genetic inheritance, Richards and Ponder found that the lay concepts of heredity strongly linked with the concepts of social dependence [18]. The amount of genetic material shared with aunts and uncles, for instance, was underestimated, while the amount shared by parents and children was generally correctly estimated.
- *Physical similarity.* Genetics practitioners are very familiar with the belief that the genetic condition in the family is linked to a physical characteristic [18]. In a study of families referred for genetic services [19], there was evidence that families brought their own lay knowledge about both the cause of the condition or the inheritance pattern to the session. Where the "scientific" explanation of a genetic condition conflicted somewhat with the family experience of the condition, families reverted to their own explanations in the longer term. Even where they could explain the scientific mechanism, this was not always integrated into their understanding of their own situation. For example, a woman whose son had a chromosomal abnormality was able to describe the chromosomes, but she had more uncertainty about the cause of her son's condition, wondering if she had caused it by her health behaviors (e.g., not drinking enough milk) late in the pregnancy. She was obviously still seeking certainty about the cause of her son's condition, and this need had not been satisfied by the explanation about chromosomes provided by the genetic counselor.

Appraisals of and Emotional Responses to Uncertainty

Appraisals are made initially based on lay knowledge, and then later upon information acquired through interactions with health-care providers. Lazarus [20] describes three types of appraisals persons make: *relevancy, congruency, and coping skills.* These types of appraisals can impact family communication about genetics. To illustrate this, we offer examples regarding alpha 1-antitrypsin deficiency (AATD). People with the severe form of this condition are likely to develop emphysema, with a younger age of onset in smokers. Additionally, babies with the condition have a 10%–20% chance of developing liver disease.

Relevancy appraisals have to do with how pertinent uncertain information is to an individual. For example, Margaret, a woman in her forties, found out that her sister, a long-time smoker, has tested positive for the deficiency. After searching for information on the condition on the Internet, Margaret makes an appraisal that this genetic information is irrelevant to her because she does not smoke, and thus she does not become engaged in family discussions about the condition, nor does she seek a specialist's opinion.

However, if a person makes an appraisal that the information is relevant, she will then make an appraisal of whether the uncertainty (e.g., whether she might also have the condition) is *congruent* with her goals. If, in the above example, Margaret were a smoker, and appraised the information as relevant, she then would consider whether the information was congruent with her goals. For instance, if Margaret already had wanted to quit smoking, she may see this information about her sister's status as another reason to quit smoking. If Margaret did not desire to quit smoking, the genetic information would be incongruent with her goals.

When information is appraised to be relevant and incongruent, the final appraisal made has to do with *coping skills*. Using our example, if Margaret, a smoker who did not want to quit, found out about her sister's test results, she will then consider how she might cope with the uncertainty of not knowing her own status, perhaps choosing to avoid family functions or not take her sister's calls.

Clearly, these appraisals are associated with emotional responses. In the above example, Margaret as a smoker would likely have a negative emotional response (e.g., fear or anxiety) that would affect her communication with her family about this issue. It is also possible that uncertainty regarding genetic information might produce positive emotional responses, such as providing hope that a late-onset condition may not manifest. However, it is likely that the complicated situations of genetic diagnosis may produce a mix of emotional responses, as in the following case.

Case Study 1: Mixed Emotional Responses to Uncertainty

When Lynn and Tom had their first child, Alex, he seemed to be a healthy baby. At about 6 weeks old, he was discovered to have two inguinal hernias as well as an umbilical hernia, and a surgery was scheduled. However, the surgeon felt Alex was too jaundiced and was concerned that if there was a liver problem, it may need to be corrected by surgery as well. Lynn and Tom subsequently met with a pediatric specialist who reviewed Alex's blood test results and explained to them what the possible diagnoses were. This uncertainty about the diagnosis produced a negative emotional response as Lynn and Tom considered all the consequences of the potential diagnoses. Following further tests, Lynn and Tom were told that Alex had AATD. The specialist explained that some children with this condition did better than others, and that it was unknown how the deficiency would manifest in Alex. This uncertainty, the uncertainty of prognosis, actually produced a positive emotional response in Lynn and Tom as they came to realize that it was possible that their child might do quite well.

MANAGING UNCERTAINTY

Uncertainty management theory holds that depending on their appraisals and emotional responses, persons have several choices in how to manage their uncertainty: reduce, maintain, increase, or adapt. While the discussion that follows focuses on the person receiving genetic information from a health-care practitioner, the same phenomena may conceivably occur when an individual is conveying genetic information to a family member or is the recipient.

Reducing Uncertainty

Often when people experience uncertainty that causes distress, they will try to reduce it. Webster and Kruglanski [21] developed the Need for Cognitive Closure Model in an attempt to explain the differences in individual differences to obtain information and reduce uncertainty. The need for closure motivates the individual to search for a definite answer in any situation, and this contrasts with a tolerance of ambiguity or uncertainty. The need-for-closure continuum ranges from strong motivation to total reluctance to obtain a certain answer in a given situation. The need may vary with the situation and uncertainty may be preferable where the repercussions of making a wrong decision are very serious [22]. For example, a person at risk of HD who believes that life will not be worth living if he discovers he will develop the condition may avoid genetic testing or participating in family conversations about testing. A strong need for closure may also influence the individual to stop seeking or receiving more information, if this would jeopardize his current lay beliefs, and it may also lead the person to accept less reliable information if it concurs with what he would prefer to believe. In a genetic counseling service, it is common to have clients arrive with material gleaned from the Internet. While some sources are reliable, others are more suspect. It can be frustrating for a genetics practitioner to be challenged by material from dubious sources; however, the client may prefer to believe this material if it enables him or her to retain a sense of certainty about the situation. The following case illustrates this phenomenon.

Case Study 2: Internet Information

Mary phoned the genetics office late one Friday afternoon. She was 19 weeks pregnant and had been told by her obstetrician that her fetus had been diagnosed with a chromosome anomaly, 47, XYY. The genetic counselor gave her information about the condition by telephone. Mary stressed that she wanted to continue with the pregnancy, but she was feeling unhappy about not knowing exactly how the baby would be affected. The counselor arranged to see her with her husband and a pediatrician on Monday morning. On Monday morning, Mary arrived with reams of information downloaded from the Internet. Much of this was either incorrect or exaggerated the negative aspects of the impact of 47, XYY chromosome structure on the child.

(continued)

Case Study 2: (*continued*)

However, Mary was adamant that she would have a termination of pregnancy based on the information she had downloaded. The counselor wondered whether Mary was using the information to justify her decision and so reduce the discomfort she was feeling due to uncertainty about the baby's future.

In a longitudinal study of families referred for genetic services, Skirton [23] tested the need for closure using Webster and Kruglanski's scale [21]. The overall need-for-closure scores were higher in the individuals in that study than in those reported in many other previous studies. This may indicate that those who seek genetic counseling are a self-selected group with a high need for closure. Data collected through individual semi-structured interviews with the families strongly showed that for those who presented for genetic testing, any result, even a "bad" result, was preferable to continuing to live with ongoing uncertainty [24]. However, families reported that one uncertainty was often replaced by another. For example, as mentioned in the introduction to this chapter, the client might be aware that he or she will develop the condition but not know when or how it will manifest. The need to seek certainty was emphasized by the strategies used by families in that study, which included creating some certainty in an uncertain situation, exemplified by families who had a child with an undiagnosed syndrome taking comfort from being told that the condition definitely had a genetic cause. Even being certain that there was no way with the current level of knowledge to find the answer was of help, with clients reporting that pursuing the information to the extent of their ability had given them some "peace of mind."

Maintaining Uncertainty

As discussed previously, in some cases people experience uncertainty as a positive and comfortable state. Rather than wanting to reduce uncertainty, they would rather maintain uncertainty. The following case illustrates this phenomenon.

Case Study 3: Maintaining Uncertainty

Ellen was a recovering alcoholic in her mid-thirties. A mutation causing cardiac arrhythmia—long QT syndrome—has been identified in her family and she is eligible for predictive genetic testing. She has had several electrocardiograms in the past, which have always been normal, but she knows this does not exclude the possibility that she has the mutation. During discussions with the genetics practitioner, Ellen is clearly reluctant to undertake genetic testing. She feels that she is currently coping with her risk and that if she were to learn she has the family mutation, and therefore confirm her increased risk of sudden death, she may struggle and return to drinking to manage her anxieties.

Increasing Uncertainty

In some cases, where genetic information has a strong degree of certainty, individuals may actually try to increase their uncertainty. This will happen in cases where the certain information is appraised negatively. For example, in a family in which one of two sisters has found that she has the mutation for HD—which confers an absolute risk of developing the condition—the unaffected sister may focus her communication with her affected sister on trying to increase uncertainty about the likelihood of the disease manifesting. This may be done through constantly telling her sister about new research being done and successful research fundraising efforts in an effort to increase uncertainty about the current inability to treat the disease.

Adapting to Chronic Uncertainty

In addition to trying to reduce, maintain, or increase uncertainty, it is often necessary for individuals and families to adapt to chronic uncertainty. This is particularly so in situations where family members face the possibility of adult-onset conditions (such as HD) or conditions with variable expression or penetrance. For example, a woman may know she has inherited the mutation for *BRCA1* but live with the uncertainty of whether she will actually develop a breast or ovarian cancer in the future. Individuals affected by neurofibromatosis may be aware of their condition from childhood but will be unsure as to whether they may develop tumors due to the disease. Adaptation can occur over time as persons learn to value or tolerate uncertainty, coming to realize that uncertainty is "just part of life" [5]. Adaptation may also come through changing tasks and developing structure or routine [5], for example, through participation in annual surveillance for bowel or breast cancer. Others adapt by "living life to the full" in case they develop the condition later. Fiona, a young woman at risk of HD, made sure she had one major travel adventure every year so that she would have no regrets if diagnosed later. Planning and undertaking these trips gave her life a structure that enabled her to live with the uncertainty about her future health in a positive way.

SEEKING OR AVOIDING INFORMATION

It is also important to consider how people actively seek or avoid information in order to manage uncertainty. Some clients and their families may seek a great deal of information on their genetic condition from health-care practitioners, each other, and the Internet. However, others choose to avoid information because it allows them to maintain their current state of knowledge; they prefer not knowing than to possibly hearing unwanted news [5]. For example, when a mother has been told that there is a chance that her child might have cystic fibrosis (CF), a fatal condition that affects the lungs, she may purposely avoid information until the status of the child is known [25] in an attempt to reduce uncertainty. Another mother in a similar situation may spend hours on the Internet learning everything she can in order to reduce uncertainty. Although information seeking may work, such information may also increase uncertainty, especially when the child's status is not yet known, or unexpected or unwelcome information is accessed. Alternatively, information seeking may resolve one type of uncertainty but lead to another [5]. For example, resolving an infant's CF status raises new concerns— for example, that he or she is a carrier, meaning one or both parents is a carrier, resulting in genetic testing for parents and siblings and family planning issues [25].

For many clients attending a genetics service, part of the session will focus on providing an approximation of genetic risk for themselves, relatives, or future offspring. However, some authors [13] question the integral value of risk estimations for the client, proposing that clients have more important expectations of the genetic consultation that need to be ascertained and addressed. One explanation for this is that the client may not welcome the focus on the uncertainties of his or her situation. In this situation, where the health-care practitioner feels an obligation to present an accurate appraisal of the risk, there may be a conflict between the agendas of the practitioner and the client.

It is clear that individuals take differing views on obtaining information to manage uncertainty. In clinical practice, it is common to find that some members of the family wish to have genetic testing for a condition, while relatives who are at equal risk decline such tests. As shown in the following case example, these divergent approaches can disrupt family relationships, particularly if the refusal to be tested by one family member has an impact on the testing choices of another.

Case Study 4: Information Avoiding and Family Dynamics

Nadia was one of three children born to a woman with a strong family history of breast/ovarian cancer. Nadia's mother and maternal aunt had both died of breast cancer, while her maternal grandmother had ovarian cancer at a young age. At the age of 47, Nadia also developed breast cancer. She knew of the high likelihood that she had inherited a mutation that had predisposed her to breast cancer, but she did not wish to have this confirmed. She felt that confirmation would make her more anxious about the risk of developing cancer again in the future. However, she had preventative (prophylactic) surgery to remove her ovaries. Nadia's sister Karin had three daughters. Karin was keen to have a mutation test, but she was told the result would not be as definite without information about the mutation carried by Nadia. Karin was extremely angry that Nadia was not willing to have the test for the sake of her family.

In families with a long history of a condition, certain family members may be identified as being the most likely to develop or not develop the condition. This has been termed "preselection" and is important in the context of living with uncertainty. It appears that families reduce uncertainty about the impact of the condition by allocating the role of affected or not affected according to their lay beliefs about the inheritance in the family. However, while this may be a mechanism to help the family to cope, it can be disrupted if the hypotheses prove to be incorrect.

Case Study 5: Preselection

Janine was a 30-year-old woman at 50% risk of developing HD. She was the eldest of three daughters in her family. Her mother, who was affected, was also the eldest child, as was her affected grandmother. For many years it had been assumed that Janine would develop HD and her sisters would escape it. Convinced she was just confirming what she already knew, Janine had a genetic test. The results indicated she did not have the mutation and would not develop HD. Janine herself found this difficult to accept. However, her family's reaction shocked and hurt her. Her sisters and father had to alter their beliefs, and the fact that Janine was not affected meant her sisters were confronted with their own risk. Janine felt they were angry with her for changing their perceived status, and it took several years for the family relationships to be restored.

HELPING CLIENTS AND FAMILIES MANAGE UNCERTAINTY

Many individuals and families seeking genetic health care will be living with uncertainty and may be seeking to use the encounter with the genetics practitioner to reduce that uncertainty. In addition, struggles with family communication that clients experience may be in part explained by different approaches to uncertainty and individual differences in the need for cognitive closure.

Health-care practitioners can support clients and families in managing uncertainty in the following ways:

1. *Acknowledge and work to understand the uncertainties of the situation with the client and family.* In working with clients and their families, different kinds of uncertainty may require different responses [4]. Health-care practitioners "must be ready to probe for clarification of the form(s) of uncertainty that their patients are experiencing" (p. 1813). For example, suppose a person were to make a statement to a practitioner such as "I just don't know what to make of all of this." The practitioner may want to reply by probing to better understand the

uncertainty with a clarifying question, such as "Can you say more about the part you are struggling with?"

2. *Explore the impact of living with uncertainty on the client and family.* As has been shown, it cannot be assumed that people prefer either certainty or uncertainty in a given situation. Managing uncertainty may require reorienting or changing one's perspective toward uncertainty or certainty [2]. In cases where there may be conflict among the family, talking with the client about how family members may be managing uncertainty may be helpful.

3. *Describe and discuss the options open to the client and how these might alter their knowledge of their status.* Remember that for some, the description and discussion of options may help them manage their discomfort by presenting them with concrete choices. Others may find multiple options overwhelming and that they increase uncertainty about the most appropriate course of action. Although giving information is obviously necessary, being attuned to individual differences about information and uncertainty can help the counselor to be more client-centered.

4. *Facilitate clients to access those tests that may reduce uncertainty, where this is desired.* This involves accessing the most current information about genetic testing for the condition concerned. It is not possible, given the range of genetic conditions and the rapid changes in testing, to be knowledgeable about every condition. However, current, freely available electronic resources can ensure that the practitioner can provide relevant information to ensure choice.

5. *Help clients to make a decision that takes into account that discomfort may not be relieved by the test results.* As has been described, there may be situations where a definitive result is not obtained through genetic testing. The information provided by the health-care practitioner must include any limitations of testing and the possibility that the results may not resolve the current uncertainty. Pre-test awareness of continuing uncertainty reduces unwarranted expectations. Moving beyond information provision, the practitioner can explore with the client what the experience of life after each possible outcome may feel like and raise awareness of unconscious or unreasonable assumptions the client may hold about the outcome of testing

6. *Help individuals and families adapt to chronic uncertainty.* In many cases, although some uncertainty may be reduced by testing, other uncertainty will remain. For example, a person who tests positive for the gene mutation for Lynch syndrome but may never get the disease will be dealing with chronic uncertainty for many years. Adapting to chronic uncertainty

may include *(a)* accepting uncertainty; *(b)* redefining tasks; and *(c)* developing structure and routine, building a "cocoon of certainty" to protect themselves [26] (p. 128). Where clinical surveillance (such as regular colonoscopy in the case of Lynch syndrome) for the condition is available, this can be a source of relief to clients, providing a measure of certainty for a period of time after the investigation. Even clients who are at risk for a neurological condition such as HD may find that their uncertainty is more manageable if they have an annual neurological examination.

CONCLUSION

People seeking genetic health care may be motivated by their desire to reduce uncertainty about their genetic or health status, and they bring their own knowledge and ideas about the genetic condition to the consultation. The role of the health-care practitioner involves providing families with information that enables them to integrate explanations into their own store of lay knowledge and to make appropriate choices regarding testing. The health-care practitioner also has a role in supporting clients as they adapt to living with either certainty, uncertainty, or the most likely scenario, living with both. While the impact of managing uncertainty on the communication of genetic information in families is not yet known, we suggest that people who are able to manage their uncertainty are likely to be more at ease communicating with their relatives. Uncertainty management theory may also provide insights that assist practitioners as they prepare their clients for the potential responses and needs of family members to whom they plan to convey genetic information.

REFERENCES

1. Brashers DE. A theory of communication and uncertainty management. In: Whaley B, Samter W, eds. *Explaining Communication Theory.* Mahwah, NJ: Erlbaum; 2007:201–218.
2. Brashers DE, Neidig JL, Hass SM, Dobbs LK, Cardillo LW, Russell JA. Communication in the management of uncertainty: The case of persons living with HIV or AIS. *Communication Monographs* 2000;67(1):63–84.
3. Gaff CL, Clarke AJ, Atkinson P, Sivell S, Elwyn G, Iredale R, et al. Process and outcome in communication of genetic information with families: A systematic review. *European Journal of Human Genetics* 2007;15:999–1011.
4. Babrow AS, Kline KN. From "reducing" to "coping with" uncertainty: Reconceptualizing the central challenge in breast self-exams. *Social Science and Medicine* 2000;51:1805–1816.
5. Brashers DE. Communication and uncertainty management. *Journal of Communication* 2001;51:477–497.
6. Claes E, Evers-Kiebooms G, Boogaerts A, Decruyenaere M, Denayer L, Legius E. Communication with close and distant relatives in the context of

genetic testing for hereditary breast and ovarian cancer in cancer patients. *American Journal of Medical Genetics* 2003;116A:11–19.

7. Costalas JW, Itzen M, Malick J, Babb JS, Bove B, Godwin AK, et al. Communication of BRCA1 and BRCA2 results to at-risk relatives: A cancer risk assessment program's experience. *American Journal of Medical Genetics* 2003;119C(1):11–18.

8. Hughes C, Lerman C, Schwartz M, Peshkin B, Wenzel L, Narod S, et al. All in the family: Evaluation of the process and content of sisters' communication about BRCA 1 and BRCA 2 genetic test results. *American Journal of Medical Genetics* 2002;107:143–150.

9. Babrow AS, Kasch CR, Ford LA. The many meanings of uncertainty in illness: Toward a systematic accounting. *Health Communication* 1998;10(1):1–23.

10. Brashers DE, Neidig JL, Russell JA, Cardillo LW, Hass SM, Dobbs LK, et al. The medical, personal, and social causes of uncertainty in HIV illness. *Issues in Mental Health Nursing* 2003;24:497–522.

11. Brookes-Howell LC. Living without labels: The interactional management of diagnostic uncertainty in the genetic counseling clinic. *Social Science and Medicine* 2006;63:3080–3091.

12. Skirton H. Parental experience of a pediatric genetic referral. *MCN American Journal of Maternal and Child Nursing* 2006;31(3):178–184.

13. Hallowell N, Richards MPM. Understanding life's lottery: An evaluation of studies of genetic risk awareness. *Journal of Health Psychology* 1997;2:31–43.

14. Kruglanski AW. *Lay Epistemics and Human Knowledge.* New York: Plenum Press; 1989.

15. Lau RR, Hartman KA. Common sense representations of common illnesses. *Health Psychology* 1983;2:167–185.

16. Leventhal H, Benyamini Y, Brownlee S, Diefenbach M, Leventhal EA, Patrick-Miller L, et al. Illness representations: Theoretical foundations. In: Petrie KJ, Wienman JA, eds. *Perceptions of Health and Illness.* Amsterdam: Harwood Academic Publishers; 1997:19–46.

17. Marteau TM, Senior V. Illness representations after the human genome project: The perceived role of genes in causing illness. In: Petrie KJ, Weinman JA, eds. *Perceptions of Health and Illness.* Amsterdam: Harwood Academic Publishers; 1997:241–266.

18. Richards M, Ponder M. Lay understanding of genetics; a test of a hypothesis. *Journal of Medical Genetics* 1996;33:1032–1036.

19. Skirton H, Eiser C. Discovering and addressing the client's lay knowledge—An integral aspect of genetic health care. *Research and Theory for Nursing Practice: An International Journal* 2003;17(4):339–352.

20. Lazarus RS. Relational meaning and discrete emotions. In: Scherer KR, Schorr A, Johnstone T, eds. *Appraisal Processes in Emotion: Theory, Methods, and Research.* New York: Oxford University Press; 2001:37–67.

21. Webster DM, Kruglanski AW. Individual differences in need for cognitive closure. *Journal of Personality and Social Psychology* 1994;67:1049–1062.

22. Kruglanski AW, Freund T. The freezing and unfreezing of lay-inferences: Effects on impressional primacy, ethnic stereotyping, and numerical anchoring. *Journal of Experimental Social Psychology* 1983;19:448–468.

23. Skirton H. Assessing the need for certainty in users of a clinical genetic health service. *Journal of Advanced Nursing* 2006;55(2):151–158.
24. Skirton H. The client's perspective of genetic counseling—A grounded theory study. *Journal of Genetic Counseling* 2001;10(4):311–329.
25. Dillard JP, Carson CL. Uncertainty management following a positive newborn screening for cystic fibrosis. *Journal of Health Communication* 2005;10:57–76.
26. Merry U. *Coping with Uncertainty: Insights from the New Sciences of Chaos, Self-organization, and Complexity.* Westport, CT: Praeger; 1995.

9

ATTRIBUTIONS AND PERSONAL THEORIES

MARION F. McALLISTER & CHRISTINA M. SABEE

When unexpected or unusual things happen, such as the diagnosis of a genetic condition, people develop attributions and personal theories about their causes. These may influence communication both within the family and outside it. Understanding the relationship between attributions, behavior and emotions can assist the health-care practitioner to facilitate adjustment and consequently enhance communication.

It is natural for people to seek explanations for how and why things happen to them, especially when those things are distressing. People from families affected by genetic diseases or conditions are likely to have faced both unexpected and distressing events—events that were just not part of "the plan." These people are unlikely to come to a clinic as blank slates, waiting for their health-care practitioner to explain to them why a disease or condition has occurred in their family. Often they will come to a clinic with ideas of their own about why they, their children, or other relatives have been so afflicted and hope that their practitioner can help them.

Attribution theory may provide a framework to help health-care practitioners understand better how this process occurs. Attribution theory posits that individuals will seek and construct explanations (attributions) for the causes of events [1]. In making those attributions, individuals may also experience emotions that are related to their attributions, which may,

Authors contributed equally to this chapter and are listed alphabetically.

in turn, influence how they communicate with other people about the family disease or condition, including how they communicate with their relatives. In this chapter, we will describe attribution theory and how it could help us understand family communication in the context of genetic diseases or conditions. We will use attribution theory as a framework to understand how family members talk about family diseases and conditions, or are influenced in their talk by those diseases and conditions. Finally, we will make some suggestions about how practitioners may use attribution theory to develop interventions to help family members communicate more effectively with each other.

ATTRIBUTION THEORY

Attribution theory describes how people search for causal attributions when unexpected, or unusual, things happen and especially when bad or painful things happen [1]. The more distressing events are, the more a person would be motivated to find a causal attribution [2]. Attribution theory predicts that people who have had, for instance, a baby born with lots of problems or a parent diagnosed with a late-onset genetic condition, would be strongly motivated to make causal attributions for these distressing events. We can expect, therefore, that by the time many of these people meet with their health-care practitioner, they may have developed their own explanations for why these events occurred. Some may hold these beliefs only tentatively; others may hold them quite strongly. Because there is such a strong underlying motivation for people to develop attributions for causes of events, understanding the kinds of attributions made could help practitioners better work with their clients toward understanding the family condition and help them better communicate about it with each other.

Causal attributions are made along certain dimensions that describe the different aspects of a causal frame. In this chapter, we will discuss three dimensions—locus, controllability, and stability—that fit well into explanations of motivation for behavior which may result from certain attributions and emotions that are associated with those attributions [1]. Along a continuum of the *locus dimension*, peoples' attributions could be more internal or external. Locus describes the location of the cause and is often thought of as the "who is to blame" dimension. For instance, a person might feel that his diagnosis of lung cancer was due to his own lifestyle choices, such as smoking (internal), or he might feel it is due solely to his environment, such as living in a smoggy city (external).

People also make attributions along the *controllability dimension*, which describes how much control they believe they or others had over the event. Because people are generally unable to control their genetic makeup, a "genetic" attribution for a particular disease is most likely placed at the uncontrollable end of the controllability continuum. However, if a person believes that the disease is caused by environmental factors, the person perceives that someone did have control over the environment and could have repaired or prevented the environmental hazard. Such an attribution would be placed at the controllable end of the continuum.

Finally, people also make attributions along a *stability dimension*, which describes how changeable the person perceives the cause to be over time. It is unlikely that one's genetic makeup would change over time, so one's genetic inheritance could be conceived as a stable cause, although the risks associated with it may be perceived as changeable over time. However, lifestyle choices or environmental hazards might be changeable, or unstable, causes.

In each case, when people make attributions about the cause(s) of a family condition, they are likely to do so from their own unique understandings of the world and their individual experiences. This was illustrated in one qualitative study of the hereditary cancer syndrome Lynch syndrome in which families were offered genetic testing. Family members were found to develop personal theories of inheritance (PTIs). These PTIs could be considered as a form of attribution, because they were used by the participants in this study to explain the pattern of cancers in their family and to predict whom in the family will inherit the mutation or develop cancer [3, 4]. Different family members may have different experiences of the same cancers in the family, and when they affect family members that an individual is emotionally and proximally close to, they may seem more salient to that individual than other cancers in the same family. This may influence how individuals interpret the family history of cancer, the attributions that they might make, and consequently who is believed to be at highest risk in the family, despite contrary genetic explanations. The context in which attributions are made and discussed is integral to the way in which people frame their situations, and consequently how they communicate about those situations.

In the remainder of this chapter, we will explore different aspects of attribution theory and family communication through discussions of examples and cases. While the theory does not change from case to case, in order to better understand individuals' attributions and their subsequent motivations, it is important to explore those attributions from the perspectives of people in different situations. We will first work through the dimensions of attribution theory, then discuss the relationship between attributions and family communication, and finally pose a model through which to consider approaching genetic counseling as a form of attributional therapy.

Locus Dimension

The locus dimension indicates where the cause for an event lies. In many cases, the way that individuals situate their attributions along the locus dimension can significantly influence how they communicate with their close relatives. The "fundamental attribution error" describes the observation that people have a tendency to misattribute *intentions* in the actions of other people [5]. Specifically, when people attribute an event as caused by another (e.g., John neglected to invite me to the party), to commit the fundamental attribution error is to assume intention (e.g., John purposely did not invite me), and reason (e.g., John must be angry with me, not like me, etc.) where neither assumption may be true (e.g., John forgot or accidentally misplaced the invitation). However, whether or not the locus of a given causal attribution is correct, it nonetheless influences the subsequent motivations for behavior and emotions of the person who makes the attribution [1], and it is further related to the goals the person develops for communication [6] and the perceptions that the person has of his or her communication partners [7].

Attributions can affect family communication. To illustrate this, we offer two examples in the following paragraphs. First, we discuss the attributions that parents may make in relation to their children's behavior and learning problems; secondly, we discuss the attributions (adult) children may make in relation to their parents' genetic status.

We turn to fragile X syndrome as an exemplar for attributions relating to children's behavior. Fragile X syndrome is an inherited condition causing developmental delay, attention deficit and hyperactivity, autism, and some characteristic facial and other physical features. Inheritance of fragile X syndrome is complex, but as a general rule, the condition is inherited by boys from their unaffected carrier mothers. However, female carriers can show mild features of the condition. Fragile X syndrome is often diagnosed by pediatricians, and the family may not be referred to a genetics clinic or offered genetic counseling if they are not planning any further pregnancies. Boys with full fragile X syndrome may have significant developmental delay and behavior problems. However, their female carrier sisters may also exhibit some features of the condition, such as behavior problems and difficulties with schoolwork, but these girls may not be investigated for this if their symptoms are mild, especially if the family is not involved with a genetics clinic. According to attribution theory, if parents of these girls are unaware of the possibility of fragile X as an explanation for their daughters' behavior problems and difficulties with schoolwork, they may be motivated to search for another cause. The parents are likely to make their own attributions and may perceive that they have unexpectedly failed at something that is very important to them—the ability to produce a "perfect" or "normal" child, especially in the context of having a boy severely affected by fragile X syndrome.

Attribution theory may help us to better understand this situation. Without understanding the condition that their daughter has, parents may be likely to make internal attributions along the locus dimension about her behavior and intention. "My daughter is always naughty and does not try to behave," suggests that the location of the cause is within the young girl, and that the young girl has control over it. This explanation does not include some uncontrollable force (a particular condition) that might be affecting her behavior. Furthermore, her parents may commit the fundamental attribution error when no other cause is known. Sentiments such as "My daughter is misbehaving intentionally," "My daughter is old enough to know better," or "My daughter is looking for attention" all suggest that the young girl is willfully misbehaving or underperforming in school. These attributions may cause parents to have unrealistic developmental expectations for their daughter, lack of empathic awareness of their daughter's emotional needs, and may increase the risk of child abuse. Parents report feeling angrier and more likely to use power-assertive parenting strategies (providing their child with no motivation to change his or her behavior except the avoidance of punishment) when they perceive that her misbehavior is internally caused and intentional, or when they believe that she always behaves like this, even when she is old enough to "know better" [8]. In this way, parents' attributions for their child's behavior can bias their judgments, causing them to have inappropriate developmental expectations and to blame their child inappropriately for "bad" behavior.

The parents of more than one child with features of a condition like fragile X syndrome may have a very difficult time managing their children's behavior. They may recognize that their son has a condition that causes his severe behavior and learning problems, but they may be less generous toward their daughters, who show only mild features of the condition (and thus may not be diagnosed), if they are not aware of all the possible manifestations of fragile X syndrome. If not supported appropriately, the parents may be at risk for depression. Depression may lead to even less charitable attributions for their daughters' below-average schoolwork and behavior problems on successive occasions. Depressed parents may be less attentive to their child's behavior, less likely to regulate their own behavior over time, and may as a result exacerbate their child's behavior problems, creating a downward spiral [8]. Understanding these attributions and their consequences (i.e., the parents' motivations and emotions) may help health-care practitioners in supporting families struggling with communication difficulties.

Our second example of attribution is also about parents and children, but it relates more specifically to the ways in which the locus dimension may affect the parent–child relationship. Adult children who learn that their parent carries a gene mutation or has developed a genetic condition may feel that their parent's genetic status puts them at a risk that has external and uncontrollable attributes. Placement of attributions along the locus dimension may interact with placement of attributions along the controllability dimension to influence whom they blame for their condition—their parents, themselves, or fate. Rarely will adult children who believe that their genetic condition or their genetic risk is caused by a gene mutation inherited from one of their parents "blame" that parent. However, the emotions surrounding these attributions may be influenced by the prior relationship—a parent is usually only blamed if the person already has a poor relationship with that parent and is looking for one more excuse to blame that parent for everything. Most people who believe that their genetic condition is transmitted from one or both of their parents accept this as having not been under the control of the parent(s). Anger and blame may still be experienced in this context, but it is more likely to be nonspecific in its direction or to be directed at "fate" or another existential force. However, a strained parent–child relationship may become more strained if children begin to "blame" estranged parents for carrying the gene mutation. This may motivate adult children to block needed family communication depending on the severity of the condition and the relationships that adult children have with siblings. Working through those emotions may be difficult for adult children and may affect their own decisions to participate in genetic testing and continued communication with their parents about the genetic condition.

From the parents' perspective, finding out that they may be a carrier of a late-onset genetic condition commonly causes emotional turmoil related to their own risk of developing the condition, as well as guilt about the possibility that they may have transmitted the condition to their children. Attribution theory provides a framework with which to understand and describe this situation. The theory predicts that internal, controllable attributions lead to feelings of guilt [1]. Parents who receive information about their genetic status may experience greater guilt, in comparison to those who are not parents, some of which reflects a conflict between their own needs and the needs of their children.

The Controllability Dimension

The controllability dimension refers to whether an attributed cause is perceived as controllable either by the individual or some outside force. Attributions to uncontrollable causes, such as a "gene" in the family over which one has no control, could lead to emotions such as frustration, anger, helplessness, or hopelessness [1]. While some individuals may find comfort in a genetic explanation, as they may feel that it absolves them from guilt, others could find themselves experiencing strong negative feelings when they realize there may be little that they can do to prevent a condition from developing or recurring, short of deciding not to have children. Questions such as, *Can anyone change my or my loved one's situation?* and *Do I have any control over the recurrence of this condition?* become important to those seeking information about their health. A sense of control may be so central to those individuals at genetic risk that it may in itself be one of the greatest benefits provided to them by the options genetic counseling and genetic testing could provide [9, 10].

As mentioned above, the locus and controllability dimensions may interact to influence the emotions experienced by individuals when they make a causal attribution (Table 9.1). Controllability, for that reason, can sometimes be a difficult dimension to identify. Therefore, we outline the four different combinations that controllability can have with locus to highlight some of the emotional responses most commonly associated with each.

Individuals may make attributions that are both internal and controllable. Typically, when someone feels in control of a situation, his or her emotions are more hopeful in nature. For example, consider a man who has assumed that he will develop colon cancer at a young age, because

Table 9.1 Locus and Controllability Dimensions and Their Relationship with Emotions

	Locus: Internal	*Locus: External*
Controllable	Hopeful, possibly frustrated with prior behavior	Angry (directed), frustrated
Uncontrollable	Helpless, at risk for learned helplessness behavior, depressed	Angry (undirected), depressed

of his strong family history of colon cancer. Because of this assumption, he has not looked after his body well, and has had a poor diet. Upon finding that although he is at significant risk for developing colon cancer on account of his family history, it is not inevitable, and that dietary interventions may reduce his risk, he may feel disappointed in himself for not having taken better care of his body in the past, but also hopeful that perhaps he can change things for the better. Thus, even when there are negative emotions associated with internal and uncontrollable causes, there is usually a way to frame them in a hopeful way if an individual believes that he or she has personal control over the situation.

Individuals who make attributions that are both internal and uncontrollable run the risk of feeling negative emotions without that hopefulness. In fact, individuals may find themselves feeling helpless about their situation [10] because there is "nothing they can do" to change it. Individuals who repeatedly make internal and uncontrollable attributions (e.g., I just can't do it) are described as suffering from "learned helplessness" that may become a life orientation [10, 11]. Individuals who become depressed or hopeless about their situations (e.g., I know I will inherit this debilitating disease) may find those emotions spilling into other aspects of their lives. Things might "not matter anymore" if an individual feels like his or her health will be uncontrollably affected in the near future. While only a minority may experience this extreme of negative emotions, it is important for health-care practitioners to be sensitive to the possibility of this pattern of responses in their work because it may adversely affect family communication about a genetic condition.

Individuals who make external attributions feel slightly differently about their attributions along the controllability dimension. Those who make external, uncontrollable attributions may feel depressed and frustrated about their situations, and if they feel anger about it, they may have no clear place to direct their anger. Because such attributions are closely associated with the notion that "it was fate" because no one could have known or changed the situation, and the individual was not at fault, those making external and uncontrollable attributions may find themselves in a position of uncertainty, which is commonly encountered in individuals at genetic risk. Certainly, some people who focus on fate or luck as causes of the disease-related events in their family may believe that these things are stable (e.g., I just have bad luck) or unstable (e.g., It just wasn't my time), but many of these will experience associated difficulties in directing their emotions and feeling comfortable with their situations. Experiencing anger around these attributions may affect both an individual's well-being and their family relationships [12]; thus, practitioners should pay careful attention to individuals and family members making external and uncontrollable attributions.

Attributions along the controllability dimension are related to a variety of emotions. When controllable causes of adverse events are also attributed as external, individuals making those attributions are likely to feel angry because someone or something has control over the cause, even though the individuals making the attributions may have no control.

Case Study 1: External Control

A woman, Joan, was referred to the cancer genetics clinic because her mother died from cancer of the colon in her early thirties, when Joan was a child. Joan explained that her mother had grown up near a nuclear power station, and that the family has believed for the last 30 years that her mother's cancer and premature death were caused by the infamous leak from that nuclear power station in the early 1970s. Her mother's cancer was attributed to an external, controllable cause, which resulted in a deep-seated anger in Joan that had influenced her political beliefs. Because of this attribution, she was motivated to be very active in the anti-nuclear power movement in her youth, and she continued to be a local representative for the Green party, taking a militant anti-nuclear stance.

Joan's health-care practitioner took a detailed family history, and at his request, Joan communicated with her maternal relatives, from whom she had become estranged when her father remarried, to collect some further information about her maternal family history. She discovered that her maternal grandmother had developed cancer of the uterus in her fifties, and a maternal uncle had developed cancer of the colon in his sixties, and so the practitioner could make a diagnosis of Lynch syndrome in the family. Joan may initially have trouble accepting a possible genetic explanation for her mother's early-onset colon cancer, which for 30 years she had attributed to the leak from the nuclear power station. Because of her initial external and controllable attribution, she may be resistant to regular screening colonoscopies.

Joan may be more likely to comply with screening recommendations if the practitioner addresses, acknowledges, and discusses Joan's strong beliefs about the cause of her mother's cancer and the effect this had on her life. Careful attention to discussing these explanations with Joan, and understanding her initial resistances, may be critical to making sure that she communicates with her siblings about their own genetic risk for developing cancer.

The Stability Dimension

Stability refers to how likely a cause is to change over time. For individuals and families making attributions about their genetic risk, placement along the stability dimension will influence perceptions of their own risk for a genetic condition. While there may be many ways to think about this, in this section, we focus on age and its relationship to the kinds of attributions that patients and families make along the stability dimension.

BRCA1 is a gene that is associated with very high risk of developing early-onset breast cancer, as well as significant risk of developing ovarian cancer in women, when mutated. A woman who carries a BRCA1 mutation will not be at the same level of risk for developing breast and ovarian cancer over her lifetime. She will be at very low risk for both cancers until she is in her late twenties. She will be at highest risk for developing breast cancer between the ages of 30 and 50 years. Once she reaches 50 years of age, her risk of developing breast cancer will begin to approach that of other women of the same age in the general population, although her risk of developing ovarian cancer will only begin to be significant when she is over 50 years of age.

However, if her mother died from ovarian cancer at the age of 51, when she was only 16 years old herself, her fear of ovarian cancer may be overwhelming. Operating from a PTI, she may "place" her risk of developing ovarian cancer at the stable end of the spectrum, and she may feel that this risk is high all the way through her adulthood. As a result, she may feel much more vulnerable to ovarian cancer than to breast cancer, even at the age of 35, when her objective risk of developing ovarian cancer is low and her objective risk of developing breast cancer is high.

On the other hand, if her mother developed breast cancer at 38 years of age, when she was 19 years of age, she may focus much more on the very early age of her mother's diagnosis. She may "place" her risk of developing breast cancer at the unstable end of the spectrum and feel extremely vulnerable to breast cancer in her mid-thirties, as she approaches the age at which her mother was diagnosed with breast cancer. Furthermore, when she reaches her 39th birthday, she may feel that she is no longer at risk—she may feel that she has lived past the "magic" age.

Understanding and acknowledging the attributions that people make about the causes of disease in their family is likely to help health-care practitioners move them toward a more realistic perception of their risk. In particular, understanding that the attributions that individuals make may be strongly influenced by their PTIs should alert practitioners that personal and family experiences may influence behavior as much and perhaps more so than the practitioner's explanation of risk. In the case of BRCA1, this may in turn influence their risk management behavior, which could ultimately reduce their risk of dying from cancer.

THE IMPACT OF ATTRIBUTIONS AND EMOTIONS ON FAMILY COMMUNICATION

The attributions that individuals make may influence their emotional state, which in turn may influence their motivation and behavior [1], and consequently the relational communication they have with family members. In this section, we discuss several important emotions related to the types of attributions that individuals make about diseases and conditions, and how they may influence family communication.

Learned Optimism and Helplessness

Earlier in the chapter, we discussed learned helplessness as a possible consequence of making consistent internal and uncontrollable attributions for adverse events. Those who find themselves with particularly challenging health situations risk falling into the habit of feeling like they have little control or ability to change their situation. While coping with a genetic condition in the family is a difficult situation for any individual, those who fall into patterns of learned helplessness may exacerbate this situation by becoming an emotional and sometimes physical burden on their families, which will influence how family members communicate with each other. A person who feels helpless about an existing or possible future diagnosis of a genetic disease may find herself communicating about other aspects of her life in the same way. An individual who decides, for instance, that quitting smoking is unnecessary at this point in life because he will likely die of the family disease sooner than the tobacco would kill him may frustrate his family members who believe that he would feel better physically and emotionally if he were to stop that habit.

Learned optimism, on the other hand, is a similar pattern, or life orientation, but it may require some effort and professional help to achieve. Seligman [13] proposed that individuals who adopt an optimistic approach experience better psychological and physical well-being in their lives. When people find themselves in potentially hopeless situations, it may be important for family members and health-care practitioners to help them better understand those aspects of their lives that they can control, and to discourage them from making negative assumptions regarding aspects of their lives that they cannot control. By helping them to change their attributions, health-care practitioners may also help them take a more healthy perspective in their motivations.

Self-Blame

In many cases, perceived self-responsibility results in feelings of guilt [1]. Spinal muscular atrophy (SMA) is a genetic condition characterized by muscle weakness, multiple congenital contractures, and difficulty feeding and swallowing. The disease can be fatal in early childhood, and there is no cure. In one example, a mother whose son was diagnosed with SMA shortly after birth experienced her son's death when he was less than 6 years old. She felt guilty because she believed that she caused her son's condition by eating shellfish, which made her violently ill, when she was pregnant with him.

When health-care practitioners confirmed the diagnosis of SMA by genetic testing, they provided the woman and her husband with an appropriate explanation of recessive inheritance. The practitioners may have hoped to relieve her feelings of guilt by explaining that her son's condition was not caused by anything she did in her pregnancy, but by gene mutations inherited from both his carrier parents, over which she had no control. When practitioners addressed her pre-existing causal attribution in making this explanation, they could call their intervention a form of "attributional therapy." What they did was to shift her belief about the controllability of her son's condition. They changed the causal attribution from an internal, controllable one to an internal, uncontrollable one. There is some suggestion in attribution theory that attributions to internal, uncontrollable causes can result in feelings of shame [1], but in many cases, the understanding of the situation could help the person feel less guilty about her own actions and better prepared for the future. Interestingly, Meiser et al. [14] found that members of families with a high density of bipolar disorder felt that having a genetic explanation for the condition in the family was likely to decrease the stigma associated with the condition. In effect, the genetic explanation changed the attribution for the disease away from the individual toward a genetic cause.

PRACTICAL ADVICE AND APPLICATIONS
Attribution theory provides an explanation for many of the ways in which individuals and families perceive genetic risks. It is important to reiterate, however, that although attributions are individual explanations for causal events, they are not always accurate, informed, or correct. In some cases, the attributions for events that individuals make might seem counterintuitive to health-care practitioners. Attributions are personal and often they become integrated into an individual's worldview. Changing them may take some time but also may provide those individuals with knowledge and peace of mind that could help them to adjust more positively to the family condition, thus improving the effectiveness with which they communicate with their at-risk relatives about the family condition.

LAY MODELS OF INHERITANCE AND PERSONAL THEORIES OF INHERITANCE
In addition to making attributions about events that have already occurred, attribution theory also tells us that people make predictions about the future based on the causal attributions that they make in the present [2]. There is some evidence that individuals at genetic risk also make predictions about who in the family will develop the family condition, based on their attributions for the pattern of disease in their family. For instance, PTIs, which seem to be specific to individuals rather than shared in families, may draw on the pattern of cancer in an individual's family and lay models of how physical and other characteristics are inherited in families [3, 4]. Personal theories of inheritance have been found to be related to co-inheritance of cancer with some other physical feature in the family, such as build or sex [3, 4]. Interestingly, the information used to construct these theories was influenced by the quality of relationships in the

family. Individuals may feel that the cancers experienced by those who are geographically and emotionally closer to them are also more salient to them. Personal theories of inheritance may not be held by all family members, but they may be more likely held among family members who are intensely engaged with (anxious and worried about) their risk [3, 4]. Thus, individual PTIs are dependent on context and emotional responses, and they may be very powerful because they are informed by vivid personal experience of life-changing events affecting close family members.

Some individuals may continue to hold a PTI, even after they have been given an explanation of the Mendelian model of inheritance [3, 4]. Other researchers have also found that people seem to be able to hold apparently conflicting beliefs about the causes of the disease in their family [15, 16]. Individuals can repeat an explanation of the genetic model of inheritance given in genetic counseling, but still use a PTI to predict who in the family is most likely to inherit the family mutation or develop cancer [3]. Attribution theory might provide one explanation about why the genetic model, in some cases, does not provide the information that an individual may need. Attribution theory tells us that people make predictions about the future based on their causal attributions. In fact, perhaps the need to gain some control over the future by enabling such predictions is the reason why causal attributions are sought. But the genetic model, based on probabilities, does not enable accurate prediction to be made in the absence of a genetic test. Personal theories of inheritance provide a means of predicting the future with greater certainty, and hence control, than the genetic model. This could be one explanation for the persistence of these models after genetic counseling.

GENETIC COUNSELING AS A FORM OF ATTRIBUTIONAL THERAPY

When family members make attributions for their family history of disease, or when they construct PTIs to help them move beyond uncertainty, they may inaccurately assess their own and other family members' risks through the attributions they have made. The term *attribution(al) therapy* has been used to describe a counseling intervention sometimes used to treat learned helplessness and depression, which uses cognitive-behavioral therapy to help people develop more realistic explanatory styles. In some ways, genetic counseling could be considered a form of attributional therapy, where the aim is to help clients to achieve two very different outcomes:

1. More realistic attributions about the genetic condition in their family, thus facilitating correct identification of, and ideally communication with, their at-risk relatives
2. More adaptive adjustment to the genetic condition in their family

The first outcome is achieved when health-care practitioners help individuals to understand the role that the family condition may play. For example, the family that had a daughter who may be mildly affected by fragile X syndrome may have started out blaming their own parenting methods or blaming their daughter for bad behavior or poor schoolwork. However, understanding that a genetic condition is underlying their daughter's learning and behavior problems can help the parents reassess their earlier attributions for their daughter's problems. Practitioners can anticipate the need for reframing these attributions and explicitly ask clients to describe the kinds of attributions they may have made before providing a scientific explanation, so that their explanation can take account of previous misunderstandings. Practitioners can even go further than this and talk with clients about how they might change their perspectives or perhaps their own behaviors in response to the genetic information.

In the example of the woman whose son died from SMA, health-care practitioners explained that SMA is a recessive condition, and the parents were both confirmed as carriers of SMA, confirming a 25% recurrence risk in every future pregnancy that the couple might have. The information about the cause of SMA, the inheritance pattern, and the genetic risks associated with future pregnancies may have helped achieve the first outcome for this woman of a more realistic attribution about the genetic condition in her family. This, of course, changes the mother's attribution from an internal, controllable cause to an internal, uncontrollable cause. Although this may relieve her feelings of guilt and self-blame for her son's death, it also runs the risk of plunging her into helplessness and hopelessness when she thinks about future pregnancies.

In this example, more can be offered, addressing the second potential outcome given above: more adaptive adjustment to the genetic condition in their family. Health-care practitioners were subsequently able to offer prenatal testing to this woman and her husband in future pregnancies. This could provide the couple with an important opportunity to regain control over their future. First, it was important for the woman to realize that her controllable actions were not the cause of her son's death. Second, concerns about SMA being an uncontrollable risk in future pregnancies could be mitigated by offering early prenatal genetic testing.

This degree of control cannot always be provided, because genetic testing is not always either possible or acceptable. Where it is not, interventions to foster more adaptive adjustment to the genetic condition in the family may still be possible. If health-care practitioners are sensitive to the range of possible emotional consequences to any changes they may have made to the individuals' attributions for the family condition, then they may be able to offer interventions to help them better understand and manage their emotions.

WORKING WITH PERSONAL THEORIES OF INHERITANCE
If individuals are using PTIs to predict who in their family may inherit a genetic mutation, or develop the family disease, and if these beliefs are persisting after they are given an explanation of the genetic model of inheritance, it is possible that this may influence who they decide to inform in the

family about risk. Health-care practitioners tend to rely on clients to inform other at-risk family members, because it is usually considered unethical for practitioners to approach clients' relatives directly. This is considered particularly important for dominantly inherited conditions such as Huntington disease, X-linked conditions, and chromosome translocations where many family members may be at risk. It is particularly important in conditions such as hereditary breast and ovarian cancer and Lynch syndrome, for which many family members may also be at risk and interventions to reduce risk are available; thus, communication about risk in the family could save lives. Not all at-risk family members are told about their risk [17, 18], and family dynamics may be one reason for this. There is evidence that individuals do deliberate before communicating genetic risk information to relatives, and that making sense of risk may be part of this process. However, the degree to which PTIs influence this has not been investigated.

While future investigations into understanding the nature of PTIs and their impact on family communication is needed, health-care practitioners can address some of the issues associated with family communication and PTIs by specifically raising them with clients in their discussion of attributions. One way of doing this would be to ask clients if they have any ideas of their own about who in the family is most likely to develop the family condition and why they believe this to be the case. This information can then be appropriately incorporated into the practitioner's scientific explanation, addressing any misunderstandings directly. Even if the client does not believe a family member is at risk, if the family member fits certain risk criteria as outlined by the practitioner then discussion should include the client's willingness to talk with this person.

CONCLUSION

Understanding why distressing things have happened in their family is important for individuals who may be at genetic risk. Whether the attributions stem from their own theories (PTIs) or their health-care practitioner's explanations, the different ways in which individuals might go about understanding why a disease or condition occurred in their family can foster myriad emotions that together influence the ways in which they communicate with their families. While always important, when conditions are genetic, family communication can become a life or death matter. Considering their practice as a form of attributional therapy may provide practitioners with a helpful framework. A practitioner's ability to foster appropriate attributions, address the strong emotions that may be associated with those attributions, and work with those attributions to facilitate appropriate family communication about risk is essential. Specifically addressing attributions and helping people to reframe inappropriate attributions through attributional therapy may be important in helping them effectively adapt to the genetic condition in their family.

REFERENCES

1. Weiner B. *An Attributional Theory of Motivation and Emotion*. New York: Springer-Verlag; 1986.
2. Taylor SE, Lichtman RR, Wood JV. Attributions, beliefs about control, and adjustment to breast cancer. *Journal of Personality and Social Psychology* 1984;46:489–502.
3. McAllister M. Predictive genetic testing and beyond: A theory of engagement. *Journal of Health Psychology* 2002;7(5):491–508.
4. McAllister M. Personal theories of inheritance, coping strategies, risk perception and engagement in hereditary non-polyposis colon cancer families offered genetic testing. *Clinical Genetics* 2003;64:179–189.
5. Heider F. *The Psychology of Interpersonal Relations*. New York: John Wiley; 1958.
6. Sabee CM, Wilson SR. Students' primary goals, attributions and facework in conversations about disappointing grades. *Communication Education* 2005;54:185–204.
7. Sabee CM, Bylund CL, Imes RS, Sanford AA, Rice IS. Patients' attributions for health care provider responses to patients' presentation of Internet health research. *Southern Communication Journal* 2007;72:265–284.
8. Wilson SR, Whipple EE. Attributions and regulative communication by parents participating in a community-based child physical abuse prevention program. In: Manusov V, Harvey JH, eds. *Attribution, Communication Behavior, and Close Relationships*. New York: Cambridge University Press; 2001:227–265.
9. Shiloh S, Berkenstadt M, Meiran N, et al. Mediating effects of perceived personal control in coping with a health threat: The case of genetic counseling. *Journal of Applied Social Psychology* 1997;27(13):1146–1174.
10. McAllister M, Payne K, Nicholls S, MacLeod R, Donnai D, Davies L. Patient empowerment in clinical genetics services. *Journal of Health Psychology* 2008;13(7):887–897.
11. Dweck CS. *Self Theories: Their Role in Motivation, Personality and Development*. Philadelphia: Psychology Press; 2000.
12. Guerrero LK, LaValley AG. Conflict, emotion and communication. In: Oetzel JG, Ting-Toomey S, eds. *The Sage Handbook of Conflict Communication*. Thousand Oaks, CA: Sage; 2006:69–96.
13. Seligman M. *Learned Optimism: How to Change Your Mind and Your Life*. New York: Simon & Schuster; 1998.
14. Meiser B, Mitchell PB, McGirr H, Van Herten M, Schofield PR. Implications of genetic risk information in families with a high density of bipolar disorder: An exploratory study. *Social Science and Medicine* 2005;60:109–118.
15. Weil J. Mothers' postcounseling beliefs about the causes of their children's genetic disorders. *American Journal of Human Genetics* 1991;48:145–153.
16. Shiloh S, Berkenstadt M. Lay conceptions of genetic disorders. *Birth Defects: Original Articles* 1992;28:191–200.
17. Clarke A, Richard M, Kerzin-Storrar L, et al. Genetics professionals reports of non-disclosure of genetic risk information within families. *European Journal of Human Genetics* 2005;13:556–562.
18. Gaff C, Clarke A, Atkinson P, et al. Process and outcome in communication of genetic information within families: A systematic review. *European Journal of Human Genetics* 2007;15:999–1011.

10

COMMUNICATION GOALS AND PLANS

Jennifer A. Samp, Melanie Watson, & Amanda Strickland

Although people may intend to convey genetic information to relatives, they do not always act on this. Planning is an important step, and it is facilitated by identifying the thoughts and intentions a person has regarding communication. The goal-plan-action sequence provides a useful framework for health-care practitioners who wish to develop greater insight into goals and planning processes.

The detection and assessment of genetic mutations may have implications for the health and well-being of an entire family. Therefore, the disclosure of genetic risk information to relatives is essential. Yet a common struggle for health-care practitioners is that most individuals are willing to fully disclose genetic risk information to family members, but they often fall short of this goal. The inability of a family member to fully disclose genetic risk information is not an artifact of laziness or neglect. Rather, other concerns may constrain or make more difficult the process of fulfilling an intention to share genetic histories. Decisions about disclosing genetic information are sometimes limited by other concerns relating to the general dynamics of family interaction, or how knowledge of particularly negative or troublesome information may negatively affect family members. For example, a woman may intend to share the results of genetic tests with family members but may find herself constrained by equally important concerns to protect certain family members from upsetting or disturbing information. A host of relational and individual concerns may be relevant to the decision to disclose genetic information;

thus, the task of prioritizing and expressing multiple concerns to others can be both frustrating and overwhelming.

Little research has acknowledged the role of individuals' thoughts, experiences, and intentions on decisions about how and when to communicate with family members about sensitive information [1], in particular with regard to decisions about sharing health-related information. However, more generalized cognitive-based approaches to communication suggest that intentions or plans for how one will communicate with others are reflective of an initial process of goal setting. Goals are broadly defined as desired end states toward which people strive [2]. Accordingly, we assume here that individuals in possession of genetic information are able to project or desire certain personal or relational effects that come through the sharing of the information (or not) with family members. Further, it is widely recognized that the intention to pursue a particular goal is constrained by other concerns that focus on the needs of a communicator or on the desires of a message recipient [3]. Given that intentions to disclose genetic information are frequently driven and/or constrained by a variety of self-, other-, and relational-oriented concerns, this chapter reviews theory and research on the goal-plan-action (GPA) process and explains the utility of considering work on GPA to better understand the multiple cognitive and behavioral processes related to the communication of genetic information to family members. In short, the GPA sequence specifies that a person's goal to communicate (or not) (the "G") stimulates cognitive activity to access goal-related information that informs the formation of plans (the "P"), which lead to some communication or action (the "A"). Figure 10.1 depicts the elements of the GPA sequence.

While Dillard [4] coined the phrase "GPA sequence" in his seminal theoretical work on the process of goal-driven communication in persuasive situations, here we use the term *GPA* to refer to the broader corpus of work focused on the pursuit of particular goals via communication. This chapter reviews the core assumptions underlying the GPA sequence and identifies how GPA Theories may inform health-care practitioners of possible ways to facilitate the process of communication between family members. A case study involving the disclosure of hereditary breast and ovarian cancer (HBOC) risk information to relatives is presented to relate the theoretical concepts underlying the GPA sequence to practice.

Case Study

Jane Jones is 42 years old and the mother of three children: Amy (18 years), Adam (15 years), and Sarah (12 years). Jane has a family history of breast cancer; her mother died from the condition when Jane was in her late teens and Jane was diagnosed with breast cancer at the age of 37 years. She found the diagnosis of breast cancer very difficult to deal with, but since her successful treatment Jane is feeling more positive. Nonetheless,

Jane is concerned about her risk of HBOC). Jane has genetic counseling and learns that HBOC has a dominant inheritance pattern. At the end of the consultation, she is offered *BRCA1/2* genetic testing to see if a gene mutation can be identified. Jane feels this information will be helpful and proceeds with testing. When available, the results indicate a *BRCA* mutation. Jane immediately decides to tell her younger sister Wendy of the *BRCA* mutation. However, Jane does not know if, when, and how to tell her children. Jane and Wendy discuss her guilt of having possibly passed the *BRCA* mutation onto her children. Jane desperately wants to protect her children from worry and ill health. Jane decides with her husband to withhold the information from her two youngest children for the time being, but she plans to inform her eldest daughter, Amy.

In addition, Jane and her husband discuss disclosing this information to other family members. Jane and her sister-in-law have a strained relationship. Further, Jane's brother has recently been diagnosed with prostate cancer; thus, she does not feel it is the right time to inform her brother, sister-in-law, or nieces.

Risk disclosure of HBOC has been described as one of the most complex areas for carriers because they are faced with deciding if, when, and how to tell relatives (including children) about their genetic status [5]. As the case study illustrates, following through with intentions to tell family members about genetic information is influenced by a host of factors. While most individuals are inclined to inform family members about their HBOC risk more so than coworkers or friends, some find it difficult to reveal such negative information [6]. Moreover, learning that one is a carrier of a genetic disorder has been suggested to pose a threat to how one experiences the parental role [7]. As shown in this example, individuals dealing with genetic conditions are faced with issues such as how to manage the disclosure of the genetic information to family members, including their children. Clearly, these decisions are multifaceted, in large part due to an individual's desire to share information while balancing the interests of other family members.

We now turn to examine how intentions, as influenced by goals, both influence and constrain messages in general, and more specifically to family members about genetic information. While we focus our examples on the case study about HBOC, the GPA process is assumed to capture cognitively influenced communication behaviors across most interactions ranging from acquaintances to intimate others. Therefore, the GPA sequence applies to any situation where an individual is faced with disclosing (or not disclosing) genetic information to family members. In turn, we by no means suggest that our application of the GPA sequence is limited to communication decisions about particular genetic issues.

THE NATURE OF GOALS IN INTERACTION

Goals are the cornerstone of most of our social interactions [2]. A goal is some desired end or state of affairs that an individual desires to attain or maintain [8]. For example, as a mother of three children, Jane has a goal for her children "to be healthy." Of course, merely thinking about this goal is not enough to achieve her desired end. The achievement of a goal requires some sort of action designed for attainment. Planning consists of producing one or more mental models detailing how a goal might be achieved through interaction [9], the product of which results in observable behavior. Also, Jane's goal for her children requires her to communicate her plans with both her husband and her children. Desires become *interaction goals* when communication and coordination with another is required for goal achievement [10].

While most theories focus on general concepts related to the GPA sequence in persuasive interactions, goal and planning processes are certainly relevant to an understanding of family interaction. As Wilson and Moran [11] note, the interdependence of family members naturally requires that each family member influence the others' goals and plans. Further, the particulars of family norms, expectations, or behaviors make goal pursuit within a family a complex task as members seek to pursue their own interests while balancing the interests of the family as a unit. For example, research has found that individuals often perceive that it is their "duty" as a family member to share genetic information with relatives [12]. Yet this duty conflicts with a desire to protect relatives from particularly harmful and difficult information. Further, familial norms about disclosure also impact the decision to reveal genetic risk information to family members [13]. If it is normative for a family to disclose very little about their lives, the decision to reveal genetic information may be difficult.

Types of Goals

The range of goals that an individual may pursue is vast and diffuse and may reflect a variety of intentions. Considering the *content* or focus of a particular desired end state, researchers have identified three distinct general types of goals people seek to achieve through interpersonal communication (Fig. 10.1) [8]. One general class of goals reflects *self-presentation* or *identity* goals, which reflect concerns about the image of "who we are" and how we want to be perceived by others. We pursue *relational* goals by working to develop, maintain, or neglect particular relationships. A third general category of goals reflects *instrumental* concerns, which involve obtaining some sort of tangible resource, getting others to do us a favor, or to accomplish some sort of task. In the case study, Jane may have a goal to convey her genetic information in a confident, self-sufficient, and self-interested manner; such intentions may reflect a *self-presentation* or *identity* goal. If she wishes to maintain an open and honest relationship with her children and sister in order to maintain family cohesion, Jane may have a *relational* goal. Or Jane may possess a goal that reflects an *instrumental* concern, such as acquiring emotional support from a friend or relative. The genetic literature has found that women with HBOC often actively seek out the support of their sisters [14], yet research to date has not examined the nuanced ways that patients go about seeking support, their decisions about with whom to share information, the results of disclosure, or importantly, the disclosure of other genetic conditions with an explicit focus on goals.

The selection of a particular goal may be informed by prior experiences within the family [15, 16]. Such familial influences impact the disclosure of genetic information. For example, Forrest et al. [11] observed that individuals faced with a decision about sharing genetic risk information were more likely to share the information if their families had a pre-existing norm of open and disclosive communication, compared to those from families who had a more guarded or avoidant style of communication. Other research suggests that family members may perceive that they are required to disclose genetic information as a service to family members. Part of the burden may be due to the psychological stress associated with having a disease [17]. Or the perceived duty to share information may come from familial exposure to a genetic illness. With regard to cancer, the term *cancer burden* has been used to describe the individual's experience of the family history of cancer and the emotional burden of witnessing relatives with cancer who have undergone treatment [18]. However, such a burden is likely present when coping with any family illness, particularly when the illness has genetic implications. Further, the particular type of genetic information to be disclosed may influence communicative intentions. For example, research suggests that individuals find it easier to communicate with family members about HBOC than Huntington disease [19], in part due to the public's greater familiarity with HBOC and its manifestations [16]. Indeed, in relation to Huntington disease the existence of family secrets and unknowing relatives has been well documented [19]. Research to date has not explored the variations in communication intentions by other illnesses. Nonetheless, health-care practitioners can better identify a client's goals by exploring his or her experiences with the condition and previous experiences of information sharing within the family, while keeping in mind the particular genetic issue to be disclosed.

HOW GOALS FUNCTION

While the content of a goal is defined by the focus of the desired end state to be pursued, goals may have different *functions* within an interaction. Unlike the three content types, different types of functions can coexist within one goal. This is illustrated in Figure 10.1. In part, functionality is defined by how a goal relates to other concerns in terms of *specificity, importance, co-occurrence,* and *difficulty.* We now turn to review each of these functions with an eye toward identifying their implications for working with individuals faced with decisions about disclosing genetic information to family members.

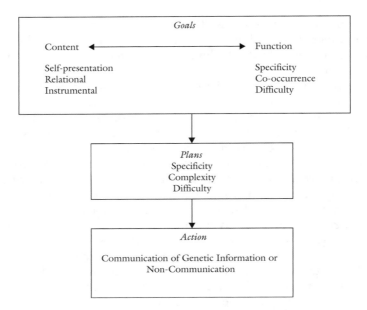

Figure 10.1   The goals-plan-action sequence.

Goals Are More or Less Specific

Individual goals exist at many levels of *specificity* and are assumed to operate within a "goal structure." As part of this structure, goals are organized hierarchically, such that higher level goals subsume other lower level goals. Higher level goals may also be termed *superordinate* or *distal goals* [20] or *motives* or *needs* [21]. These goals are abstract. For example, Jane has an abstract goal to "protect her children." Higher level goals are pursued via a variety of lower level *basic* goals. Basic goals are more proximal, concrete, and facilitate specific behaviors that are pursued in the service of attaining more abstract, higher level goals [10]. As the case study describes, Jane pursued the higher level goal of protecting her children by pursuing a specific lower level goal of withholding her *BRCA* test results from her two youngest children. The pursuit and achievement of a goal is more likely if the lower level goal is in line with (and less likely to be in conflict with) higher order goals [22]. Further, clear attainable goals produce higher levels of performance than general intentions [23].

Because specific goals are easier to achieve than abstract concerns, it is important for health-care practitioners to facilitate the identification of specific communication goals related to information disclosure. For example, if a person identifies a goal to "tell someone about my diagnosis," a practitioner can assist the individual in developing more specific goals that will facilitate informing family members, including specific goals related to whom the information will be disclosed (e.g.,

I will tell my Aunt), when the disclosure will occur (e.g., I will meet with her by next Tuesday), and how the information will be delivered (e.g., I will be self-assured). By breaking up abstract goals into more specific goals, practitioners can help individuals overcome a seemingly impossible-to-achieve abstract intention.

Goals Are More or Less Important

Goals may also be defined and organized in terms of their *importance*. Importance reflects the particular value or salience of a goal relative to other goals [24]. Dillard [4] observed that individuals are able to articulate several goals that are *relevant* to an interaction, yet a host of goals are easily prioritized. For example, individuals faced with a recent genetic diagnosis may wish to pursue the self-interested concern of sharing the information to immediately "get it off my chest," yet they may also be sensitive to the fact that it may be important to wait until a family member is sufficiently prepared to hear the news.

Important goals are motivating and energizing. The occurrence of an important goal directs cognitive processing resources toward the pursuit of that goal [25], and this encourages the production of behaviors structured toward the realization of that goal, in place of other behaviors that are not directly related to the most important goal [26]. In other words, deciding that a goal is important engages cognitive efforts to pursue the goal as well as to stay committed to its pursuit [27]. Therefore, although an individual may have a goal to share genetic information, if it is more important to preserve the well-being of a family member, a direct disclosure of one's genetic history may be put off in favor of the best interest of the family member, and in turn, general family functioning.

Health-care practitioners can help individuals prioritize their concerns, thereby facilitating the process of managing genetic information. Given that important goals motivate action, practitioners may enhance disclosure by helping people to identify their goals and to distinguish particular goals by importance. By doing so, the practitioner can have a better sense of what an individual views as a priority when communicating (or not) with family members.

Goals Frequently Co-Occur and Change in Priority

Individuals may possess self-interested, relational, and instrumental (i.e., content-related) goals simultaneously, or some goals may be more relevant and important than others at particular points in an interaction [28]. While sometimes an important goal drives an interaction consistently throughout the entire interaction, research by Dillard [8] and Samp and Solomon [24, 26] advanced that important goals may be displaced by other concerns. Across a series of studies, participants were asked to engage in an interaction and then write about what they wanted to achieve during the interaction. Subsequently, they were asked to rate a variety of interaction goals.

Sometimes participants rated other goals as more important than the one they reported initially wanting to achieve in the interaction. While the act of communication is often framed by an instrumental goal such as providing information, changing another's attitude, or problem solving [29], the degree to which a given goal influences communication content is situationally bound, particularly in family relationships. Specifically, people commonly pursue self-interested concerns, even while in close relationships [26]. Yet the binds of the family relationship coupled with the needs of a family member may result in individuals pursuing goals that benefit the family member at the expense of their own personal desires. For example, the pursuit of a goal to discuss genetic risk with a family member may be interrupted by the realization that the information recipient is too emotional to understand the information presented at the time [30]. In such cases, an other-focused goal of providing emotional support or comfort to the family member may be more important than sharing information out of a concern that introducing stressful information may negatively impact the mental health of the individual. Or the decision to not disclose the genetic information may be driven by more temporary concerns that an initial emotional reaction by the recipient of the information may impede a complete understanding of the genetic disclosure and its implications.

That goals change and may displace one another during interaction highlights that goals may serve different functions during interactions. Guided by this assumption, Dillard's [4, 7] GPA Model distinguishes between primary and secondary goal functions. *Primary goals* define the focus of an interaction and answer the question, What is going on here? *Secondary goals* shape and constrain what people say as they go about pursuing a primary goal. Dillard et al. [3] identified five categories of secondary goals: *(1)* identity goals, which reflect desires to act consistently with one's beliefs; *(2)* interaction goals, or desires to maintain a positive image, saying things that are relevant and appropriate, and protecting the image of the other person in the interaction; *(3)* relational resource goals, which reflect desires to maintain relationships; *(4)* personal resource goals, which reflect concerns about maintaining one's time, money, or safety; and *(5)* arousal management goals, as reflected in concerns to reduce anxiety or nervousness. While primary goals define what an interaction is about, secondary goals "pull" the conversation by constraining what people say. For example, Jane's primary goal of informing her eldest daughter, Amy, of her genetic risk may be constrained by secondary-level concerns. While Jane wishes to protect her daughter from the distress and anxiety such information may arouse (arousal management), she may not feel she has the personal resources to support her daughter (personal resource goals) while she comes to terms with her own genetic diagnosis and risk. Because certain goals may not be pursued out of the interest of other concerns, health-care practitioners should work with clients to identify their ideal goals and those goals that can likely be achieved given other concerns.

Goals Are More or Less Difficult to Achieve

Another functional property of goals is their *difficulty*. The difficulty of goal pursuit may be defined by one's anticipated performance in satisfying a given goal or by the operation of multiple important goals. First, goal difficulty may be defined according to perceived performance in goal pursuit. For example, Ford [31] argued that individuals possess personal agency beliefs which reflect the perceived probability of goal attainment. Two types of beliefs define personal agency beliefs: context and capability. Context beliefs reflect the perceived responsiveness of the environment, such as controllability [32]. Capability beliefs concern perceptions of those resources (time, effort) that individuals have to achieve a given goal. Such beliefs are conceptually similar to the concept of self-efficacy [20]. In the context of family communication about genetic information, intentions to communicate with family members may be met with barriers, including the following: having little or no contact with family members; being emotionally distant with family members; divorce, remarriage, and family rifts; reluctance to discuss sensitive issues with biologically and/or socially distant relatives; problems in understanding or explaining concepts such as genetic inheritance; and assuming that other relatives will pass on this information [18]. Such barriers may all inform context beliefs relevant to goal achievement. Context beliefs may also concern perceptions of how a relative may respond to potentially sensitive and upsetting information about genetic risk. Capability beliefs would concern such issues as lack of confidence in oneself in being able to explain genetic concepts. Considering the case study, Jane's reluctance to inform her brother and nieces may be borne out of uncertainty about whether male relatives ought to be told about genetic testing and uncertainty regarding whether her nieces are at risk. This may be further compounded by a tendency of aunts or uncles not to speak to nephews and nieces and or a sense that they do not have the authority to do so. A health-care practitioner can facilitate dissemination of the risk information by identifying those relatives at risk in both pre- and post-test counseling sessions, while providing both verbal and written explanations of genetic inheritance to share with their relatives.

Goal difficulty may also be defined in terms of the number of goals that an individual attempts to pursue. The pursuit of multiple, rather than single goals, may be a complex task for individuals as they try to manage multiple concerns [26]. When multiple goals are important, each important goal is assumed to drive the activation of concepts in memory that are relevant to a given goal. Thus, the greater the number of goals that are deemed important, the greater the diversity and number of activated concepts that will be afforded prominence throughout an interaction. The need to pursue several goals should drive speakers to attempt to realize all of their important concerns within messages. As such, Samp and Solomon [26] observed that when multiple compatible goals are important, speakers enact longer messages than when singular concerns are important. Further, the information contained in messages is more redundant, as speakers attempt to highlight information relevant to important goals.

Difficulty in goal attainment may occur as individuals attempt to communicate their intentions as well. For example, Roloff and colleagues [33, 34] argued that resistance from another increases the difficulty of realizing influence goals. Samp and Solomon observed that communicators faced with disagreeable or difficult partners respond by enacting longer messages in order to increase the likelihood of goal achievement despite opposition. Thus, both situational contexts and conversational partners can make goals more or less difficult to achieve.

A health-care practitioner can facilitate a client overcoming the difficultly associated with the pursuit of a difficult goal by acknowledging and exploring the complexity and the moral dilemmas that the individual responsible for transmitting information may be experiencing. For example, Jane may be overwhelmed by the responsibility of informing more distant relatives when she is coming to terms with her own diagnosis and the impact on her immediate family. Feelings of guilt and blame may affect family relationships and hinder communication about genetic risk [16]. Furthermore, in studies of HBOC families, psychological defense mechanisms such as denial have been suggested as strategies employed by men to minimize the emotional impact of the risk to themselves and their daughters [35]. The practitioner could explore feelings and thought processes as well as strategies for alleviating this burden by possibly employing other key family members to support information sharing within the family, such as Jane's sister Wendy.

PLANNING TO PURSUE GOALS VIA COMMUNICATION

No matter the type of goal or collection of goals pursued, goal-relevant knowledge must be available in one's memory to guide the process of goal pursuit. Goal-plan-action theories commonly assume that goals stimulate planning processes designed for goal achievement [9]. *Plans* are purely cognitive; they reflect information amassed in memory about the preconditions, contingencies, and actions that may facilitate goal pursuit and achievement [9, 36]. Our knowledge of plans may come from a variety of sources, including our own prior experiences, observing how others have pursued goals, imagining hypothetical interactions, or following recommendations from others [9]. *Planning* refers to the psychological and communication processes involved in recalling, generating, selecting, implementing, modifying, and negotiating plans [10]. While planning how to implement a goal occurs to some extent before an interaction [9], quite a bit of planning occurs during an interaction as participants define and negotiate their plans together [37].

Just as there are a variety of goals, so too are there many types of plans that vary in specificity, complexity, and difficulty. Complex plans include more actions, more diversity or behavior, and more contingencies than simple plans [38]. Such multifaceted plans may have their benefits. For example, Waldron and Lavitt [39] found that individuals enrolled in a "welfare to work" program had more success at finding a job when their plans for their job search were specific and contained several contingencies. However, plans that are *too* complex may be a hindrance for individuals, as they may be seen as too difficult to sufficiently execute [9].

Some plans may not be appropriate for every circumstance. Read and Miller [40] suggested that plans are developed with the following considerations in mind: What goals does a situation easily afford? What are the rules and roles associated with the situation? Is the pursuit of the goal and its associated behaviors socially acceptable? In family contexts, the answers to such questions may be embedded in family norms for behavior. For example, according to Baxter, Bylund, Imes, and Scheive [41], families can be distinguished by how a family's communication environment treats the establishment and enforcement of "rules." Families high in *expressiveness* value individual decision making; therefore, parents set few rules, do little to sanction rules that are in place, and children display little compliance to rules. Families high in *structural traditionalism* emphasize conformity to the family unit and adhere to a rigid rule structure set in place by authority figures. Families high in avoidance actively seek to avoid unpleasant discussions. In a study of parental social control of adolescents' healthy lifestyle choices, Baxter et al. [41] had 164 student–parent dyads report on the family rules about healthy behavior. Their results indicated that adolescents from expressive families did not comply with family rules for healthy lifestyle choices. Thus, a "one-size-fits-all" plan cannot be applied across all families in all situations.

When planning conflicting responsibilities in disclosing genetic information, individuals may assess their family members' receptivity to the information as well as their vulnerability [19]. In addition to exploring previous experiences, health-care practitioners can generate health-related hypothetical scenarios and interactions for clients to work through planning a family interaction in a relatively "safe" environment. Hypothetical scenarios and interactions aim to explore how certain family members may react and enable the family member to prepare for a variety of possible outcomes of an interaction and develop contingency plans. Thus, using such hypothetical scenarios provides a "test run" of potential plans that may be enacted in similar circumstances. Discovering that a family member may find information to be useless, unpleasant, upsetting, or likely to be rejected should inform future attempts at sharing information with family members [43].

STRIVING, MONITORING, AND REVISING
GOALS AND PLANS

Of course, we are not always conscious of our goals and plans. In some instances, people may behave without any clear goal in mind [44]. This is often the case in routine interactions. While we may not think about our goals and plans all of the time, we have a frequent, although fleeting, awareness of our goals and plans during conversations [45]. For example, Wilson, Morgan, Hayes, Bylund, and Herman [46] had 42 mothers recall a 10-minute play interaction with one of their young children. Of the over 2000 thoughts recalled, over 21% involved goals, plans, or obstacles. Further, goals embedded in routine behaviors may also rise to consciousness when there is a disruption to the status quo.

Challenges to Goals and Plans

While individuals may be able to engage in goal pursuit and achievement with relative ease, some goal pursuit is frequently challenged, or even thwarted. Sometimes goals are thwarted when individuals realize that goal pursuit is not proceeding satisfactorily [37]. However, goal pursuit may also be challenged during an interaction with another. As noted earlier, Roloff and colleagues [33, 34] observed that resistance from another increases the difficulty of realizing influence goals. In a study of the interactions of 49 romantically involved couples, Keck and Samp [23] observed that individuals moved from pursuing relationally oriented goals when conversational partners acted self-interested and less relationally oriented. Applying this finding to the context of disclosing genetic information suggests that those who talk with family members in a pro-relational fashion that acknowledges the needs of the family or the conversational partner will only be effective in pursuing such messages when their intentions are acknowledged and reciprocated by the conversational partner. If a family member responds to a pro-family message with a focus on his or her own interests, integrative family-oriented efforts will fail, as those faced with a perceived rejection of relational efforts often turn to focus on their own needs. Other research suggests that the experience of having a conversational partner block a goal-related plan encourages individuals to focus on their own needs, at the expense of a conversational partner [26]. Applying these findings to the case study, suppose that Jane pursues a plan that focuses on the needs of her family above her own concerns. In the process of acting on her plan to protect the family from her "bad news," her husband emphatically states that he believes that all of the family should be informed about the HBOC risk—even Jane's sister-in-law. Faced with a husband who does not agree with Jane's plan, it is likely that Jane will then focus on her own needs in order to protect herself from the "threat" presented by her husband's opposing view. Tensions may also arise between Jane and her husband if they hold different views about when children should be told of their risk [47].

When a goal or plan is challenged, there are several potential outcomes. First, an individual may continue a current plan of action toward goal pursuit. Second, an individual may increase his or her efforts in pursuing that goal. Alternatively, an individual may temporarily disengage from goal pursuit, or abandon that goal altogether [20]. Berger [48–50] conducted a series of studies in which individuals' plans were experimentally disrupted. This research has found that when individuals possess plans that anticipate potential failures and specify contingent actions, these persons are able to move more quickly to the pursuit of alternative plans compared to those who did not anticipate objections. Further, Berger's research has identified that when faced with the need to revise a plan, individuals are more likely to revise specific, lower level plan-related behaviors rather than general "plans for action" because specific plan alterations require less cognitive demand than revising more general plan elements. Berger labeled this pattern the "hierarchy principle" and suggests that when attempting to disclose information to others, individuals should at least initially persist in the pursuit of a general plan by revising more specific components of a plan. For example, in Jane's attempt to inform her eldest child about her *BRCA* gene results, she may pursue a plan that involves an indirect approach to revealing her mutation-positive *BRCA* gene results, such as discussing a family friend's recent *BRCA* genetic diagnosis. If it becomes clear to Jane that her daughter does not understand why she is discussing her friend's diagnosis, the hierarchy principle suggests that Jane will not abandon her plan to inform her daughter of the *BRCA* diagnosis; rather, Jane will select another means of sharing her information.

In short, it is important for health-care practitioners to recognize that individuals may have multiple goals. Previous experiences and the communicative interaction influence the plans employed for goal attainment. One of the main findings in the literature on the disclosure of genetic risk information is that disclosure is not a distinct event; rather, it is a process that involves distinct phases over time [5, 51] That the goals, plans, and actions to communicate about genetic risk information can unfold during an unlimited timeframe with unanticipated results suggest that follow-up counseling sessions may be needed to facilitate the diffusion of information within a family and to help to identify and overcome communication barriers.

CONCLUSION

Many complexities constrain the disclosure of genetic risk information. Goal-plan-action sequence can provide a theoretical framework in which to explore such complexities. Given the multifaceted nature of the disclosure process, it is hard to make practical universal recommendations for health-care practitioners. Nonetheless, by understanding the processes that underpin the disclosure process, practitioners may be able to address genetic risk disclosure issues associated with family communication. Some key practice points are presented in Table 10.1. Certainly, future

Table 10.1 Key Practice Points

Assessing Goal-Related Processes
- Identify those family members at risk.
- Explore motivations for information sharing.
- Identify important concerns (goals) and less important concerns about communicating.
- Identify multiple concerns that may constrain communication.
- Identify possible conflicts of roles or responsibilities.
- Provide literature for the diagnosed and or relatives.
- Identify other key family individuals who may help with dissemination.

Assessing Planning-Related Processes
- Explore individual experiences with the condition.
- Explore previous experiences of information disclosure with the family.
- Identify existing family norms for communication.
- Explore the perceived options that the client views for managing genetic risk information.
- Identify how the client will respond to roadblocks in disclosure and/or misunderstandings.

Assisting with Ongoing Support and Management
- Offer contact or appointments with relatives to facilitate communication.
- Encourage flexibility in communication options.
- Explore hypothetical interactions to facilitate the communication process.
- Schedule multiple sessions to review progress on feelings about and reactions to the disclosure process.

research is required to elucidate goal-directed activity and planning processes within family communication, and in particular, in situations focusing on health issues within the family. Practitioners can address some of the issues associated with family communication within the theoretical framework of GPA. In particular, they can specifically address potential goal conflicts, assist with the planning stages of disclosure, and support the ongoing management of this genetic risk information within the family. Helping people understand their motivations, intentions, and plans for managing genetic information has the potential to benefit both the individual faced with managing genetic information, as well as the broad network of members within the fabric of a family.

REFERENCES

1. Koerner AF. Social cognition in family communication. In: Roskos-Ewoldsen DR, Monahan JL, eds. *Communication and Social Cognition: Theories and Methods*. Mahwah, NJ: Erlbaum; 2007:197–216.
2. Kellermann K. Communication: Inherently strategic and primarily automatic. *Communication Monographs* 1992;58:288–300.
3. Dillard JP, Segrin C, Harden JM. Primary and secondary goals in the production of interpersonal influence messages. *Communication Monographs* 1989;56:19–38.

4. Dillard JP. A goal-driven model of interpersonal influence. In: Dillard JP, ed. *Seeking Compliance: The Production of Interpersonal Influence Messages*. Scottsdale, AZ: Gorsuch Scarisbrick; 1990:41–56.

5. Clarke S, Butler K, Esplen MJ. The phases of disclosing BRCA1/2 genetic information to offspring. *Psycho-oncology* 2008;17(8):797–803.

6. Smith KR, Zick CD, Mayer RN, Botkin JR. Voluntary disclosure of BRCA1 mutation test results. *Genetic Testing* 2002;6(2):89–92.

7. McConkie –Rosell A, DeVellis B. Threat to parental role: A possible mechanism of altered self-concept related to carrier knowledge. *Journal of Genetic Counseling* 2000;9:285–302.

8. Dillard JP. Goals-plans-action theory of message production: Making influence messages. In: Baxter LA, Braithwaite DO, eds. *Engaging Theories in Interpersonal Communication: Multiple Perspectives*. Thousand Oaks CA: Sage; 2008:65–76.

9. Berger CR. *Planning Strategic Interaction: Attaining Goals through Communicative Action*. Mahwah, NJ: Erlbaum; 1997.

10. Wilson SR. *Seeking and Resisting Compliance: Why People Say What They Do When Trying to Influence Others*. Thousand Oaks, CA: Sage; 2002.

11. Wilson SR, Morgan WM. Goals-plans-action theories: Theories of goals, plans, and planning processes in families. In: Braithwaite DO, Baxter LA, eds. *Engaging Theories in Family Communication: Multiple Perspectives*. Thousand Oaks, CA: Sage; 2006:66–81.

12. MacDonald DJ, Sarna L, Giger JN, Servellen GV, Bastani R, Weitzel JN. Comparison of Latina and non-Latina White women's beliefs about communicating genetic cancer risk to relatives. *Journal of Health Communication* 2008;13(5):465–479.

13. Forrest K, Simpson SA, Wilson BJ, Teijlingen EV, Mckee L, Haites N, et al. To tell or not to tell: Barriers and facilitators in family communication about genetic risk. *Clinical Genetics* 2003;64(4):317.

14. Hughes C, Lerman C, Schwartz M, Peshkin BN, Wenzel L, Narod S, et al. All in the family: Evaluation of the process and content of sisters communication about BRCA1 and BRCA2 genetic test results. *American Journal of Medical Genetics* 2002;107:143–150.

15. Keenan KF, Simpson SA, Wilson BJ, et al. 'It's their blood not mine': Who's responsible for (not) telling relatives about risk? *Health, Risk, and Society* 2005;7:209–226.

16. Wilson BJ, Forrest K, van Teijlingen ER, McKee L, Haites N, Matthews E, et al. Family communication about genetic risk: The little that is known. *Community Genetics* 2004;7:15–24.

17. Foster C, Watson M, Moynihan C, et al. Genetic testing for breast and ovarian cancer pre- disposition: Cancer burden and responsibility. *Journal of Health Psychology* 2002;7:469–484.

18. Tercyak KP, Hughes C, Main D, et al. Parental communication of BRCA1/2 genetic test results to children. *Patient Education Counseling* 2001;42:213–224.

19. Cox SM, Mckellin, W. There's this thing in our family: Predictive testing and the social construction of risk for Huntington disease. *Sociology of Health and Illness* 1999;21(5):622–646.

20. Bandura A. Self-regulation of motivation and action through internal standards. In: Pervin LA, ed. *Goal Concepts in Personality and Social Psychology.* Hillsdale, NJ: Lawrence Erlbaum Associates; 1989:19–85.

21. Kuhl, J. Volitional mediators of cognition-behavior consistency: Self-regulator processes and action versus state orientation. In: Kuhl J, Beckmann J, eds. *Action Control: From Cognition to Behavior.* New York: Springer-Verlag; 1985:101–128.

22. Maes S, Gebhardt W. Self-regulation and health behavior: The health behavior goal model. In: Boekaerts M, Pintrich P, Zeider M, eds. *Handbook of Self-regulation.* San Diego, CA: Academic Press; 2000:343–368.

23. Bandura A, Cervone D. Self-evaluative and self-efficacy mechanisms governing the motivational effects of goal systems. *Journal of Personality and Social Psychology* 1983;45:1017–1028.

24. Samp JA, Solomon DH. Communicative responses to problematic events in close relationships II. *Communication Research* 1999;26(2):193.

25. Srull TK, Wyer RS. The role of chronic and temporary goals in social information processing. In: Sorrentino RM, Higgins ET, eds. *Handbook of Motivation and Cognition.* New York: Guliford Press; 1986:503–549.

26. Samp JA, Solomon DH. Toward a theoretical account of goal characteristics in micro-level message features. *Communication Monographs* 2005;72(1):22–45.

27. Gollwitzer PM. Goal achievement: The role of intentions. In: Stroebe W, Hewstone M, eds. *European Review of Social Psychology* (Vol. 4). London: John Wiley & Sons; 1993:141–185.

28. Keck KL, Samp JA. The dynamic nature of goals and message production as revealed in a sequential analysis of conflict interactions. *Human Communication Research* 2007;33(1):27–47.

29. Cody MJ, Canary DJ, Smith, SW. Compliance-gaining goals: An inductive analysis of actor's goal types, strategies, and successes. In: Wiemann J, Daly J, eds. *Communicating Strategically.* Hillsdale NJ: Lawrence Erlbaum Associates; 1994:33–90.

30. Dillard JP, Shen L, Laxova A, Farrell P. Potential threats to the effective communication of genetic risk information: The case of cystic fibrosis. *Health Communication* 2008;23(3):234–244.

31. Ford ME. *Motivation Humans: Goals, Emotions, and Personal Agency Beliefs.* Newbury Park, CA: Sage; 1992.

32. Austin JT, Vancouver JB. Goal constructs in psychology: structure, process, and content. *Psychological Bulletin* 1996;120(3):338.

33. Roloff ME, Janiszewski CA. Overcoming obstacles to interpersonal compliance: A principle of message construction. *Human Communication Research* 1989;16:33–61.

34. Roloff ME, Janiszewski CA, McGrath MA, Burns CS, Manrai LA. Acquiring resources from intimates: When obligation substitutes for persuasion. *Human Communication Research* 1988;14:364–396.

35. McAllister MF, Gareth D, Evans R, Ormiston W, Daly P. Men in breast cancer families: A preliminary qualitative study of awareness and experience. *Journal of Medical Genetics* 1998;35:739–744.

36. Wilensky R. *Planning and Understanding: A Conceptual Approach to Human Reasoning.* Reading, MA: Addison-Wesley; 1983.

37. Waldron VR. Toward a theory of interactive conversational planning. In: Greene JO, ed. *Message Production: Advances in Communication Theory.* Mahwah, NJ: Lawrence Erlbaum Associates; 1997:195–220.

38. Berger CR, Bell RA. Plans and the initiation of social relationships. *Human Communication Research* 1988;15:217–235.

39. Waldron VR, Lavitt MR. "Welfare-to-work": Assessing communication competencies and client outcomes in a job training program. *Southern Communication Journal* 2000;66(1):1.

40. Read SJ, Miller LC. Inter-personalism: Toward a goal-based theory of persons in relationships. In: Pervin LA, ed. *Goal Concepts in Personality and Social Psychology.* Hillsdale, NJ: Lawrence Erlbaum Associates; 1989:413–472.

41. Baxter LA, Bylund CL, Imes RS, Scheive DM. Family communication environments and rule-based social control of adolescents' healthy lifestyle choices. *Journal of Family Communication* 2005;5(3):209–227.

42. Hamilton RJ, Bowers BJ, Williams JK. Disclosing genetic test results to family members. *Journal of Nursing Scholarship* 2005;37:18–24.

43. Claes E, Evers-Kiebooms G, Boogaerts A, Decruyenaere M, Denayer L, Legius E. Communication with close and distant relatives in the context of genetic counseling for hereditary breast and ovarian cancer in cancer patients. *American Journal of Medical Genetics* 2003;116A:11–19.

44. Langer E. *Mindfulness.* Reading, MA: Addison-Wesley; 1989.

45. Greene, JO. Evanescent mentation: An ameliorative conceptual foundation for research theory and message production. *Communication Theory* 2000;10:138–155.

46. Wilson S, Morgan W, Hayes J, Bylund C, Herman A. Mother's child abuse potential as a predictor of maternal and child behaviors during play-time interactions. *Communication Monographs* 2004;71(4):395–421.

47. Peterson SK, Watts BG, Koehly LM, Vernon SW, Baile WF, Kohlmann WK. How families communicate about HNPCC genetic testing: findings from a qualitative study. *American Journal of Medical Genetics* 2003;119C:78–86.

48. Berger CR. Processing quantitative data about risk and threat in news reports. *The Journal of Communication* 1998;48(3):87–106.

49. Berger CR, Karol SH, Jordan JM. When a lot of knowledge is a dangerous thing: The debilitating effects of plan complexity on verbal fluency. *Human Communication Research* 2006;16(1):91–119.

50. Berger CR, Knowlton SW, Abrahams MF. The hierarchy principle in strategic communication. *Communication Theory* 1996;6:111–142.

51. Gaff CL, Collins V, Symes T, Halliday, J. Facilitating family communication about predictive genetic testing: Proband's perceptions. *Journal of Genetic Counseling* 2005;14(2):133–150.

11

FAMILY COMMUNICATION PATTERNS

Ascan F. Koerner, Bonnie LeRoy, & Pat McCarthy Veach

Editors' Note: Similar to earlier chapters, a theoretical approach to family communication—Family Communication Patterns—is presented here. However, the authors add novelty by also considering how family communication patterns can affect different aspects of the counseling process. A model of genetic counseling, the Reciprocal Engagement Model (REM) [1], forms the foundation for describing how genetic counselors can work effectively with patients and families with different communication patterns. Although the REM is a model of genetic counseling, many of its tenets have relevance to other health-care practitioners, and awareness of Family Communication Patterns is likely to be helpful to a broad spectrum of practitioners.

For communication to be successful, the participants need to assign similar meaning to each others' messages and behaviors. In families, shared understanding is affected by the degree of openness and frequency of communication (conversation orientation) and the extent to which authority shapes meaning (conformity orientation). The resulting family communication patterns affect interactions with health-care practitioners, as well as many family processes. Insight into these patterns can lead to strategies to work more effectively with different family types.

THE RECIPROCAL ENGAGEMENT
MODEL OF GENETIC COUNSELING

Historically, two predominant models describing genetic counseling practice are the "education" model and the "counseling" model [1]. Recently, a new model has been developed based on ideas generated during a consensus meeting of genetic counseling program directors in North America. The Reciprocal Engagement Model (REM) [2] includes elements of both education and counseling and describes how these elements mutually interact within the genetic counselor–patient(s) relationship. The model includes many aspects of the education and counseling model but provides the bigger picture of the genetic counseling process. According to the REM model, "Genetic counselors contextualize scientific facts within the intrapersonal, interpersonal, and cultural identities of a given patient and her or his family…" [2]. Five *tenets* form the basis of the REM model:

Tenet 1: *Genetic information is key.* Genetic counseling involves a unique content, namely, provision of genetic knowledge intended to inform patients. Genetic counselors generally believe that "being informed is better than being uniformed" [2]. They must determine which information is most pertinent for a given patient and also how to communicate that information in a way that is comprehensible and useful for the patient and family members. A major goal of this tenet is that "patient family dynamics are understood by counselors and patients" [2]. An understanding of family dynamics helps the genetic counselor determine how best to share appropriate information with various family members.

Tenet 2: *Relationship is integral to genetic counseling.* The relationship formed between the patient and genetic counselor is the conduit for information provision and decision making. One goal for realizing this tenet is that genetic counselors know "how to intervene in order to build rapport and foster communication" [2]. Communication occurs between the genetic counselor and patient, the counselor and family members, and patient and family members. Genetic counselors strive to maintain open and honest communication among all of these parties. Within sessions, they may provide feedback regarding the flow of communication and any perceived communication barriers. There is the recognition that respecting individual autonomy involves helping patients understand how a decision is affected by and has an effect on the family.

Tenet 3: *Patient autonomy must be supported.* This tenet derives from a belief that patients know best what they should do. Genetic counselors value family contexts—family values and practices—and they attempt to work to the extent possible within each patient's family context. Genetic counselors strive to promote individual- and family-directed decisions. In order to achieve these goals, genetic counselors must assess and understand each patient's family dynamics and respect family members' varying perspectives. Genetic counselors adopt a collaborative role with patients and families but do not determine decision outcomes.

Tenet 4: *Patients are resilient.* Genetic counselors assume that most patients and families have the requisite strength to hear and use genetic information to make difficult decisions. Therefore, it is important that genetic counselors acknowledge patient/family strengths, help patients and families adapt to their situation, and encourage them to draw upon coping strategies that have worked for them in prior crisis situations.

Tenet 5: *Patient emotions make a difference.* Affect is an influential force in patients' and their family members' communication and decision-making processes. Genetic counselors aim to assess patients' and family members' emotional responses and help them understand how their feelings influence their decisions.

According to the REM model, genetic counselors tailor their approaches to various families by considering four basic questions: *(1)* What do the person and family members know? *(2)* What do the person and family members think and feel about the information I am presenting? *(3)* How might the person and family members use this information to make decisions, manage a condition, and/or cope with their situation? and *(4)* How do my own values, biases, feelings, and previous experiences affect both my communication of information to all involved parties and the nature and quality of the relationship I establish with them?

THE CENTRALITY OF FAMILY IN GENETIC COUNSELING

Despite its inherent focus on family, a defining characteristic of genetic counseling is that it is grounded in an individual-centered Western medical view of the counseling and decision-making process. This view assumes that the patient makes sense of her or his medical situation and decisions about the course of action largely as an independent person. This view is consistent with much of Western psychological counseling and medical traditions with their focus on individual health and individual privacy and autonomy. An individualistic perspective, however, is inconsistent with the large body of research that describes "sense making" as a social phenomenon [3] as well as research showing that actual behavior and behavioral intention are affected by those around us, and especially close others

[4]. The reality is this: it is not possible to talk to a person about genetics without talking about family.

The REM discussed above represents at least a partial departure from this individual-centered view of counseling in that it recognizes the importance of the counselor–patient relationship in the counseling process (tenet 2). Further, it explicitly acknowledges that individuals are members of families and that how they think and feel about the information provided in genetic counseling is affected by their family relationships (tenet 1). As such, family members are recognized as participants rather than mere bystanders in the counseling process. It therefore follows that genetic counselors should take the family and family dynamics into consideration when preparing for and conducting genetic counseling. What the REM does not provide, however, is an explication of what counselors need to know about the family and family dynamics that are most likely to affect counseling processes and outcomes. To provide exactly this type of information is the purpose of the remainder of this chapter. First, we will describe a theory of family communication that addresses both sense making and decision making in families. Then we will delineate how family communication affects each of the five tenets of the REM, and finally, we will give examples of how genetic counseling may play out in families that have different communication styles.

FAMILY COMMUNICATION PATTERNS THEORY

Human communication is a symbolic activity. This means that the connection between a symbol (e.g., word or gesture) and its meaning relies on the consensus of the people using the symbols rather than being the result of some inherent quality of the symbol itself. As a result, the meaning of words and gestures is forever fluid and changing, and the meaning of messages and behaviors is inherently ambiguous. This fluidity forces communicators to assign meaning by making assumptions about themselves, others, and their relationships, as well as about the social context in which an interaction takes place. Thus, for communication to be successful, communicators must be able to assign similar meaning to each others' messages and behaviors; that is, they need to share a social reality, or at least understand each other's.

One theory that is built around the notion that families create a shared social reality and that links specific communication behaviors in families to a wide range of family and child outcomes is Family Communication Patterns Theory [5–10]. This theory is based on the assumption that creating a shared social reality is the most basic function of family interactions, that a shared social reality is necessary for families to function, and that the ways in which families establish shared social reality define family relationships. According to Family Communication Patterns Theory, families create a shared reality through two communication behaviors: conversation orientation and conformity orientation, which also define families' communication patterns. Conversation orientation refers to open and frequent communication between parents and children with the purpose of co-discovering the meaning of symbols and objects that constitute social reality. This orientation is associated with warm and supportive relationships characterized by mutual respect and concern for one another. Conformity orientation, in contrast, refers to more restricted communication between parents and children in which those in authority, typically the parents, define the meaning of things, and thus social reality, for the family. This orientation is associated with more authoritarian parenting and less concern for the children's thoughts and feelings.

Theoretically orthogonal, these two orientations define a conceptual space with four family types. Consensual families are high on both conversation orientation and conformity orientation. Their communication is characterized by a tension between interest in open communication and in exploring new ideas on the one hand, and pressure to agree and to preserve the existing hierarchy of the family on the other hand. Family members resolve this tension by listening to one another but also explaining one's own values and beliefs with the expectation that other family members will adopt one's belief system. Members of these families are usually well adapted and satisfied with their family relationships.

Pluralistic families favor conversation orientation over conformity orientation. Their communication is characterized by open, unconstrained discussions that involve all family members and a wide range of topics. Family members do not feel the need to control one another and accept differences of opinion, although they also explain their own values and beliefs to others. Family members tend to be independent and autonomous and to communicate persuasively, and they generally are satisfied with their family relationships.

Protective families emphasize conformity over conversation orientation. Their communication is characterized by an emphasis on obedience to authority and by little concern for conceptual matters. Those in authority, usually a parent, decide for other family members and see little value in explaining their reasoning to them. Rather, they state their beliefs and values in the form of rules and expect others to follow them. Family members learn to place little value on family conversations and to distrust their own decision-making ability. As a consequence, they often are very susceptible to influence by authority figures, such as doctors and counselors.

Laissez-faire families are low on both conformity and conversation orientation and as a result do not always share a social reality. Their communication is characterized by few, usually uninvolving interactions. Members of laissez-faire families are emotionally distant from one another, and they have little interest in the thoughts and feeling of other family members. Family members learn that there is little value in family conversation and that they have to make their own decisions. Because they do not receive much support from family members, they come to question their decision-making ability and also are susceptible to influence from outside the family.

Family communication patterns have been associated with a number of family processes, such as conflict resolution [11], confirmation and affection [12], family rituals [13], and understanding [14], as well as with child-related outcomes, such as communication apprehension [15], conflict with romantic partners [11], resiliency [16], children's mental and physical health [17], and externalization of adopted children [18].

FAMILY COMMUNICATION PATTERNS AND THE RECIPROCAL ENGAGEMENT MODEL

Because family relationships are usually the most intimate and most enduring interpersonal relationships people have, the ways in which families communicate internally affect the sense and decision making of an individual and the extent to which family members are part of the decision-making process. That is, family communication patterns affect both the counselor–client relationship and client decision making and consequently should be taken into consideration during genetic counseling. To explicate the impact of family communication patterns on genetic counseling, it helps to take another look at the five tenets describing the counseling process outlined in the REM and to consider how they are affected by family communication patterns.

The first REM tenet states that genetic information is central to the genetic counseling process. Thus, the "what" and "how" of genetic counseling are driven to a large extent by the information that counselors provide and the realities and probabilities of genetics. An assumption about this genetic information on which the whole counseling process rests, but that is usually unstated, is that the information is objectively true and that the person understands the information and believes it to be true. This assumption, however, fails to consider the fact that families construe their own social reality, which might be less influenced by objective medical facts than by internal family processes and relationships.

For example, a genetic test might establish a parent as a carrier of a certain gene mutation and the objective probability of passing on that copy of the gene to any given child is 50%. Yet for family members, accepting the idea that the parent could carry that gene mutation, much less pass it on to his or her child, is inconceivable, because it fundamentally violates the role that the parent has in the family as protector and provider. In other words, this information is inconsistent with the social reality of that family and accepting it would require family members to change their belief systems about their most central relationships. In such cases, it is much easier for the patient to ignore or to discount the "objectively true" information provided by the practitioner. Similarly, some families generally do not regard outside sources of information, such as health-care practitioners and medical tests, as truthful and reliable. Rather, they rely on the family or specific family members to determine the accuracy and meaning of information they receive from the outside. In such circumstances, a consultation based on the assumption that the patient shares the same reality with the practitioner might not be very successful, because the practitioner operates in a reality fundamentally different from that of the patient.

Family communication patterns affect how families create the social reality in which they operate. Conversation orientation is associated with an open engagement of the external world and the willingness to evaluate outside sources of information based on the quality of their arguments. It is also linked to warmer, more cohesive, and more supportive familial relationships and families that confront, rather than isolate themselves from, outside challenges. In short, families high in conversation orientation are likely to accept information provided by health-care practitioners and to share social reality with them. Conformity orientation, by contrast, is associated with a more internal focus when engaging the external world and less willingness to critically engage external information. Although generally obedient to authority figures, information provided by outside sources needs to be interpreted and/or validated by family authorities. As such, the influence outsiders have on families is mediated by authority figures within the family. In short, although families high in conformity orientation are likely to comply with practitioners' requests, ironically they are also more likely to operate in a social reality divergent from that of the practitioner.

The second REM tenet states that relationships are integral to the counseling process, including those between patient and counselor and between patient and the patient's family. Both of these relationships are affected by family communication patterns. This is obvious for family relationships, whose closeness, warmth, openness, and the mutual influence that family members have over one another are determined by how they communicate with one another. Less obvious, but equally important, is the effect that family communication patterns have on relationships with outsiders, such as counselors and other health-care practitioners. Not only do family communication patterns affect how family members regard outsiders and the information they provide, but they also influence the type of relationship they have with them.

For example, persons with families that are high in conversation orientation are used to discussing and exploring the meaning of things with others. They view facts presented to them as well as the opinions of others about these facts as information they can use to arrive at their own understanding of the situation. These people are most likely to perceive the genetic counselor as a partner in the decision-making process and are most persuaded by facts and evidence. Individuals stemming from families high in conformity orientation, by contrast, are less experienced in making sense of facts and other information through discussion. They are, however, attuned to how those in authority interpret information. Depending on whether their family is open or closed, they are most likely to either perceive the counselor or other health-care practitioner as an authority figure to be followed or as an outsider to be mistrusted. In either case, practitioners who structure their sessions based on an assumption that their relationship is that of a socially equal provider of information will be much more effective with people from conversation-oriented families as opposed to those from conformity-oriented families.

The effects of family communication patterns on the third REM tenet, that patients are autonomous decision makers, is similar to the tenet concerning relationship between counselor and patient. Both in regard to their relationship with the counselor and with their families, people from high conversation-oriented families are fairly autonomous in their decision making. They will be clearly influenced by information and opinion from both, but they are accustomed to making decisions based on the quality of arguments rather than the social status of others. Regardless of their conversation orientation, however, people from families high in conformity orientation are used to orienting themselves toward, and adopting the views of, those in authority. Given the medical context in which genetic counseling usually takes place, the counselor is often perceived to be such an authority. Despite the counselor viewing patients as autonomous decision makers, patients might very well perceive themselves as subordinate and therefore motivated to comply with what they think the counselors want them to do.

The fourth REM tenet, that patients are resilient, also is affected by family communication patterns. Specifically, research [16] has shown that families high in conversation orientation are more flexible in adapting to changes in their circumstances and therefore are much more resilient than families low in conversation orientation. Thus, while it is probably true that all individuals and their families display some resilience in their adaptation to illness and disease, some are much more resourceful and resilient than others. Counselors capable of recognizing which families are more versus less resilient are more likely to provide genetic counseling effectively.

Finally, the last REM tenet, that patient affect is relevant in the counseling process, also is influenced by family communication patterns. People from families high in conversation orientation are more open about their emotions and are generally more responsive to their family members' emotional needs. Consequently they are better at realizing, expressing, and discussing their own emotions. Members of these families are also attuned to each other's emotional needs and willing and capable of providing and receiving emotional support. People from families high in conformity orientation, by contrast, have learned to express their emotions in ways that do not upset the family hierarchy. For most family members, this means that they are not very practiced at expressing emotions, in particular negative affect and distress. They also are not very accustomed to providing and using emotional support. They are very good, however, at masking their true affect and appearing composed and in control, even when their internal emotional experience is quite upsetting. Consequently, health-care

Table 11.1   Communication and Decision Making in the Four Different Family Types

Consensual (high conversation orientation, high conformity orientation)
Family communication is open, warm, supportive, and cohesive. The family is open to the outside and enjoys making new experiences. Decision making is collaborative and involves all family members. Families like to come to a consensus that takes everyone's positions into account. The interest of the family as a group is of the highest priority. Problems are solved by creating unique solutions based on all available evidence.

Pluralistic (high conversation orientation, low conformity orientation)
Family communication is open, warm, and supportive of individual differences. The family is open to the outside and enjoys making new experiences. Decision making is individualized and based primarily on the concerns of those directly affected. Group decisions are often based on majorities, not necessarily consensus. The concerns of the individuals are of the highest priority. Problems are solved by creating unique solutions based on all available evidence.

Protective (low conversation orientation, high conformity orientation)
Family communication is restricted and not particularly warm and supportive. The family is suspicious of outside influences and does not enjoy changes in their customs and habits. Decisions are made by family members in authority (parent or grandparent), but all family members are expected to comply with the decision. The interests of the family as a group are of the highest priority. Problems are usually solved by relying on social rules and norms or the counsel of authority figures.

Laissez-faire (low conversation orientation, low conformity orientation)
Family communication is restricted and often characterized by a disinterest or emotional coldness toward others. The family is not very cohesive, and family members are often unaware of what others are doing and how they feel. Decisions are made usually by individuals in isolation from other family members. The interests of individuals are of the highest priority. Problems are usually avoided, but if action has to be taken, it is often based on advice stemming from outside the family.

practitioners have to realize that people have varied emotional responses and also vary in how they communicate their affect. Those who understand the family communication backgrounds of their patients will be better equipped to evaluate how patients may display and manage affect.

ASSESSING FAMILY COMMUNICATION PATTERNS

In research, Family communication patterns usually are assessed with questionnaires or through observation. Given the time constraints of health-care consultations, such assessment is impractical. Nonetheless, because people are usually quite aware of how their families communicate, it is possible to arrive at a reasonable assessment of their family types through a few pointed questions about who is in their families and how they communicate with one another. Alternatively, people might be given brief descriptions of each family type and asked to identify their own family (see Table 11.1). Equipped with this information, health-care practitioners can use their knowledge of how family communication patterns affect sense making and decision making to conduct their sessions to match each individual's communication style.

Illustrative Cases

We conclude this chapter with four hypothetical cases demonstrating the effects of family communication patterns on the genetic counseling process. In each case, family communication patterns affect how individuals and their families approach genetic testing and the role that they allow the counselor to play in their decision making. By adapting their approaches to the particular family communication patterns, genetic counselors are able to provide counseling consistent with their professional obligations and enable their patients to make decisions optimal to their needs and circumstances.

Case Study 1: Consensual Family

Jeff and Julie come to neurology clinic with their first child, 5-year-old Robbie. Robbie recently started showing signs of muscle weakness. The neurologist, suspecting Duchenne muscular dystrophy (DMD) based on examination and the pediatrician's clinic notes, orders genetic testing. Inherited in an X-linked recessive fashion, DMD is a severe disorder, meaning that if confirmed, Julie is at risk for being a carrier and if so, all of her sons, but not daughters, are at a 50% percent risk of being affected. Her daughters are at a 50% of being carriers. Moreover, Julie's sisters and other maternal family members may also be at risk for having affected sons. Affected children are likely to be wheelchair bound by early adolescence and to die in early adulthood.

During counseling, Robbie's parents appear appropriately concerned, sit close together, and are supportive of each other's comments. They look at each other a lot and occasionally joke to release tension. Both parents have called their respective families to gather family medical history information and are able to use this information to answer all of the genetic counselor's questions. To their knowledge, no one in their families had been diagnosed with a neuromuscular disease, and their families were waiting to hear from them after the visit today. The discussion indicates that Jeff, Julie, and Robbie have the support of a loving family.

In the context of the consensual family communication pattern, the genetic counselor's role is that of an objective information provider. Consensual families are very supportive and make their decisions collaboratively while considering information from the outside. Due to their high conformity orientation, however, there is the possibility that these families construct subjective social realities that do not correspond to objective reality. For example, in the family Jeff's father is considered the most knowledgeable family member, and he is convinced that Robbie's symptoms are due to childhood vaccinations. In this case, it is unlikely that the family will accept a solely genetic explanation of the disease. The effective counselor will involve all family members' views in the decision-making process while providing forthright and complete information about DMD, the genetics involved, and available courses of actions. Most of all, the counselor will trust the family to be resilient and to arrive at the best course of action for themselves.

Case Study 2: Pluralistic Family

Judy is a 32-year-old woman requesting chromosomal testing because she is a potential carrier of a chromosomal translocation. Her brother Joe and his wife had a premature baby that died a few weeks after birth due to a chromosome abnormality: an unbalanced reciprocal translocation. The unbalanced chromosome translocation caused the baby to have multiple birth defects, including a severe heart defect. Chromosomal testing on the baby's parents revealed that Judy's brother Joe carries a balanced translocation, which also explained a 3-year history of infertility and miscarriages that he and his wife experienced before the birth of the baby. The translocation puts Judy, her sister Sarah, as well as her parents and their extended families at risk for also carrying a translocation. Without testing, there is no way to know who is a carrier.

After learning of his condition, Joe, Judy, and their other sister Sarah sat down with their parents and discussed what this means for everyone in the family. Judy decided that she wanted to be tested because she and her husband were ready to start a family and wanted to be informed about their risk before a pregnancy. Sarah, on the other hand, decided not to pursue testing because she is not currently in a relationship. Judy's mother was undecided about testing and wanted to wait for Judy's test results before making a decision.

This open communication and independent, rational decision making is typical of pluralistic families. The genetic counselor's role is primarily as a source of objective information about genetics and the individual risks family members face. Because of their independence, family members sometimes have difficulty appreciating the consequences their actions have for other family members, so counselors should make sure that these consequences are discussed. Generally, however, this family type is the one that allows genetic counselors to act most in line with the individual-centered counseling model.

Case Study 3: Protective Family

Susan is a 25-year-old woman who is at risk for the fatal, neurodegenerative condition Huntington disease (HD). Her mother recently died of HD at age 62 after first showing symptoms at age 41. Susan's maternal grandfather, two of her maternal aunts, and one maternal uncle were all affected with the disease. Susan has two older sisters (ages 36 and 27, respectively). Neither Susan nor her sisters are symptomatic. Susan recently married and comes to genetic counseling to learn if there are any recent advances in treatment or any way to prevent having an affected child without being tested. She is interested in genetic testing, but she is afraid that her family will reject her for this decision. She is adamant that she does not want her child to suffer with this disease as have so many of her family members. Susan reports that her husband feels the same way, but he was unable to come to clinic with her. Further complicating the situation is the fact that Susan and her husband very much want a child, but they want the child to be biologically their child. They are not interested at this time in discussing the options of donor egg or adoption.

In the context of Susan's family, Susan is the baby. Susan's oldest sister, Claire, took on the maternal role for Susan and her sister as their mother's illness progressed, and she is now the matriarch of the family. Claire does not want anyone to be tested for HD because there is no treatment for the disease and she does not see the point in knowing. The sisters are very interdependent and being at risk for HD is the glue that binds them. They spend a lot of time together and talk a lot about HD, including which of them will get the disease, what it will look like, and who will care for whom. They watch their cousins and discuss who looks like they are starting to have symptoms. All three talk about dealing with whatever adversity comes their way and being there for one another.

This type of family provides the greatest challenge to genetic counselors who view the patient as an autonomous decision maker. In this particular case, the counselor needs to recognize the tremendous influence the family, and the older sister in particular, has on Susan's decision making. Given Susan's desire to start a family with her new husband and her goal of ensuring that her baby does not have the HD-causing gene, getting tested seems to be a reasonable solution for Susan. However, it has the potential to seriously disrupt her relationships with her sisters, on whom Susan depends for a large part of her identity. Consequently, for Susan there are significant social costs associated with getting tested. In addition, because of her older sister's opposition to testing and her dominant role in the family, Susan will not make a decision unless the counselor actively takes part in the decision-making process and clearly directs Susan to think through her choices.

Susan came to clinic stating that she wants a child that is genetically hers, but she does not want the child to have the gene mutation. She also stated that she is interested in testing and that the information would be useful for her but that her family would not understand this decision. In this case the counselor could be directive in asking Susan to think about what she is really saying. One approach would be for the counselor to say something like, "If you did not have to worry about the consequences of your decisions from your family, what would you do?" The counselor could then take the discussion in the direction of, "Let's talk about why you are not doing this and the consequences for you and your husband and your new family." Such a directive approach (directing what Susan needs to think through) is likely to work, because conformist families are susceptible to influence from authority figures. In this context then, the counselor in essence is pointing Susan in the direction of the decision she wants to make and providing support for that decision. Not taking a strong stance likely will result in Susan not making any decision that works for her and her reproductive goals.

To make this decision requires that the counselor accepts this responsibility and thoroughly understands all of Susan's values and the consequences of each available action. The competent counselor will explore these issues in depth during counseling sessions offer all options, including those that Susan may not have thought of such as using preimplantation genetic diagnosis with or without disclosing Susan's status, donor egg, adoption, and so on, and also provide the necessary emotional support to Susan. It is important to note here that it is possible that the greatest risk to Susan is that she will lose her identity and her family. This may be too great of a risk for her to take, but this should come out in the discussion.

Case Study 4: Laissez-Faire Family

At week 12 of their first pregnancy, Mike (38 years old) and Angie (39 years old) come to genetic counseling to discuss prenatal screening and testing options. The counselor takes the family medical history to assess genetic risks for the baby. Mike's father died of colon cancer at 42, and three other members of his paternal family had colon cancer before age 50. The family history suggests that Mike's risk for colon cancer could be as high as 50% but that also means that his baby and his siblings are at risk as well. Thus, the counselor's goals expand beyond informing about prenatal testing to include informing Mike and Angie about Mike's cancer risks.

The counseling session is characterized by very restricted communication, which is typical for laissez-faire families. Mike, who has no primary care physician and has not had a physical exam in years, has never had a colonoscopy. He is also not willing to obtain medical records to confirm the diagnosis of cancer in the family. He says his family does not talk about the cancer at all, and he believes no one is interested in talking about it. Angie knew that Mike's father had died of cancer, but she did not know about the other affected family members. When she expresses concern, Mike tells her not to worry. He says that all families have something, so this is "no big deal."

In laissez-faire families, individual family members make decisions very much autonomously from other family members but are susceptible to influence from outsiders with authority, such as the counselor. Their preferred mode of problem solving, however, is avoidance and denial. Thus, it is important to recognize that the patient is unlikely to take any action unless the genetic counselor exerts direct influence on the patient. To do so responsibly, counselors have to determine for themselves what actions might be in the best interest of the patients and their families by thoroughly discussing their values and goals with them. In particular, the counselor needs to explore with the patients how other family members likely would be affected by individual decisions, because members of these families often have difficulty considering how their behaviors affect others. In addition, given that members of laissez-faire families are poor at requesting and providing emotional support for one another, the counselor has to be a source of emotional support for family members. For this family, Mike has not considered that if he develops cancer and does not survive, his wife is a single mom and his baby does not have a father. The role of the counselor is to help Mike consider this possible outcome and strategize ways to prevent this from happening.

CONCLUSION

In this chapter, we have argued that genetic counseling as currently practiced and conceptualized in the REM is based on a view of the patient as an autonomous decision maker and that objective medical facts and probabilities comprise a major part of sessions. Although the REM acknowledges variability due to patient and counselor individual characteristics and familial and cultural backgrounds and experiences, it lacks specificity regarding the complex interplay of these factors. One salient factor concerns the extent to which genetic counselors and patients share similar social realities. We have argued that families do create their own social realities that influence how they make sense of "objective" information from the outside and how they relate to outsiders, such as genetic counselors. We have introduced Family Communication Patterns Theory as a model explaining how families make sense of their environments and how family members relate to outsiders. Furthermore, we have delineated how communication patterns define different family types—each with its own set of challenges for the counselor. Finally, we provided hypothetical examples of the type of adjustments counselors might make in their approach to counseling in order to work more effectively with members of various family types. Clearly, our recommendations are based on our theoretical understanding of how family communication and genetic counseling interact, and not on empirical evidence and applications of our model. As such, they are currently suggestions more so than recommendations. We hope, however, that we have instilled in the reader an appreciation of at least the possibility that family communication patterns play an important role in the genetic counseling process—and potentially the consultations of other health-care practitioners—and a willingness to adapt how one counsels to whom one counsels.

REFERENCES

1. Kessler S. Genetic counseling is directive? Look again. *American Journal of Human Genetics* 1997;61(2):466–467.
2. McCarthy Veach P, Bartels DM, LeRoy BS. Coming full circle: A Reciprocal-Engagement Model of genetic counseling practice. *Journal of Genetic Counseling* 2007;16:713–728.
3. Berger PL, Luckmann, T. *The Social Construction of Reality: A Treatise in the Sociology of Knowledge*. Garden City, NY: Anchor Books; 1966.
4. Cialdini RB, Trost MR. Social influence: Social norms, conformity, and compliance. In: Gilbert DT, Fiske ST, Lindzey G, eds. *The Handbook of Social Psychology* (4th ed.). Boston: McGraw-Hill; 1998:151–192.

5. Fitzpatrick MA, Ritchie LD. Communication schemata within the family: Multiple perspectives on family interaction. *Human Communication Research* 1994;20:275–301.

6. Koerner AF, Fitzpatrick MA. Toward a theory of family communication. *Communication Theory* 2002;12:70–91.

7. Koerner AF, Fitzpatrick MA. Understanding family communication patterns and family functioning: The roles of conversation orientation and conformity orientation. *Communication Yearbook* 2002;26:37–69.

8. Koerner AF, Fitzpatrick MA. Communication in intact families. In: Vangelisti A, ed. *Handbook of Family Communication.* Mahwah, NJ: Erlbaum; 2004:177–195.

9. Koerner AF, Fitzpatrick MA. Family communication patterns theory: A social cognitive approach. In: Braithwaite DO, Baxter LA, eds. *Engaging Theories in Family Communication: Multiple Perspectives.* Thousand Oaks, CA: Sage; 2006:50–65.

10. Ritchie LD, Fitzpatrick MA. Family communication patterns: Measuring interpersonal perceptions of interpersonal relationships. *Communication Research* 1990;17:523–544.

11. Koerner AF, Fitzpatrick MA. Family type and conflict: The impact of conversation orientation and conformity orientation on conflict in the family. *Communication Studies* 1997;48:59–75.

12. Schrodt P, Ledbetter AM, Ohrt JK. Parental confirmation and affection as mediators of family communication patterns and children's mental well-being. *Journal of Family Communication* 2007;7:23–46.

13. Baxter LA, Clark CL. Perceptions of family communication patterns and the enactment of family rituals. *Western Journal of Communication* 1996;60:254–268.

14. Sillars A, Koerner AF, Fitzpatrick MA. Communication and understanding in parent-adolescent relationships. *Human Communication Research* 2005;31:103–128.

15. Elwood TD, Schrader DC. Family communication patterns and communication apprehension. *Journal of Social Behavior and Personality* 1998;13:493–502.

16. Fitzpatrick MA, Koerner AF. Family communication schemata: Effects on children's resiliency. In: Dunwoody S, Becker LB, McLeod D, Kosicki G, eds. *The Evolution of Key Mass Communication Concepts: Honoring Jack M. McLeod.* Cresskill, NJ: Hampton Press; 2005:113–136.

17. Schrodt P, Ledbetter AM. Communication processes that mediate family communication patterns and mental well-being: A mean and covariance structures analysis of young adults from divorced and non-divorced families. *Human Communication Research* 2007;33:330–356.

18. Rueter MA, Koerner AF. The effect of family communication pattern on adopted adolescent adjustment. *Journal of Marriage and Family* 2008;70:715–727.

12

ETHICAL
PERSPECTIVES

SAMANTHA J. LEONARD & AINSLEY J. NEWSON

Despite the best of intentions, a person may not always share genetic information with at-risk family members. This chapter presents an ethical analysis of this situation and explores the responsibilities of health-care practitioners to help individuals share with relatives the potential health benefits arising from their consultation.

In debates over communication of genetic information within families, much existing literature has focused on the concepts of the "duty to warn" of a genetic risk and considerations of when it may be acceptable or even required to breach confidentiality [1–3]. The questions posed have tended to focus on those circumstances in which a family member has explicitly or actively refused to pass on information to a relative—so-called active nondisclosure of genetic information. Empirical research into this issue has tended to focus on professional experiences of this problem and their attitudes towards it [4, 5]. However, as research has also shown, the acute dilemma arising when a person explicitly refuses to disclose a genetic risk to relatives occurs only rarely in practice [6]. A more common and potentially more intractable problem arises when it becomes apparent that a proband has not passed on genetic information to family members, despite the best of intentions. This problem has been referred to as *passive nondisclosure* [7].

In this chapter, we present an ethical analysis of the communication of genetic information within families, as applied to the problem of passive nondisclosure. This issue gives rise to several ethical questions. For example, to whom should genetic information belong: the individual or the family? What role should clinical genetics services play in facilitating disclosure? What should be done when, instead of refusing to disclose, a person states an intention to disclose but never quite manages to do so? How can the presumption in favor of disclosing genetic information be weighed against the presumption of the "right not to know"? We tackle these questions in the following text and put forward some points for consideration in overcoming this difficult issue in practice. We focus first on clinical genetics services and then on other health-care services.

We begin by outlining a case study and describing some of the types of genetic information that can give rise to the above issues. We then outline the ethical significance of the presumption of confidentiality and how this presumption is challenged by the nature of genetic information. The health-care practitioner perspective is then discussed, followed by deliberation on some of the parameters to the debate over family communication, such as four models of ownership of genetic information, ethical issues surrounding different methods of disclosure, and the "right not to know." We conclude by suggesting some of the implications and challenges for practice that will arise if the problem of passive nondisclosure is to be resolved. Throughout this chapter, we will refer to the hypothetical case of Anne as an illustration of how the issue of passive nondisclosure can arise in practice.

Case Study

Anne is referred to the genetics service by her colorectal surgeon because she has been found to have bowel cancer in her late twenties, and her mother had died of bowel cancer in her early forties. She undergoes counseling and has genetic testing. She is found to have a mutation in the *MSH2* gene, known to cause the condition Lynch syndrome, which predisposes to bowel and other cancers. Anne has a maternal half-sister aged 17. Her mother also had an older sister who died in an accident at age 29 but who had two children who are now in their forties.

When the issue of genetic testing for her family is raised, Anne states that she will tell her half-sister and will "probably" tell her cousins, whom she does not know all that well. However, she is concerned that this may raise worries for them, and as they are in their late forties and have not yet developed cancer, she does not think they will have inherited the *MSH2* gene mutation. A year later, the service learns that Anne has not yet taken any steps toward disclosure to either her half-sister or cousins.

This scenario is illustrative of this not-uncommon problem [8]. Should we try to ensure Anne tells her half-sister and cousins, and if so how? Might her relatives be harmed through receiving this information, and how should we weigh this factor against the potential benefits this information may have? We will address these questions further, but we will first review the ethical justification for maintaining confidentiality.

CONFIDENTIALITY IN THE CLINICAL RELATIONSHIP

Under a traditional medical model of the health-care practitioner–patient relationship, Anne's decision about whether to share medical information with her family would be left up to her. All the information she gained in her consultation would be confidential, and there would be no expectation or obligation on the practitioner to ensure that relevant information reaches her relatives. However, she could decide to share this information if there was a perceived significant risk of harm to traceable relatives. This presumption of confidentiality remains a fundamental (although not absolute) principle governing modern health care. Two rationales underscore this value. First, we value our autonomy and privacy. Medical information is very personal, and maintaining control over who we share this with is an important part of our right to self-determination. Second, confidentiality is an important, if not essential, component of the practitioner–patient relationship. Patients require assurance that their information will remain confidential in order to maximize full disclosure of clinical information. If people were concerned their details might be shared, they may delay seeking medical advice or avoid it altogether. Under some circumstances it is possible to breach confidentiality, but the applicability of these to passive nondisclosure of genetic risk is uncertain.

There can be little doubt that some form of recognizable ethical code governing confidentiality is vital for the formation of a practitioner–patient relationship, but how far does (and should) such a code extend? Some have argued that confidentiality is an absolute obligation, which must not be transgressed in any circumstances, as any transgression will lead to its irrevocable breakdown [9, 10]. Some have also claimed that transgressions are morally indefensible on any basis, given that the harms that the transgressor intends to prevent are always "only" potential, whereas the harm to the patient of breaking confidentiality in terms of loss of trust and of privacy are actual harms in every instance of a breach [9].

It is well-recognized that genetics practitioners are in the unusual position of holding medical risk information about individuals who are not "their" clients. So if Anne does not share information with her family, the genetic service faces a decision over whether to breach or maintain confidentiality (assuming that they have enough information to track down her relatives). If a decision is made to breach, there is a risk of an adverse effect on their relationship with Anne or even legal liability (see Chapter 13). Maintaining Anne's confidentiality will mean that her relatives remain ignorant of their risk and the possible steps they can take to reduce it. The significance of this will vary according to the type of genetic condition, but in cases like that of Anne, her relatives are left ignorant of being at high risk of a condition for which their risk could be reduced.

Anne's case demonstrates a particular kind of scenario not uncommon in clinical practice. She has not voiced any intention to withhold genetic information from her relatives, but nonetheless a year later her relatives remain unaware of their risk of inherited cancer. Passive nondisclosure can occur for a variety of reasons, which we discuss further in the text that follows. A further problem is that when information is passed on to family members, it may be incomplete or inaccurate [11].

These issues raise a complex question: what (if any) should the role of a genetics service be in ensuring that family members are informed of their risk of genetic disease?

TYPES OF INFORMATION THAT MAY BE REVEALED BY GENETIC TESTING

Before discussing ethics and passive nondisclosure, we will note that there are some genetic conditions that are not going to be of relevance to other family members. To this end, it is neither necessary nor desirable that genetics services be involved in disseminating all kinds of genetic information to families. For example, where a genetic condition has arisen de novo in a particular individual it would be inappropriate to undergo familial dissemination because that condition would not be present in family members (apart from any offspring that patient may have).

There are, however, three other categories of genetic conditions with a potential impact on family members. The first and arguably most relevant are those genetic conditions that are treatable if detected early and fatal if detected late. The paradigmatic example for this group is familial cancers such as familial adenomatous polyposis. The second category includes those conditions that are not preventable or treatable, but for which advance knowledge offers individuals the chance to make life and reproductive decisions they otherwise would not have made, such as Huntington disease. Lynch syndrome arguably sits between the first and second categories, although it may be reconceived as fitting into the first category as screening methods improve. The third category includes conditions that will have no health consequences for the relative but will potentially affect their offspring, as is the case with many chromosome translocations.

The particular category that a condition falls into is likely to influence the weighing up of risks and benefits arising from passing on information to relatives. In the first category, there is a clear benefit to relatives, who will be able to avoid or ameliorate their genetic health risks if they choose to do so. In the second and third category, the information will not have a direct impact on the health of the relatives but will allow them the freedom to make important life decisions with the benefit of advance knowledge. Considerations of passing on information do, however, also have to be weighed against the presumption of the "right not to know," which we discuss in the text that follows. Also of relevance are the models of ownership of genetic information within families.

MODELS OF OWNERSHIP OF GENETIC
INFORMATION WITHIN FAMILIES

There are two broad models relating to ownership of genetic information, summarized in Table 12.1. The first is the traditional model of medical information that we have described above. In this model, the client is the "owner" of her genetic information. Anne would be able to choose whether she told her relatives and she cannot be coerced into disclosure. The health-care practitioner should not breach confidentiality and share this information with Anne's family members unless the practitioner has strong reasons for doing so, in line with other generally accepted breaches of medical confidentiality.

It is, however, difficult to see how the traditional interpretation of confidentiality can be in the client's interests. Anne may well assume confidentiality; however, if she decides that she wants to withhold information from her relatives, she may discover that it is a moveable feast: it applies only as long as it is not needed. If there are interested parties (e.g., her relatives), and Anne has decided that she requires confidentiality to protect herself against their interests, then her treatment team might decide to breach her confidentiality.

This situation is additionally not wholly in the interests of genetics practitioners. It is left to their discretion to decide whether to violate the practitioner–patient relationship, which Anne would assume to be sacrosanct, or to protect it and knowingly allow Anne's relatives to remain ignorant of their risk. Genetics practitioners will be left out on an "ethical limb"; the practitioner has to make the decision, but either way, the media, professional organizations, or the courts may dictate that the wrong decision has been made.

In the second "joint account" model of ownership, genetic information is viewed as belonging to the family with all members having equal rights of access, much like holders of a joint bank account [12]. The presumption is that the information will be shared with the family (perhaps anonymously, insofar as this is possible), unless there are strong reasons for not doing so [13]. The genetics practitioner would have to believe that the risk of harm to the client from sharing the information would

Table 12.1 Models of Ownership of Genetic Information

Model Name	Defining Feature
Traditional model	Confidentiality assumed unless good reason to breach.
Joint account model	Family ownership assumed unless good reason to withhold information from relatives.
Genetic unity model	Genetic information that applies to the family belongs to the family—position made clear before testing so no breach of confidentiality necessary.
Family comity model	Genetics practitioners take active role in promoting the notion of sharing information with family.

be greater than the risk to family members of remaining ignorant of the genetic condition in the family.

Both models lead to dilemmas for the genetics practitioner. In the first, if the client does not pass on information, the practitioner holds information about relatives that could allow preventative action but is unable to warn them. She must decide whether to risk her relationship with her client and breach confidentiality to warn relatives that are previously unknown to the service. Under the "joint account" model, the same dilemma arises. Although there is a presumption that information will be shared with the family, if a client fails to do so, the practitioner must still decide whether to breach confidentiality. This model could be seen as a balance between the desire to protect the practitioner–patient relationship and to allow people at risk of genetic disorders access to appropriate intervention. Alternatively the practitioner–patient relationship could still be threatened by the practitioner's ability to divulge information at her discretion, and some people would not receive appropriate medical help because the practitioner may decide against disclosure.

Alternative Approaches: Genetic Unity and Family Comity

The limitations with the traditional and joint account models may be overcome to some extent by either the genetic unity (GU) or family comity (FC) models. In the GU approach, it is acknowledged and explicitly explained to all clients that genetic information is inescapably familial, and as such that it must be communicated to family members. The GU model goes beyond the joint account model in that the genetics consultation and any testing are only continued if the client agrees that the genetics service can share genetic test information with family members as necessary. The relative merits of the different methods of sharing information with family members will be considered later in the text, but here the assumption is that clients like Anne will inform their at-risk relatives themselves, unless they decide that they would prefer the genetics service to contact relatives directly.

The GU approach avoids the dilemma of choosing between breaching confidentiality or allowing relatives to remain unaware of their risk. Anne will be informed at the outset of the intention to share genetic information, so that she can decide whether to proceed with the consultation. Her family members have the guaranteed chance to benefit from having access to their risk information. This approach encourages openness about genetic conditions and has the potential to reduce stigmatization.

The GU approach therefore emphasizes the fact that our DNA differentiates us from other species and unites us in our own. This commonality is an opportunity to bring society closer together. By assenting to clients not informing their relatives of their genetic risk, and preventing genetics practitioners from informing named individuals, society gives credence to the idea of genetic shame and allows people to deny others access to appropriate health care.

The FC approach also builds on the two alternative models of ownership of genetic information [14]. It offers a means by which to conceive of genetic information within families, balancing individual notions of autonomy with those drawn from more relational or communitarian ethical theories, which conceive of the self in relation to others, including a sense of familial responsibility [3, 15]. Comity can be defined as "considerate behavior towards others" and FC reflects the fact that genetics practitioners already encourage clients to disclose, as well as evidence that family members consider a sense of responsibility when deciding to disclose. It also reflects the U.K. Human Genetics Commission's proposal for a concept of "genetic solidarity and altruism" [16] and Doukas' concept of a "family covenant" [17]. So like GU, the FC approach requires us to recognize that we share common genetic bonds. Under a FC approach, genetics practitioners would be required to have detailed discussions with clients regarding implications for relatives. To this end, both the GU and FC approaches could help ameliorate the difficulties caused by passive nondisclosure through ensuring that family members have a stake in all genetics consultations from the outset.

The GU and FC approaches are subject to several difficulties. First, under GU some people may decide not to come forward for or proceed with genetic testing if they feel that they will then have to inform relatives about a genetic risk. It has been argued that as neither the family members nor the individual benefits if the individual does *not* proceed with testing, this type of approach would lead to less people being helped than if confidentiality was maintained [10]. However, others have provided a consequentialist calculation to argue that for each person who decides to proceed with genetic testing, it is likely that multiple people will benefit, and so it is questionable whether less people would be helped by this approach [18].

A second objection is that those people that do proceed may feel coerced to share the genetic information in order to get the medical advice they are seeking. In response, one can argue that the justice principle can also be invoked. That is: to receive genetic counseling, the client must use information about his or her family to ensure accurate provision of genetic counseling. It is therefore only fair that other family members should receive some benefit in return for having their information used. [12]

A third problem is that it is unclear what timeframe for disclosure would activate either GU- or FC-informed action. As Anne has still not informed her family after a year, does this justify the genetics service becoming involved? We will return to this point below. A final concern is how GU and FC will be able to work within the current practical institutional and resource constraints of clinical genetics services. Resolving this issue is beyond the scope of this chapter. However, we believe that if there is general commitment to this approach, then practical resolutions are not beyond the realm of possibility.

THE ROLE OF GENETICS SERVICES: HOW SHOULD RELATIVES BE CONTACTED?

We have discussed that adopting a joint account, genetic unity, or family comity model of genetic information may assist in mitigating the problem of passive nondisclosure of genetic information to relatives. These models do so by ensuring clients like Anne are aware of the importance of familial communication from the outset of their contact with genetics services. Yet even under such a model, as the case of Anne illustrates, a declaration of an intention to inform relatives of a genetic risk is no guarantee that disclosure will take place. Indeed, empirical evidence suggests that at-risk relatives are routinely not informed of their risk by the family member seen, despite the absence of a conscious decision to withhold information [7].

Passive nondisclosure can occur for a variety of reasons, including disengagement with relatives, a lack of understanding of the importance of the information, or wanting to protect relatives from potentially bad news [7]. Qualitative evidence also suggests that emotional rather than biological ties will influence who is told about a risk in the family [7].

This gives rise to an interesting yet vexing question: what role (if any) should genetics services take in ensuring that relatives are contacted? Current practice tends to reflect a more traditional model of medical confidentiality. Often the client is advised that there are family members who may also be affected by the genetic risk information, and that they should let them know of this risk. In the United Kingdom, for example, family members who receive a communication from a relative can then go to their general practitioner for referral to a genetics service. This form of relative contact can be termed "family mediated contact" [19]. A difficulty with this approach is that as some family members live in areas covered by different genetics services, and some may choose not to find out any more about their genetic risk, it is virtually impossible to determine whether all relevant family members have been informed.

An alternative approach, which would reflect the models of ownership akin to genetic unity, is one where the genetics service will assume greater practical and moral responsibility for ensuring that relatives are informed of their genetic risks. However, there has been anxiety about assuming a duty for care of relatives for a number of reasons. There are concerns that declaring a duty to inform relatives could lead to a legal obligation to do so. Indeed a legal case in one U.S. state has suggested that practitioners do have a duty to disclose information to relatives, which is not discharged merely by warning the patient [20]. This legal duty would place a significant burden on genetics services to track down and contact relatives (often a difficult and time-consuming process), with the risk of legal action if this fails. Furthermore, there are concerns about the potential harm to relatives of being informed that they are at genetic risk, without allowing them the opportunity to choose to remain ignorant of this risk—an issue we discuss further later in this chapter.

Let us assume that a clinical or legal duty to inform relatives would not be desirable. There may be valid reasons for not warning that need to be taken into account when deciding to be more proactive in informing relatives to overcome passive nondisclosure. However, some responsibility to do as much as is reasonably possible, within the constraints of budgets and time, might be acceptable. What form would this responsibility take, and what would be the best way to ensure that relatives are informed? A method of relative contact consistent with this approach is "direct contact" [19]. Under this model, Anne would provide names and addresses of relatives whom the genetics service knows to be at risk, and the genetics service would then send them letters, inviting them to come for counseling. Such a practice would have to be acceptable under the privacy or data protection laws of the relevant jurisdiction. Furthermore, letters would be carefully worded to provide enough information for relatives to make a decision about whether or not they want to learn more, without creating unnecessary anxiety [21].

A potential issue with direct contact is that it could inadvertently cause harm through a "blanket" approach to contacting relatives. Although two large studies of direct contact have not revealed any evidence of harm to relatives, and there were no complaints about the method of contact used [11, 21], this should be borne in mind. Godard et al., for example, have commented that "...the physician cannot presume to have complete and accurate information about the patient's family history and interpersonal dynamics, about how information may be received by his [sic] relatives. In some cases, providing genetic information to family members could do more harm than good" [22] (p. 109).

To mitigate any potential for harm, an alternative to direct contact is a form of "partnership model," which reflects recent thinking on models of the doctor–patient relationship [23]. In this model, the genetics service will work with Anne to decide how each relative should be contacted. This model also favors the genetic unity approach, and so the familial nature of genetic information will be explained during initial counseling. At-risk relatives will be identified from the pedigree provided by Anne. For each relative, Anne will be asked whether she feels comfortable contacting the person directly, or whether she would prefer the genetics service to write a letter to her relatives. This allows room for both Anne's experience of her family but also the practitioner's knowledge. If particular barriers to communication are identified, such as a concern that a particular relative might not cope with the news, then the counselor will use his or her experience to help Anne decide whether the relative really would not derive benefit from being given the opportunity to learn more about his or her genetic status. Partnership is a more proactive approach than much current practice, but it allows for greater flexibility. It will appropriately utilize Anne's expert knowledge of her family but will also minimize the chance of passive nondisclosure.

THE RIGHT NOT TO KNOW

We have so far suggested that passive nondisclosure is problematic and that a more proactive role for health care providers could be considered— perhaps adopting a partnership model—to ensure that relatives can be informed about their genetic risk, at least for the first category of genetic conditions described above. However, this position contains an implicit premise: that it is generally good for relatives to be told that they may be at genetic risk. We should not assume that relatives, if they were aware of a genetic risk, would always want to find out more about it. Anne is already aware that she may have a *MSH2* mutation and she has actively sought medical advice. Her relatives may have an entirely different set of attitudes and beliefs.

This dilemma means we must consider a common concern that arises when contacting relatives: the "right not to know" one's genetic status [24–27]. There are two senses of this right: the right not to know one's exact genetic status, and the right not to know that one is at risk at all. While most would support the first sense (with some exceptions [28, 29]), the second is more contested. The right to remain in complete genetic ignorance is based in considerations of autonomy or privacy [30]. The right may therefore be violated if a relative is contacted to be told of a familial genetic risk. Takala and Häyry, for example, have argued that it could be harmful to inform people that they are at risk of any genetic disorder, regardless of whether it is preventable [31].

The argument is that if autonomy gives us a right to find out information about ourselves, it also gives us a right not to find out information about ourselves. Husted has argued that we should adopt two conceptions of autonomy, one "thick" and one "thin" [32]. Thin autonomy is, broadly speaking, an ability to make choices with full access to information. The person making the choice has no "defects in reasoning" [32] (p. 59) and can control his or her desires. On this account, receipt of unsolicited information about genetic risk will enhance autonomy, as information will facilitate decision making and the formation of short- and long-term goals. The thick conception of autonomy, on the other hand, adds another dimension. It can be seen as a longer term project to achieve self-determination and self-definition [32] (p. 61). We are shaped by the decisions we make and the actions we take throughout our lives—these decisions and choices collectively make us who we are. Providing a person with unsolicited information about genetic risk (i.e., taking away a decision to remain in complete ignorance of a familial risk) may diminish the self-determinative component of the person's autonomy. This is because providing a person with information about genetic risk could undermine his or her ability to make his or her own decisions (e.g., whether to remain in ignorance), and it could also be seen as paternalistically deciding what is best for another person. Even though we may not condone providing people with definitive information about their genetic status against their will, autonomy may still be undermined by providing broad information about genetic risk. Therefore, to protect the thick conception of autonomy, information about genetic risk should not be disclosed to otherwise ignorant relatives.

There is a fundamental problem with this argument in that no one can autonomously decide not to know something in advance if he or she does not know what it is that he or she is choosing not to know about [24]. One of Anne's relatives may indeed decide that he would never want to know that he had a familial risk of bowel cancer. Yet how many of us would make these kinds of wishes known to our relatives in advance? Genetic illnesses are individually rare, and so it is unreasonable to expect people to give serious consideration to their risk of different categories of genetic illness. This decision to remain in ignorance may also have been made without important knowledge about screening and other interventions, which Anne's relatives may wish to know about.

To argue that information about genetic risk should be withheld could also be subject to claims of "genetic exceptionalism," that is, treating this information as somehow different to other medical information merely because it is genetic. This is because we routinely find out about general risks to our health by way of family communication or incidentally acquired knowledge of our relatives' general health status; much of which has implications for other family members.

Therefore, even strong advocates of the right not to know must concede that at most the right not to know is a consideration to be taken into account when deciding whether to inform someone of his or her risk, rather than an absolute principle [33]. If knowledge of a genetic condition confers little obvious benefit to the recipient, then the right not to know may supersede the right to know. However, in situations in which a reasonable person could be judged to have a significant interest in knowing his or her risk, there is a prima facie presumption in favor of providing a choice as to whether to confirm genetic status.

If we accept that the right to remain in complete genetic ignorance is illogical and is usurped by a presumption in favor of knowing, we must take care in two respects. The first is to ensure that any information passed on to relatives (whether by the family, directly, or in partnership) is drafted in such a way so as to not cause undue panic, alarm, or harm. The information should stipulate that a test is available and allow a relative who might be interested to contact a health-care practitioner for further advice. But it should not provide specific individualized risks or provide too much negative information about the condition in question. Names should not be shared unless permission has been given. Second, in situations like that of Anne, where she is generally willing to disclose but is worried about how her cousins may react, concerns about relatives' well-being should be listened to and taken seriously. The benefits and possible harms in disclosing should be discussed with Anne, as she will have far better knowledge of the relatives in question than the genetics service. However, the genetics practitioner's experience with family disclosure and knowledge of how family members may react should not be ignored. Discussion with Anne will allow practitioners to see what action should be taken, on balance.

IMPLICATIONS AND CHALLENGES FOR CLINICAL PRACTICE

From the discussions above, it may be concluded that there are ethical justifications in taking a more proactive approach to help ensure that family members are told of their genetic risk, where there is on balance a benefit to them in doing so. Patterson et al. reflect this attitude when they write, "Because genetic information has implications for families as well as individuals and because prevention is a realizable goal, our sense of professional responsibility has now expanded beyond the individual to include other family members as well" [34] (p. 2101).

A change in practice, however, would have far-reaching and potentially over-burdensome implications for clients and genetics practitioners. The first implication is that there would need to be a shift in approach from the more traditional doctor–patient model to a more family-centered model, with clients being informed of this early on during the consulting process. Enhanced public education about genetic issues and their familial nature may assist with this process, so that people come for genetic counseling with some expectation that this will have implications for their wider family.

A more proactive approach involving discussion with clients about how each family member will be informed, and looking at potential barriers and strategies for overcoming them, will lead to increased demand on resources, mainly in terms of a need for more face-to-face contact. There may also be a need for specific training for health-care practitioners involved in counseling to enable them to feel comfortable with taking a more proactive role in identifying and discussing barriers and strategies.

As discussed above, consideration will also have to be given to the involvement of the genetics service in developing the information that is passed along to relatives. Evidence about the quality of information that is currently passed on by clients of genetic services suggests that there is a legitimate need for some oversight of this information rather than merely ensuring that relatives are informed. A recent study of dissemination within families in the context of *BRCA* gene testing showed that 55% of relatives were not or were only slightly aware that a predictive genetic test for the condition was available, even after relatives had reported passing on information [35].

It is also likely that taking a more proactive approach will lead to more people coming forward for genetic testing. For example, Suthers et al.

found that within 2 years of a mutation being found in an individual, 23% of relatives had their mutation status determined when contact was family mediated, whereas 40% did so when the contact was direct [21]. This will have implications for genetics services, who will need to provide counseling and testing for those who seek it. In those conditions for which screening is available to prevent or detect a condition, such services will also need to be prepared to cope with this increased demand.

Overall, we would argue that a more proactive approach has the potential to work well as a preventative form of medicine, identifying conditions and allowing for early treatment. Having genetics practitioners taking a lead will also ensure that policies and guidelines are developed using a "bottom-up" approach, whereas if nothing is done it is increasingly likely that legal considerations will dictate the process [34]. It will also enable people to make life decisions and derive the maximum benefit from the clinical genetics service.

Of course clinical genetics services are not the only avenue by which genetic testing is done, which raises the question of what role other health-care practitioners could take in helping to support family communication. Genetics services are in a slightly different position to other specialties because they routinely inquire about and record details of relatives, and genetic consultations are usually set up to allow for discussion of the implications for family members. The structure of consultations in other specialties, which often need to be of shorter duration, may make it difficult for other practitioners to spend the length of time required for explaining the implications for each family member, and for counseling patients to assist them in contacting relatives. It may be that practitioners working outside of clinical genetics have less opportunity to be proactive in assisting patients to contact their relatives, and so the ethical requirements for them to do so are less clear. If this is the case, their role could be to identify the familial nature of the condition and to refer the patient to a clinical genetics service where appropriate, therefore taking a positive step toward enabling relatives to be contacted. This interaction with clinical genetics services is a situation which is occurring with increasing frequency as more and more genetic conditions are recognized across a wide range of specialties.

CONCLUSION

In this chapter, we have argued that genetic information is inherently familial and that health-care practitioners, particularly those working in clinical genetics services, have the potential to do even more to assist individuals to share the potential health benefits arising from their consultation with their relatives, where appropriate. While confidentiality is undoubtedly important, there are alternative ways in which genetics can be conceived of in families, which do not necessarily involve breaching confidentiality. We have supported a partnership model for dissemination of information, which emphasizes a process of negotiation and discussion between clients and genetics practitioners. This model supports concepts of genetic information as familial, such as the genetic unity approach. The right not to know one's genetic risk is a powerful one and this should not be overlooked, but equally powerful is the ethical consideration of providing relatives with choices, particularly for those genetic conditions where there is an opportunity to prevent significant harm. Now the challenge is to work in a multi-disciplinary way to discuss and develop models of working that allow health-care practitioners to best care for clients and their families, within the constraints imposed by the financial and practical aspects of the health system. If a more proactive role is considered helpful and viable within such constraints, then passive nondisclosure of genetic information may be dramatically reduced. Throughout this chapter, we will refer to the hypothetical case of Anne as an illustration of how the issue of passive nondisclosure can arise in practice.

REFERENCES

1. Lacroix M, Nycum G, Godard B, Knoppers BM. Should physicians warn patients' relatives of genetic risks? *Canadian Medical Association Journal* 2008;178(5):593–595.
2. Offit K, Groeger E, Turner S, Wadsworth EA, Weiser MA. The "duty to warn" a patient's family members about hereditary disease risks. *Journal of the American Medical Association* 2004;292:1469–1473.
3. Bell D, Bennett B. Genetic secrets and the family. *Medical Law Review* 2001;9:130–161.
4. Wolff K, Brun W, Kvale G, Nordin K. Confidentiality versus duty to inform-an empirical study on attitudes towards the handling of genetic information. *American Journal of Medical Genetics Part A* 2007;143(2):142–148.
5. Falk MJ, Dugan RB, O'Riordan MA, Matthews AL, Robin NH. Medical geneticists' duty to warn at-risk relatives for genetic disease. *American Journal of Medical Genetics Part A* 2003;120A:374–380.
6. Clarke A, Richards M, Kerzin-Storrar L, et al. Genetic professionals' reports of nondisclosure of genetic risk information within families. *European Journal of Human Genetics* 2005;13:556–562.
7. Gaff CL, Collins V, Symes T, Halliday J. Facilitating family communication about predictive genetic testing: Probands' perceptions. *Journal of Genetic Counseling* 2005;14:133–140.
8. Crawford GC, Lucassen AM. Disclosure of genetic information within families: A case report. *Clinical Ethics* 2008;3:7–10.
9. Kottow MH. Medical confidentiality: An intransigent and absolute obligation. *Journal of Medical Ethics* 1986;12:117–122.
10. Kipnis K. A defense of unqualified medical confidentiality. *American Journal of Bioethics* 2006;6:7–18.
11. Aktan-Collan K, Haukkala A, Pylcvänäinen K, et al. Direct contact in inviting high-risk members of hereditary colon cancer families to genetic counselling and DNA testing. *Journal of Medical Genetics* 2007;44:732–738.

12. Parker M, Lucassen A. Genetic information: A joint account? *British Medical Journal* 2004;329:165–167.

13. Skene L. Patients' rights or family responsibilities? Two approaches to genetic testing. *Medical Law Review* 1998;6:1–41.

14. Davey A, Newson A, O'Leary P. Communication of genetic information within families: the case for familial comity. *Journal of Bioethical Inquiry* 2006;161–166.

15. Gilbar R. Communicating genetic information in the family: The familial relationship as the forgotten factor. *Journal of Medical Ethics* 2007;33:390–393.

16. Human Genetics Commission. *Inside Information: Balancing Interests in the Use of Personal Genomic Data.* London: Department of Health; 2002.

17. Doukas DJ, Berg JW. The family covenant and genetic testing. *American Journal of Bioethics* 2001;1:3–10.

18. Duncan R, Newson A. Clinical genetics and the problem with unqualified confidentiality. *American Journal of Bioethics* 2006;6:41–43.

19. Newson AJ, Humphries SE. Cascade testing in familial hypercholesterolaemia: How should family members be contacted? *European Journal of Human Genetics* 2005;13:401–408.

20. Safer v. Pack, 677 A.2d 1188 (NJ Superior Court, Appelate Division; 1996).

21. Suthers GK, Armstrong J, McCormack J, Trott D. Letting the family know: Balancing ethics and effectiveness when notifying relatives about testing for a familial disorder. *Journal of Medical Genetics* 2006;34:665–670.

22. Godard B, Hurlimann T, Letendre M, Egalite N. Guidelines for disclosing genetic information to family members: From development to use. *Familial Cancer* 2006;5:103–116.

23. Bergsma J. *Doctors and Patients: Strategies in Long-Term Illness.* Norwell, MA: Kluwer Academic Publishers; 1997:14–15.

24. Andorno R. The right not to know: An autonomy based approach. *Journal of Medical Ethics* 2004;30:435–440.

25. Wilson J. To know or not to know? Genetic ignorance, autonomy and paternalism. *Bioethics* 2005;19:492–504.

26. Räikkä J. Freedom and a right (not) to know. *Bioethics* 1998;12:49–63.

27. Wilcke JR. Late onset genetic disease: Where ignorance is bliss, is it folly to inform relatives? *British Medical Journal* 1998;317:744.

28. Harris J, Keywood K. Ignorance, information and autonomy. *Theoretical Medicine and Bioethics* 2001;22:415–436.

29. Rhodes R. Genetic links, family ties and social bonds: Rights and responsibilities in the face of genetic knowledge. *Journal of Medical Philosophy* 1998;23:10–30.

30. Laurie G. *Genetic Privacy: A Challenge to Medico-legal Norms.* Cambridge, England: Cambridge University Press; 2002.

31. Takala T, Häyry M. Genetic ignorance, moral obligations and social duties. *Journal of Medical Philosophy* 2000;25:107–113.

32. Husted J. Autonomy and a right not to know. In: Chadwick R, Levitt M, Shickle D, eds. *The Right to Know and the Right Not to Know.* Aldershot, England: Ashgate; 1997:55–68.

33. Laurie G. Commentary on the right not to know: An autonomy based approach. *Journal of Medical Ethics* 2004;30:439–440.
34. Patterson RD, Robinson LD, Naftalis EZ, Haley BB, Tomlinson GE. Custodianship of genetic information: Clinical challenges and professional responsibility. *Journal of Clinical Oncology* 2005;23:2100–2104.
35. Sermijn E, Goelen G, Teugels E. The impact of proband mediated information dissemination in families with a BRCA1/2 gene mutation. *Journal of Medical Genetics* 2004;41:e23.

13

LEGAL PERSPECTIVES

Loane Skene & Laura Forrest

Health-care practitioners are subject to laws that govern their practice. Privacy legislation is relevant to practitioners, considering their role in communicating directly with at-risk relatives of their clients. A broadly similar approach to privacy legislation has been adopted internationally. This chapter describes and illustrates the legal complexities and offers a structure to guide decision making.

Deciding what information, if any, should be disclosed to family members after a genetic test is not easy and, as alluded to throughout this book, health-care practitioners can face challenging situations when information is not conveyed. Practitioners are required to act such that they obey the pertinent laws when responding to these situations. After a short discussion of the variety of responses within families when information is offered, this chapter describes the complexities arising from privacy legislation. This chapter does not, of course, offer legal advice to practitioners but serves to highlight the complexities that arise from legislation and raise awareness of issues that may need to be considered within the practitioner's own country's legal system. An example of one legal system is given in illustration, namely Australian law. We explore when it is legally justifiable for health-care practitioners to breach confidentiality when a person's genetic test results are significant for other people, especially close blood relatives. Although the Australian law is primarily used as an example, U.S. law is considered on some issues. The duties of health-care practitioners are not always clear, but it is suggested that they might follow the procedures listed in Table 13.1 (at the end of the chapter), which also highlights the potential legal risk if information is disclosed without consent.

The genetic test results referred to here may be from living or deceased people, or from death or autopsy results, cancer or other genetic registries, deposits of stored tissue, research studies, and other sources. Genetic test results include those of adults, who may or may not be symptomatic, and also of children, since genetic conditions are often first recognized in infancy. The text therefore refers to communication by adults on their own behalves and by parents (as the decision makers for children[1]) to family members.

PRACTICAL MATTERS IN DISCLOSING GENETIC INFORMATION

There have been a number of interesting empirical studies concerning people's responses to the receipt of genetic information, especially relatives who have not sought a genetic test themselves. Although one might assume that relatives would want to know about their own genetic risks, especially if the risk can be avoided or minimized by having the information so that they can act on it, that is not always the case. For example, in research on families affected by hemophilia, Boddington and Gregory investigated "how people deal with information that is difficult to handle" and "mak[ing] truth king [as in accounts of autonomy]...may not fully respect the range of human interests" [1]. Quoting from their interviews with family members, the authors said that striving for "integrity," people make "disparate choices," sometimes seeking to "control" their lives and their "notion of family" through ignorance [1].

The range of reactions from family members is well illustrated by a recent empirical study undertaken by one of the authors, Laura Forrest [2]. She interviewed people recently diagnosed with a genetic condition, and also some family members, about their response to the genetic diagnosis. She made a number of significant findings.

First, the initial reaction of the person receiving the diagnosis was (not surprisingly) based mainly on his or her own (or child's) health issues, not the significance that the diagnosis may have for relatives. Many of the people who were interviewed described being given the genetic diagnosis as a traumatic experience. For example, Ava (pseudonyms used to preserve anonymity), whose son was diagnosed with adrenoleukodystrophy, recalled, "The first 2 weeks, I just [lay] in bed and cried. Between the hours of seven and seven I got up and I was on remote control and did what I needed to do but as soon as the children were back in bed, I was curled up in my bed in the fetal position just thinking...this cannot be happening to my child."

Most of the people Laura interviewed contacted close family members soon after getting the news. However, they did so in an ad hoc manner, and their purpose was to seek comfort themselves, not to warn the relatives of their own genetic risk. For example, Nicole, whose daughter was diagnosed with cystic fibrosis, said, "I'm from a close family and maybe right at that time, I was more concerned about her [daughter's] health anyhow, more than worrying about my brothers and their children."

Thus, coping with their own medical and social issues, people often consider informing other family members to be a burden. Both they and health-care practitioners indicated that there is a greater role for genetic practitioners in informing family members of their risks.

On the other side, some relatives seemed uninterested and even hostile when told about a family risk. Another empirical study shows that relatives often do not seem to want genetic information. One Australian cancer genetic service regularly sends letters directly to relatives of people who have had genetic tests (with the consent of those people), offering to share "important health information" with them. Although the letter states that "A member of your family has been found to have an inherited tendency to develop cancer [and]...there is therefore an increased chance of you developing cancer," 50% of the recipients in the 8-year study period (812 letters) did not respond to the letters offering advice about the genetic counseling services available at no cost to themselves. The median response time was 116 days [3].

THE LAW

It is difficult for the law to take account of such a wide variation in the practices of individuals in informing relatives, and in the relatives' desire to know about genetic risks and their reactions to being offered such information when they do not want to have it. The law is formulated in general terms and, for the most part, it is based on protecting the privacy of the person who was first tested, rather than protecting the health interests of relatives who might benefit from knowing their potential risks from a familial genetic mutation.

The general principle in privacy legislation, and also in the common (or judge-made) law, is that a person's medical information is confidential and that health-care practitioners must not disclose it to other people without that person's consent, or other lawful justification, such as a statutory requirement or authorization. However, there is a generic but limited exception in the privacy legislation and also in the common law, based on two competing public interests: the public interest in protecting confidentiality, and the public interest in protecting innocent third parties and the community. This exception enables information to be disclosed in cases where it is necessary to avoid serious risks to the person or to other people (in some jurisdictions the risk must be "imminent" as well as serious).

It should be noted at the outset that, in many jurisdictions, there are professional guidelines that suggest procedures for genetic counselors and other health-care practitioners concerning the disclosure of genetic information to close family members. These guidelines have the benefit of having been developed by practitioners trained and experienced in genetic counseling. However, they do not always coincide with the law and, if there is an inconsistency between the guidelines and the law, compliance with the guidelines may not provide a defense to legal proceedings arising from a breach of confidentiality. In other words, practitioners who follow the guidelines when disclosing genetic information to relatives may still be the subject of a complaint to a privacy body or a registration board, or sued for breach of confidentiality, if the disclosure is not covered by a legal exemption. In future, guidelines may be published that have statutory force. In Australia, this was recommended by the Australian Law Reform Commission and the Australian Health Ethics Committee in their widely commended report on genetic privacy, *Essentially Yours* [4], but it has not yet been implemented.

On the other hand, family members who are not warned of their genetic risk may, in some jurisdictions, also be able to sue health-care practitioners who keep the information confidential. This is on the basis of the so-called duty to warn.

The apparently conflicting duties to keep information confidential and to warn third parties of risks that are unknown to them obviously raise problems for genetic counselors when deciding whether they should pass information on to relatives. The procedures listed in Table 13.1 may provide some guidance, including the potential legal risk where the law and the guidelines may diverge (see the table footnote). At that point, they will have to decide in each case how to proceed, weighing up the health issues for family members against the perceived legal risk. The nature and extent of the legal risk is discussed in an Australian context toward the end of this chapter.

CODES OF ETHICS AND PROFESSIONAL GUIDELINES

A number of codes of ethics and professional guidelines have been developed to assist health-care practitioners in deciding whether to inform close blood relatives about a genetic condition in their family. The codes include the World Medical Association Code of Ethics, the International Code of Medical Ethics, and the Australian Medical Association Code of Ethics. The guidelines stem from human genetics societies, bioethics committees, research institutes, and regional and national health organizations.

The codes of ethics and guidelines have significant differences with regard to the disclosure of genetic information to family members, especially when an individual seen by the genetics service refuses to inform family members of the family risk. Although they commonly state that information may be disclosed with the consent of the person tested, some codes and guidelines envisage that information may sometimes also be disclosed without the knowledge, or even against the wishes, of the person tested.

A number of organizations have produced guidelines that illustrate "exceptional circumstances" where disclosure without the person's consent is acceptable [5]. For example, the American Society of Human Genetics Social Issues Subcommittee on Familial Disclosure stipulates four conditions that permit disclosure of genetic information by health-care practitioners to family members. These include cases in which

(1) encouragement to disclose has failed, *(2)* harm to family members is serious and imminent, *(3)* at-risk family members are identifiable, and *(4)* the genetic condition is preventable or treatable.

In contrast, there are limited guidelines available for health-care practitioners when people do not refuse to disclose genetic information to family members but information is nonetheless not conveyed [6]. People often report struggling to communicate genetic information to family members. Therefore, the development of comprehensive guidelines that address the involvement of practitioners in family communication may benefit both the person seen by the practitioner and that person's relatives.

PRIVACY LEGISLATION: THE EXAMPLE OF AUSTRALIA

In Australia, there is an extensive system of privacy and health privacy legislation, both federal and state [7]. Much of it overlaps, and it is not always clear when it applies. The Australian Law Reform Commission drew attention to this issue in its recent report on privacy law in Australia and recommended that the legislation should be unified and streamlined [8]. However, that is unlikely to occur for some time, if at all, and health-care practitioners must continue to comply with state and federal laws, so far as they apply. For simplicity, the following discussion will concentrate on the law of the state of Victoria. Other Australian states and territories have equivalent provisions.

When considering the relevant privacy legislation, the context in which the health-care practitioner works is important. In Victoria, practitioners must comply with the state legislation (the Health Records Act 2001) if they work in a state institution, like a Victorian public hospital. If they work independently, they must comply with both the state and federal privacy legislation and if they work in a federal institution, they must comply with the federal privacy legislation, the Privacy Act 1988. That Act applies if the Commonwealth has jurisdiction to cover particular people or activities in Australia under the federal constitution. It does not apply to state institutions, but it does apply to people who are working in other incorporated institutions. Where the Acts are accompanied by regulations (e.g., Health Records Regulations 2002), the regulations have the same weight as the Acts themselves.[2]

These federal and state Acts have similar provisions regarding health privacy. There are sections in both Acts that impose privacy obligations.[3] Also, both Acts contain privacy principles in Schedules to the Acts (the National Privacy Principles, or NPPs, in Schedule 3 of the federal Act and the Health Privacy Principles, or HPPs, in Schedule 1 of the Victorian Act).[4] These principles augment the provisions in the sections of the Acts and have the same legal force. Note that the Acts do not apply to patients and their relatives; thus, those people are not restricted in passing information on to family members, provided this is for the purposes of their "personal, family or household affairs."[5]

Both the federal and state Acts provide exemptions for the disclosure of personal information in certain circumstances, which have recently been extended in the federal Privacy Act. When the Act was first passed, it stated that information may be disclosed where that was necessary to "lessen or prevent *a serious and imminent threat* to an individual's life, health or safety ..." (emphasis added).[6] The current Victorian Act still has the same provision.[7] However, the "serious and imminent" test raises problems in the context of genetic conditions, where a risk may be serious but not imminent. As a result of recommendations of the Australian Law Reform Commission and the Australian Health Ethics Committee,[8] the Privacy Act has been amended and a risk can be disclosed to relatives if it is "serious" but not necessarily "imminent"[9].

The amended Act now permits health-care practitioners to disclose genetic information about an individual that they have "obtained...in the course of providing a health service to the individual" where they "reasonably believe" that "disclosure is necessary to lessen or prevent a *serious threat* to the life, health, or safety (*whether or not the threat is imminent*)" of a "genetic relative of the individual"; provided that disclosure is made "in accordance with guidelines approved by the Commissioner under section 95AA" (emphasis added).[9] Note that the risk must still be serious. This amendment goes some way in recognizing the familial nature of all genetic information and the justification for sharing it among family members. However, it applies only where the information denotes a serious risk; one cannot assume that the information may be shared solely because of its familial nature.[10] Also, disclosure is permitted only to *genetic relatives.* Disclosure must not be made to other parties who may be affected by a genetic risk, such as domestic partners and people who may have a risk of infection associated with a genetic factor (e.g., the neurodegenerative condition Creutzfeldt-Jakob disease[11]), though the risk to people other than relatives may be considered in deciding whether to disclose a risk to relatives.

However, even if a health-care practitioner decides to inform a family member of a genetic risk, the person who was tested may not initiate a complaint under the Act, so no action would ensue for breach of privacy even if there was a breach of the Act. Also, even if the person tested lodged a complaint, the penalty may be relatively minor.

DISCIPLINARY ACTION: COMPLAINTS TO MEDICAL REGISTRATION BODIES

Another recourse for a person who believes that a health-care practitioner has wrongfully disclosed his or her personal information to a third party is to lodge a complaint with the practitioner's registration body. In Victoria the complaint may be lodged, for example, with the Medical Practitioners' Board of Victoria.[12] A complaint to the Board would probably allege "professional misconduct,"[13] but the fact that a practitioner has acted in accordance with professional guidelines or accepted professional practice would be relevant, though not necessarily determinative,[14] in deciding whether the complaint is justified.

COMMON LAW

In addition to facing possible complaints under privacy and disciplinary legislation, a health-care practitioner who unlawfully divulges personal information about a patient may be sued for damages in tort,[15] contract,[16] or for equitable breach of confidence.[17] Such actions would be available only if the identity of the person is apparent or can reasonably be ascertained.

There are a number of circumstances in which it is permissible for health-care practitioners to disclose information to third parties. The usual case is where the person concerned has consented, either expressly or by implication, to disclosure. However, consent cannot generally be implied where information is given to third parties, even close relatives. Another exception is if disclosure is in the public interest, which has been held to justify breaches of medical confidentiality to protect the community from a dangerous criminal,[18] an impaired bus driver,[19] or people with an infectious disease who refuse to take precautions to protect other people from infection.[20] This concept of public interest underlies the exception in privacy legislation, which has been discussed earlier, that justifies disclosure of serious genetic risks to close blood relatives. To date, however, there has been no reported Australian case in which disclosure of genetic information has been held to have been justified without consent, because no relevant case has come before the courts. Despite the changes to the privacy legislation, a genetic risk may seem to be in a different category from the more serious and imminent risks that have been considered by the courts to date (namely, violent offenders, impaired drivers, and people with infectious diseases).

Nevertheless, cases alleging breach of confidentiality at common law are very rare. In negligence actions, plaintiffs must prove that they have suffered an injury or loss (such as loss of a job), and there is rarely such an outcome in these cases, particularly of a magnitude that will meet the threshold for negligence claims after the statutory "tort law reform" introduced by amendments to the Victorian Wrongs Act 1958 . They must also prove that the injury or loss was caused by the defendant's failure to take reasonable care. If a health-care practitioner has acted in accordance with professional guidelines or peer professional practice in disclosing information to close blood relatives, that compliance is very likely to be a defense to a claim in negligence.[21] Additional legal protection could be obtained by seeking advice from a clinical ethics committee if one is available and has jurisdiction to advise on such matters.[22]

Actions in contract or in equity are not subject to the Wrongs Act, and they do not require proof of an injury or loss that meets the threshold under the Act. However, people will rarely undertake the cost and stress of litigation unless they have suffered an injury or loss. This is especially the case in Australia when the complaint procedures under the privacy legislation are free and relatively simple. Also, evidence of peer professional practice would be relevant in deciding whether a health-care practitioner had failed to take reasonable care, which would be as relevant in actions in contract as in negligence.

DUTY TO WARN

It should be noted that it is possible, if information is *not* disclosed to relatives, that the relatives might sue because they have not been warned of their own risk. Such actions have been allowed in some states of the United States, on the authority of the *Tarasoff* case, in which it was held that health-care practitioners may have a duty to warn where there is a foreseeable risk of significant harm to an identified third party.[23] The principle has been applied in cases involving a genetic risk,[24] but the cases differ on whether practitioners can discharge the duty to warn relatives by stressing to the person seen by the health-care service that he or she should warn relatives,[25] rather than the practitioner warning the person directly.[26] If there were a legal duty to warn, that would, of course, be a defense if a practitioner was sued for breach of confidentiality.

The "practical difficulties" of recognizing a legal duty to warn have been noted to include "how to define the relatives to whom the duty is owed; determining how far practitioners are required to go in seeking to contact them; and the level of advice that practitioners should give in order to discharge the duty."[27] In Australia, there has been no reported case recognizing that health-care practitioners may have a legal duty to warn relatives. The report of the Australian Law Reform Commission and the Australian Health Ethics Committee recommended that the law should not recognize a duty to warn in such circumstances.[28]

Thus, although it is possible under Australian law that health-care practitioners may have a legal duty to warn close blood relatives of their genetic risk, it would seem that, at most, the practitioner's duty could be discharged by clearly telling the person seen that he or she should pass on the information to close blood relatives.

CONCLUSIONS

Health-care practitioners need to be aware of the legislation that governs their practice and that its requirement may not be consistent with professional guidelines. Nonetheless, legislation might not provide the level of certainty practitioners seek when trying to resolve their responsibilities in the face of refusal by an individual to convey genetic information to his or her relatives. Ongoing research and discussion with health-care practitioners and the wider community is necessary to resolve the issues discussed in this chapter. Procedures that practitioners might follow in doing so are summarized in Table 13.1, with reference to the Australian law on disclosing information to family members.

Table 13.1 Summary: Disclosing Information to Family Members

Note: Professional guidelines and the law are generally similar on the first three dot points. They differ in some jurisdictions on the last dot point, which raises the most difficult legal issues. Similar procedures are suggested if a relative asks a health-care practitioner for genetic information for his or her own health care, including the need to consult the person tested first for consent, even if that is not finally determinative

- Explain to the person tested the results of the genetic test and its implications for the person and his or her own health: certainty of diagnosis and prognosis (such as the penetrance of the genetic mutation); when symptoms may be expected to appear and their nature; progress of the condition; potential treatment or other intervention, etc.
- Emphasize to the person the familial implications of the genetic information. Stress the need for him or her to inform close blood relatives if a familial risk is identified, explaining how the family could benefit from knowing the information. For example, family members may choose to be tested themselves and, if they are positive, they may undertake preventive measures to avoid or minimize their risk or, in other cases, use the information in other ways, such as reproductive decision making. Even if there is no intervention available, people may benefit simply from knowing about a family risk, but that is less straightforward. Ideally, the familial implications should be raised earlier rather than later—for example, as part of pre-test counseling.
- Help the person attending the health-care service to identify which relatives need to be informed and offer to provide a letter or other written information to assist the information process. Guidelines commonly state that the appropriate person to contact relatives, at least initially, is the person seen by the health-care practitioner. This person knows the family and is best placed to inform them. Practitioners can later provide advice and offer tests if relatives choose to be tested themselves. With proper counseling, most people will probably agree to disclose information to relatives.* In all cases, when relatives are seen, only the information that is necessary to assist diagnosis and treatment for that relative should be divulged.† This may be regarded as "familial" genetic information—the fact that a mutation exists in a family—rather than "personal" genetic information, such as another family member's mutation status (positive or negative).‡
- If the person seen indicates that he or she will not inform any other family members, you may choose to wait while he or she adjusts to the initial diagnosis and then try again to discuss approaching family members or to allow you to do so. If the person still does not agree, you will need to consider whether the familial risk is so serious that close blood relatives should be alerted to their risk. In assessing seriousness, you might consider "the degree of likelihood of having a genetic condition...[such as] a 50% likelihood of carrying a mutation of the BRCA1 gene"; and "the degree of likelihood that the genetic predisposition will lead to the actual physical manifestation of the disease."§ Other factors such as the "level of morbidity, mortality and preventability";** and the availability of any treatment or intervention may also be relevant; but note that the ALRC, AHEC report said that "the threat of harm through the exercise of reproductive choice is too remote a 'harm' to justify [non-consensual disclosure]."†† If you consider the risk to relatives is serious, and bearing in mind the possible legal risk of nondisclosure without consent, you may decide to contact the relatives with information in general terms, inviting them to contact you for further information or to seek their own testing or genetic advice. As in other cases, any information provided should be limited to what is necessary for the relatives' care, disclosing as little genetic information about the person tested or other family members as possible, and bearing in mind the possibility that the relatives will not want to know about their risk.

(continued)

Table 13.1 *continued*

* Compare ALRC, AHEC Report, para 21.73.
† The U.S. President's Commission for the Study of Ethical Problems in Medicine and Biomedical and Behavioral Research and the Ontario Provincial Advisory Committee on the New Predictive Genetic Technologies, the UK Human Genetics Commission, quoted ALRC, AHEC Report, paras 21.99, 21.102, 21.103.
‡ Skene, L. Patients' rights or family responsibilities? Two approaches to genetic testing. *Medical Law Review* 1998;6(1):1–41.
§ Lemmens, T. and Austin, L. The challenges of regulating the use of genetic information. *Isuma: Canadian Journal of Policy Research* 2001;2(3):26, 32–33, quoted in Australian Law Reform Commission, Australian Health Ethics Committee, Report 96, *Essentially Yours*, March 2003, para 21.67. Lemmens and Austin consider the test of "seriousness" problematic in its application: ibid.
**Cancer Council Victoria Cancer Council Genetics Advisory Committee, *Submission*, quoted ALRC, AHEC Report, para 21.95.
†† AHEC Report, paras 21.80–21.82.

NOTES

1. Although the term "parents" is used, either parent could generally make decisions concerning a child under 18 years of age, by virtue of their "parental responsibility" for the child: Family Law Act 1975 (Cth) ss 61B (definition),61C. Older children (perhaps 14 to 18 years old) who meet the "mature minor test" may be legally competent to make their own medical decisions without involving their parents: *Gillick v West Norfolk & Wisbech Area Health Authority* (1986) AC 112, approved by the High Court of Australia in *Health & Community Services (NT), Department of v JWB & SMB (Marion's case)* (1992) 175 CLR 218. For example, older children may be sufficiently mature to consent to the disclosure of a genetic risk identified from their test to other family members: Skene L. *Law and Medical Practice* (3rd ed.). Sydney: LexisNexis; 2008:127–136.

2. There are other provisions on privacy and privacy principles in the Information Privacy Act 2000 (Vic), and on confidentiality in the Health Services Act 1988 (Vic) s 141 and the Mental Health Act 1986 (Vic) s 120A, but those are not discussed here. The Office of the federal Privacy Commissioner also publishes privacy codes (ss 18BB-18BI), guidelines, and other information: Office of the Privacy Commissioner. Available at http://www.privacy.gov.au/. Accessed 23 December, 2008. The Victorian Health Services Commissioner also published privacy guidelines: http://www.health.vic.gov.au/hsc/

3. Privacy Act s 16B(2); Health Records Act ss 8, 21; HPP2(2)(h)(i).

4. Note that an "organization" includes individuals, see Privacy Act 1988 (Cth); ss 6(1), 6C(1)(a); Health Records Act 2001 (Vic) s 3. The federal Privacy Act also contains "Information Privacy Principles," but they apply to ministers, departments, and other government bodies: ss 6, 14, 16.

5. Privacy Act 1988 (Cth) s 16E; Health Records Act 2001 (Vic) s13.

6. Privacy Act 1988 (Cth) Sch 3, NPP 2.1(e).

7. HPP 2.2(h)(i).

8. Australian Law Reform Commission, Australian Health Ethics Committee, *Essentially Yours: The Protection of Human Genetic Information in Australia,* 2003; *ALRC Report 96,* Sydney, Australia, 2003 (ALRC-AHEC Report),

Recommendation 21–1.The full report is available at: http://www.austlii. edu.au/au/other/alrc/publications/reports/96/

9. National Health and Medical Research Council, Office of the Privacy Commissioner, Use and disclosure of genetic information to a patient's genetic relatives under Section 95AA of the Privacy Act 1988 (Cth), Guidelines for health practitioners in the private sector, effective from December 15, 2009..

10. I (L. Skene) have argued for some years that blood relatives are entitled to know familial genetic information (that a mutation exists in a family), but "personal" genetic information (a person's own status for the mutation— positive or negative) should not be disclosed without that person's consent: Skene L. Patients' rights or family responsibilities? Two approaches to genetic testing. *Medical Law Review* 1998;6(1):1–41; Skene L. Genetic secrets and the family: A response to Bell and Bennett. *Medical Law Review* 2001;9(2):162–169.

11. ALRC, AHEC Report,(note 8 above), para 21.28.

12. Health Professions Registration Act 2005 (Vic) s 3 (professional misconduct).

13. Under the Health Professions Registration Act 2005 (Vic) s 3, professional misconduct is defined to include "(a)...conduct [that] involves a substantial or consistent failure to reach or maintain a reasonable standard of competence and diligence; and (b) conduct that violates or falls short of, to a substantial degree, the standard of professional conduct observed by members of the profession of good repute or competency..."

14. The ALRC-AHEC Report (note 8 above) observes that privacy legislation and professional guidelines serve different purposes and are not always consistent: disclosure may constitute unsatisfactory professional conduct even if it complies with the guidelines: para 21.107. While this is true, such a finding seems unlikely in practice and, if it did occur, one cannot imagine a penalty being imposed on the health-care practitioner beyond, at most, a reprimand.

15. Alleging a breach of the broad duty to take reasonable care in treating the patient.

16. *Parry-Jones v Law Society* [1969] 1 Ch 1.

17. *Breen v Williams* (1996) 186 CLR 71.

18. W *v Egdell* [1990] Ch 359; [1990] 1 All ER 835.

19. *Duncan v Medical Disciplinary Committee* [1986] 1 NZLR 513.

20. AMA Position Statement, Blood Borne Viral Infections—1995. Revised 2002. Revised 2004. 2.4.4 In exceptional circumstances, where repeated attempts at counselling fail, a doctor may need to take action that will ensure notification of a patient's partner(s). However, this should be undertaken only in close consultation with the relevant State or Territory health department.

21. Wrongs Act (Vic) s 59 (1958).

22. Compare the ALRC-AHEC Report (note 8 above), para 21.96.

23. *Tarasoff v Regents of the University of California* 551 P2d 334 (1996).

24. *Pate v Threlkel* 551 P2d 334 (1976); *Safer v Pack* 291 NJ Super 619 (1996), 677. These cases are discussed by Bell D, Bennett B. Genetic secrets and the family. *Medical Law Review* 2001;9:130,149–152. Andrews L. The genetic information superhighway: Rules of the road for contacting relatives and recontacting

former patients. In: Knoppers B, ed. *Human DNA: Law and Policy.* The Hague, Netherlands: Kluwer Law International; 1997:133,136–138.
25. *BT v Oei* (unreported, Sup Ct of NSW, Bell J, November 5, 1999).
26. There is also a question of causation. Has the harm (the plaintiff's worsening health) been caused by failure to disclose the risk, or by the genetic condition? Has the nondisclosure deprived the plaintiff of a possible benefit? See Laurie G. Obligations arising from genetic information: Negligence and the protection of family interests. *Child and Family Law Quarterly* 1999;11(2):109.
27. ALRC-AHEC Report (note 8 above) para 21.49.
28. ALRC-AHEC Report (note 8 above), para 21.48.

REFERENCES

1. Boddington P, Gregory M. Communicating genetic information in the family: Enriching the debate through the notion of integrity. *Medicine, Health Care, and Philosophy* 2008;11:445–454.
2. Forrest LE. *Communicating Genetic Information in Families.* Melbourne, Australia: The University of Melbourne; 2009.
3. Armstrong J, Trott D, McCormack J, Suthers G. Letting the family know: SA experience in notifying relatives of genetic test availability. *Journal of Medical Genetics* 2006;43:665–670.
4. Australian Law Reform Commission, Australian Health Ethics Committee, *Essentially Yours: The Protection of Human Genetic Information in Australia,* 2003; *ALRC Report 96,* Sydney, Australia, 2003.
5. Godard B, Hurlimann T, Letendre M, Egalite N. BRCAs I. Guidelines for disclosing genetic information to family members: From development to use. *Familial Cancer* 2006;5(1):103–116.
6. Forrest LE, Delatycki MB, Skene L, Aitken MA. Communicating genetic information in families: A review of guidelines and position papers. *European Journal of Human Genetics* 2007;15(6):612–618.
7. Office of the Privacy Commissioner. *State & Territory Privacy Laws.* Available at: http://www.privacy.gov.au/privacy_rights/laws/. http://www.privacy. gov.au/individuals. Accessed 23 December, 2009.
8. Australian Law Reform Commission. *For Your Information: Australian Privacy Law and Practice* (ALRC Report 108). Canberra, Australia; 2008. Available at; http://www.austlii.edu.au/au/other/alrc/publications/reports/108/. Accessed 23 December, 2009.
9. Otlowski MFA. Disclosure of genetic information to at-risk relatives: Recent amendments to the Privacy Act 1988 (Cth). *Medical Journal of Australia.* 2008;187(7):398–399.

14

HELPING PARENTS
TALK TO THEIR
CHILDREN

JENNIFER SULLIVAN & ALLYN McCONKIE-ROSELL

When a genetic diagnosis has been made, parents are faced with the difficult challenge of when, how, and what to tell children who are minors about their risk while simultaneously trying to foster a healthy self-concept in their children. Families frequently turn to health-care practitioners for assistance in deciding how to have these discussions with children.

Parents[1] of children[2] with genetic disorders find that they are primarily responsible for discussing the diagnosis with their children and answering any questions they may have. Additionally, these parents need to communicate with teachers about special educational needs and to discuss the disorder with other professionals, such as developmental therapists, physicians, and other health-care practitioners [1]. Communication with the children in the family about genetic disorders takes many different shapes. Children may themselves be clinically affected and may have many questions about their own diagnosis. Children may also be currently unaffected but at-risk for developing a health concern in the future and/or face a risk of having affected children. Children, when asked, prefer being informed about genetic risk by a close relative, typically a parent [2, 3]. However, talking with children about genetic risk presents complex challenges. Questions commonly asked by parents include the following: "When should we start talking to our children about this?" "When should my children be offered testing?" and "How can we help our children deal with this information?"

227

Conveying information about genetic conditions within families in a sensitive and age-appropriate manner is important because family communication is a major determinant in how families manage tension, stress, and strain and develop or maintain family functioning, adjustment, and adaptation [4]. Families have different styles of communication, which may be influenced by both the family customs and responses to crisis as well as influenced by the meaning the family makes of the diagnosis and the importance and implications of the information. In some families, information is not openly transmitted because there are family rules about what can and cannot be said [5]. Communication about genetic information is transmitted in families typically using pre-existing communication patterns [6] (see Chapters 6 and 11 for more information).

Studies of adult children who grew up in families with genetic disorders in either a parent or a sibling have stressed the importance of good communication and being appropriately informed. Importantly, Holt [7] found that communication patterns started in childhood about Huntington disease (HD) persisted in adulthood. Bradbury et al. [8] reported that parents often either under- or overestimated their child's emotional response to learning a parent's BRCA test result. Fanos [9] reported on the misunderstandings carried from childhood in adults with siblings with cystic fibrosis and siblings of individuals with X-linked immune deficiency [10, 11]. She also found that major life decisions, such as whether to have children, were made based on this misinformation. Sparbel et al. (2008) [12] interviewed teens (ages 14–18 years) growing up in families where there had been a diagnosis of HD. These teens also emphasized the importance of open, honest communication about the diagnosis. Additionally, adolescent girls and young women from families diagnosed with fragile X syndrome when considering the possibility that they might not have been informed about their own genetic risk status, expressed a sense of betrayal of being left out of something that was not only of importance for their family but also directly involved them [13]. Thus, how genetic information is communicated in childhood may have direct implications on future communication and adjustment to the diagnosis.

When a genetic diagnosis is made, parents often turn to health-care practitioners for assistance in considering the risk to the children in the family as well as how to best communicate the information. The purpose of this chapter is to first discuss some of the barriers to communication and to review literature on how children understand medical information. Then we will present an approach, using a parent–practitioner partnership model, breaking the information down into stages, considering both the type of information that needs to be communicated and the developmental age of the child.

BARRIERS TO COMMUNICATION

Families may encounter multiple barriers to communication when they are informing relatives about genetic risk. Some of these barriers include difficulty in determining who is at risk, uncertainty about how to explain the diagnosis and its inheritance, worry over providing the wrong information, as well as concerns about when and how to inform [2, 3, 7, 14–17].

A major barrier to talking with children may be uncertainty [2] Uncertainty encompasses not only the information itself but also current and future implications for the child, how to explain it, when to inform, and what the child's ability to understand, cope, and manage the information is (see Chapter 8). Adults themselves may find genetic information emotionally upsetting, complex, and difficult to understand. Dealing with uncertainty about how to talk about a genetic diagnosis in the family requires that the parents be comfortable with the information. Furthermore, it requires the development of a staged plan for informing the children that is tailored to the needs of the family, sensitive to the family's own communication patterns, and is developmentally appropriate for the child.

Medical information in general may be emotionally charged for the family and difficult to understand. Genetic information adds the additional component of concern for others in the family who may have to face the same diagnosis or may also be at risk for having affected children. When thinking about talking with their children, parents may also remember the emotions they felt at the time of the diagnosis and may be concerned about their children feeling those same emotions.

The uncertainty about how to approach talking to their children combined with concern for their children's well-being may lead to keeping a "family secret." Family secrets, although often meant to protect a child from harm, can cause harm themselves once revealed [18]. Some family secrets are kept intentionally; others may evolve. For example, well-intentioned parents may be waiting for the "right time" to tell their child, and the difficulty in finding the words may lead to keeping a secret. The longer the secret is kept, the harder it is to reveal.

Secrets may create an environment of tension and distrust. In the absence of direct information, children may already be aware of limited aspects of the family diagnosis. For example, a child might observe the effects of chemotherapy in his mother diagnosed with breast cancer or go along with a sibling with Down syndrome to speech therapy sessions.

Children may also be brought to a medical clinic for evaluation and may draw their own conclusions about the meaning of the clinic visit. When one child in a family is diagnosed with a disorder, such as neurofibromatosis (NF; an autosomal dominant condition that mainly affects the brain, nerves, and skin), parents as well as siblings are evaluated to determine whether they also have the condition. In one family, seen in clinic for a routine evaluation, the affected child had died of a rare brain tumor related to NF. During the clinic visit, the genetic counselor obtained appropriate family and medical histories, and the geneticist completed detailed skin examinations on the children. The parents were visibly upset at the process, and their concern for their surviving children was obvious. They had not told the younger children why they were in the clinic and requested that the health-care practitioners not talk about the diagnosis when the children were in the room. During her physical examination, the 7-year-old sister turned to the genetic counselor and said, "Am I going to die too?"

If they are unable to discuss their own observations, children may misinterpret what is occurring and perceive it as more severe than the adults in their life would anticipate [19]. Additionally, without factual information, children tend to think the worst and may become concerned about their own health, even when it may not be directly affected [20]. Children may also identify tension in the family and without a discussion to help understand the problem, they may blame themselves [21]. On the other hand, some children may have almost complete factual information about the situation but lack the psychological support to contextualize and personalize the implications of that information.

INDIRECT COMMUNICATION

Children are an integral part of the communication going on all around them. Communication can be both direct to the individual for whom it is intended or communicated indirectly through overheard or unintended exposure [22], such as conversation among family members. A teenage daughter may be listening when her mother calls her sister on the phone to talk about a carrier test result. An elementary school age son may be listening to his father talking to a sibling's teacher. Children may be listening as parents talk with relatives, teachers, developmental specialists, and health-care providers. In families diagnosed with *BRCA* mutations, Tercyak and colleagues [23] found that the greatest exposure of children to genetic information was indirect, through contact with family members who were affected or who were undergoing testing themselves. In a study of how adolescent and young adult women from families diagnosed with fragile X syndrome remember learning their genetic status, one quarter of the girls who knew they were at risk to be a carrier reported learning about the inheritance of fragile X syndrome as well as their own at-risk status through overhearing "adult" conversations in medical clinics, at family gatherings, and at home [2]. Importantly, these girls did not typically ask questions about the sometimes confusing or upsetting information they had overheard. Metcalfe and colleagues [3] in their meta-analysis of family communication also reported that children often did not ask questions.

Indirect communication may include unintended verbal information and observed situational and emotional reactions. A 16-year-old adolescent remembers learning about the diagnosis of fragile X syndrome through her attendance at a medical appointment for her brothers [2]. She was 10 years old at the time.

I remember when we were at some doctor...my mom was really having a rough time with it and like I was in the office with them and she started to cry because she didn't know anything about it. Well, so at that point, she didn't think the diagnosis was necessarily a good thing, so, but I was too young to really be just like, so I was like, okay, they have Fragile X. Now we know what's wrong with them...But I felt bad for my mom because she has never been like one to break down or anything and that really took a lot out of her. So it's what I remember the most. [2]

A child may observe a parent's tearful or angry emotional response to a genetic diagnosis and be unable to determine the source of the distress. Additionally, a health-care practitioner may focus on the informational and emotional needs of the parent(s), sometimes forgetting that the children in the family may also have their own questions and concerns. Practitioners, parents, and other adult family members may inadvertently create mistrust and misunderstanding in children, if they do not consider the effect of indirect verbal and nonverbal communications as well as the children's own questions.

Although there is very limited research on what children understand about genetic diagnoses, adolescents and young adults from families diagnosed with genetic disorders have endorsed an open, honest approach to discussing the information that is consistent with a resilient communication pattern [2, 3, 7, 8]. Resilient communication is characterized by an optimistic bias, clear consistent messages in both words and actions, clarification of ambiguous information, with both truth seeking and truth speaking [21]. In general, positive open communication leads to improved family functioning [24]. To facilitate a resilient communication pattern related to genetic information with children, it is important to first consider what information a child is capable of understanding and to overcome barriers to positive conversations.

WHAT WE KNOW ABOUT TALKING WITH CHILDREN

Developmentally, children are very different from adults. Discussions with children need to be tailored to their social, emotional, and cognitive development [20]. Koopman and colleagues [25] have proposed a practical model to help identify the type of medical information that children of different developmental levels are most likely to be able to understand. According to their model, young children age 2–7 years may begin to ascribe the cause of illness to persons, places, or events in their direct surroundings. Children age 7–11 years may perceive illness and associated treatments as a punishment for perceived negative behavior, and a discussion of physiological mechanisms to explain disease might not be understood until a child is 11 years or older. However, if presented with appropriate cues (physical cues for relatedness and contagion for a contagious disease such as a cold), Raman and Gleman (2005) [26] found that children in first grade (age 6–7 years) to fifth grade (10 years) were able to understand the differences in how genetic versus contagious illnesses occur. In their study, even children under the age of 5 years were able to match physical characteristics to birth parents versus adoptive parents. They were also able to distinguish that genetic disorders had more permanency than a contagious disease. Springer [27] found that children age 4–8 years expect families to share more biological properties than unrelated people. Thus, if given the opportunity for open conversation, children can understand genetic information.

The emotional tone of conversations is as important to consider as what is said. A large part of communication is the emotional undercurrent related to the factual information being shared. Children may remember and react to what they observe and the emotions with which information is said, as much as what is said directly to them [25]. If a parent is visibly distressed when trying to talk about a genetic diagnosis, the child might associate the information about the possibility of being a carrier with the emotional upset of seeing his mother cry. Children may not understand the implications of what they are being told, but they may well remember the emotion with which it is presented [2, 28].

It is also important to contextualize what is being said and to provide concrete examples using words that are familiar to the child. Koopman and colleagues [25] suggest that when talking with children under the age of 11 years about the cause of an illness it is important to build on prior discussions, using short direct statements that are concretely tied to what the child has experienced. However, even if information is provided in a simple and straightforward manner, it may be interpreted and remembered in a different way when the child is older [29]. Therefore, repeated discussions allowing for the opportunity to ask questions and to clarify misunderstandings are critically important. Communication between parent and child involves a commitment to consider the developmental level of the child, to anticipate and "hear" the child's unspoken needs, and to act to address those needs in a timely manner.

The combination of indirect information, uncertainty, observed family emotions, and complex genetic information may be confusing to a child. It is important for families as well as health-care practitioners to consider the family environment, the family response to the diagnosis, and how genetic information is being discussed by *all* members of the family, both directly and indirectly. Direct communication with trusted adults that provides the available information, acknowledges the uncertainties, and creates an open environment that encourages questions may be reassuring to children [21]. Working together, parents and practitioners need to consider how parents and close family perceive the disorder and just as importantly, how the family describes the disorder to their child(ren), as well as to others.

AN APPROACH TO COMMUNICATING GENETIC INFORMATION TO CHILDREN

A parent–practitioner partnership focused on the commitment to the well-being of the children in the family can be the foundation on which to build the steps to a positive communication process about genetic risk information. Dunst and Paget [30] have described such a partnership model. This parent–practitioner partnership model is characterized by mutual contributions and agreed-upon roles, a desire to work together to achieve an agreed-upon goal, trust and honesty in all dealings, disclosure of pertinent information, and a parental locus of decision making regarding what is in the best interest of the family.

Communication of genetic risk information to children is not a one-time event; instead, it is a process. Health-care practitioners can partner with families to identify mutually agreed-upon goals and objectives. Families should be encouraged to utilize available resources, as well as health professionals, teachers, psychologists, and social workers, to develop a plan for their family, to take the opportunity to explore and practice what they might say to their children, and to follow up with genetic services to make sure information is up to date and correct. Practitioners can actively engage parents in an open discussion about their perceptions, both positive and negative, about their concerns for their children's reaction to the genetic diagnosis. Metcalfe et al. [3] found that the support needed by families to help children develop positive coping strategies includes education, understanding, and identifying and managing emotions.

Families may be overwhelmed by the volume of information that needs to be conveyed to their children, while health-care practitioners may be focused on the appropriateness of offering a genetic test to a minor child. There has been much debate among practitioners, ethicists, and families affected by genetic disorders about what age to offer genetic testing and what age a child should be before he or she is able to make an informed decision [31]. Talking to children about genetic risk is much more complex than deciding when or if to offer genetic testing to a minor child. It encompasses talking about the diagnosis itself and the clinical implications, learning that the disorder is inherited, learning about the possibility of being a carrier, and perhaps discovering the likelihood of having an affected child of their own. Communication to children in a family about a genetic diagnosis is a multistage process that requires different types of knowledge be shared and understood by multiple family members. Genetic counseling for families with genetic disorders requires a commitment to this process.

An approach to overcoming uncertainty about talking with children about genetic information is to take the information and break it down into stages. Each stage represents tasks that have unique implications for the child and require the communication of specific messages related to genetic risk. Considering the information in stages can be used as a framework to develop an approach that is appropriate for each member of a family and that is tailored to the medical and social implications of the disorder itself. The order in which the stages of knowledge discussed in the following sections are listed is not intended to represent an ideal order because the specific order will vary based on the disorder and the family. It is also important to consider that *understanding* and *incorporating* the various stages of knowledge is an evolving process that changes as the child matures. It is the task of all involved with the family to explore and honestly assess what a particular child may understand about each stage of knowledge and tailor the information accordingly. While it is obvious that a 3-year-old child can appreciate information at a different level than a 13-year-old child, progress is unique for each and every child and will vary based on the child's own life experience.

What's in a Name?

Often a first step in talking about a genetic disorder in the family it to name the disorder and learn to use the name appropriately, as well as to also learn about the clinical features. A name for why a brother has physical or cognitive delays can help even a young child to begin to understand a genetic diagnosis. For instance, Adam is a 3 year old with 22q13 deletion (Phelan-McDermid) syndrome and has significant cognitive and motor delays. His older brother, Tom, age 6 years, has been going to all of Adam's physical therapy appointments, and he has heard his mother talking about the exercises that help to make Adam better. Tom was very angry with Adam for not working harder on his exercises so that he could be "like everybody else." A 6 year old is developmentally likely to attribute a sibling's delayed motor skills to an observed experience (such as needing more exercise) and perceive it as fixable, as opposed to understanding the lifelong clinical consequences of a chromosome deletion.

Children will often have questions about a genetic disorder in the family: What are the implications? What do we need to be concerned about? Siblings may not understand why their brother or sister is the focus of family attention. When parents make adjustments to daily life in order to accommodate a child with medical, emotional, or physical differences, it can lead to sibling resentment or rivalry if the siblings do not have an adequate understanding [32]. Young children may also blame themselves or engage in "magical thinking" [25]. Opperman and Alant [33] found in their study of adolescent siblings (12–16 years) of children with severe disabilities that siblings often did not have sufficient information about their sibling's disability. They concluded that in order to help the unaffected sibling develop effective coping strategies it is important that they be well-informed about the disorder and its consequences. Such data reinforce the idea that knowledge of the specific genetic condition in a family is beneficial to all children in that family.

What Does "Inherited" Mean?

A second step in understanding that a particular genetic diagnosis is part of a family's medical history is to understand that biologically related family members share genetic traits. Depending on the developmental age of the child, conversations could include tangible ways that relatives look like each other to complex concepts, such as how genes are the body's blueprints and inheritance patterns. In some families, young children may have been introduced to the idea that siblings or other relatives have a particular genetic diagnosis at such an early age that its initial introduction can no longer be recalled [2]. For these children, the diagnosis, clinical features, and the fact that the condition "runs in their family" are things they have always known and are part of their own "family story." These family stories are important because they help to define the family identity as well as to make meaning of an event [34]. They also play a critical role in the process of developing a shared understanding among family members [35]. (See Chapter 4.)

The family stories can be used to help the child understand the fundamentals of inheritance. Discussions about inheritance can include who shares the same common physical traits, such as eye color, as well as cognitive abilities, such as who is good at math. These common family traits can then be extended to the clinical characteristics of the genetic disorder. For children, memorable stories of the affected and unaffected individuals are simply "family," and a genetic diagnosis becomes part of the shared family story, a part of the family culture.

Older children and teenagers may do a school project or research on the Internet on their own. It is not uncommon for teens to take an active interest in the family diagnosis and seek out information. Parents can help children manage the information by providing it to them, as opposed to allowing children to learn the inheritance and genetic risk on their own, possibly from unreliable sources. By providing the information, parents also help to develop a communication pattern that demonstrates they are willing to talk with the child and answer questions. In a partnership model, the health-care practitioner is available as a resource for the entire family. Clinic follow-up visits should not only focus on the immediate health concerns but also on the questions and future concerns of the children.

Can I Have This, Too?

For some genetic disorders, there is the possibility that the child is currently affected, will be affected in the future, or is a carrier for a genetic change. This stage is much more personal to the child than learning to use the name correctly or simply learning that a disorder is inherited. In this stage the child learns that the diagnosis is not just for other relatives but means "me, too" and the connection between general family information and individualized details specific to the child is made. There is a clear difference between a child being able to state that he has "ABC disease" and that child being able to understand the medical and psychosocial implications of such a diagnosis.

Parents may find this stage challenging because it may bring back memories of their own emotional response to first learning about the diagnosis. If these emotions were negative, parents may be concerned that their child will feel the same pain. Prior to being able to successfully discuss this level of information with a child, parents must address their own feelings. Parents may also be overwhelmed at the scale of implications for their child, including such items as the natural history of the disease, reduced fertility, or increased mortality.

Young adults and adolescents have recommended that, when informing children about their own personal genetic risk, parents provide reassurance and try to normalize the information [2]. Parents and health-care practitioners can offer reassurance through identifying actions that can be taken and help the child to accept what cannot be changed. A father with Marfan syndrome can emphasize to his affected son increased medical surveillance, including echocardiograms, in a positive manner, so that the child knows that actions are being taken to keep him and his family safe. Additionally, the identification for the child of others in the family facing the same situation can help to normalize the information. We have previously described the importance of the family genetic identity in helping to incorporate genetic information for the individual [36].

How Do We Figure Out If I Have This?

The primary goals are to help children understand, to their best developmental ability, why a particular test could be performed and what information the test may provide. Parents and health-care practitioners can individualize the information by identifying the pieces that are important for the child to know and how much information the child can meaningfully absorb. Furthermore, the child's own understanding of and curiosity about the test and access to additional information (i.e., the Internet) can serve as a guide for both immediate discussion and follow-up review at home. For some disorders, such as familial adenomatous polyposis or Marfan syndrome, a diagnostic test may have occurred at a very young age for the purposes of increased medical surveillance. For other children, it may be important to know that genetic testing is available in the future and can definitively answer their questions about their own risk.

Do I Have This, Too?

At some time, if genetic testing results are available, the information from these results should be shared with the child. The disclosure of test results can occur either at home or in a medical clinic setting. A *plan* for results discussion should be developed before a test is done. This plan should consider the specific needs, desires, and logistics of the family as well as the medical and social implications of a positive or negative genetic test. It is important to note that disclosure to a child may occur at any time after the testing is completed, and in some families, disclosing test results may occur years after the test is completed. Although this stage is very personal, if families have provided information in small pieces, the staged preparation may help reduce the emotional impact [36]. An 18 year old from a family diagnosed with fragile X syndrome describes the process in this manner:

> I think I just learned because they (my parents) would like say stuff to me over time, and I'd put it together myself....casually like this and that and here and there, and I put it together. [2]

Can I Have a Child with This?

Talking with an adolescent about her likelihood of having children who may be affected may present unique challenges. Perceptions about the enactment of the parental role and consideration of future options may occur long before actual decisions are made [37]. There is limited research on how adolescents in families with genetic disorders perceive the implications of genetic information on their reproductive options. Research has focused on female carriers of X-linked conditions or with women with Turner syndrome. Women with Turner syndrome have emphasized the sense of betrayal they felt at not being told about the reproductive implications of their diagnosis [38]. Importantly, similar to providing information about the diagnosis, the girls and young women felt that talking about reproductive options should be approached in a staged, factual manner. Adolescents from fragile X families have also stressed the importance of open, honest communication about reproductive options but have also stressed the need for the child to be old enough to comprehend the information [13]. Thus, similar to the other stages of knowledge, consideration of this stage should be sensitive to the child's needs and understanding.

CONCLUSION

Health-care practitioners should not only explore the family communication pattern with parents but also help the family to consider both what is being said directly to the child as well as what the child might have overheard. Families will vary in their ability to talk with their children about genetic risk. How genetic risk information is communicated to the children in the family is important. It is important to explore how parents are currently talking about a diagnosis and how they plan to address the information in the future. Discussions also need to be sensitive to the emotional developmental age of the child as well as the type of information that is being provided. Practitioners can engage with the family to develop a collaborative plan, considering the different genetic information stages, to provide ongoing support at critical developmental ages to facilitate good communication between the child or adolescent and the rest of the family. Table 14.1 provides a list for heath care practitioners and

Table 14.1 How Can Health-Care Practitioners Help?

Partner with the Family to Facilitate Communication

- Explore family communication patterns.
- Consider both direct and indirect communication:
  - What is being said to the child
  - What the child might have overheard or observed
- Explore the family's personal story and determine how it is being told to the next generation of children.
- Explore the family's emotional response to the diagnosis.

Facilitate Resilient Family Communication

- Identify and focus on family strengths.
- Encourage truth telling.
- Reduce uncertainty and foster confidence about the information and how to communicate it effectively.
- Facilitate the development of clear and consistent messages about the genetic diagnosis in the family, in both words and actions.
- Personalize the genetic information for a specific family.

Offer a Safe Environment for Parents

- Discuss their fears and concerns about the implications of the genetic diagnosis for their children.
- Practice what they might say to their children now and in the future.
- Work with families to identify simple definitions of complex terms and ways to approach discussions of the diagnosis with their children.

Provide Concrete Tools to Parents

Help ensure that the parents get the facts straight and are able to accurately discuss the genetics.

Plan Follow-up

Staged follow up allows for the opportunity to address misunderstandings, respond to the children's own questions, and consider the family's current educational and psychosocial needs as well as to provide anticipatory guidance.

Engage in Collaborative Problem Solving

- Anticipate potential problems.
- Be creative and encourage the family to identify and use available resources:
  - Family physician/other health-care practitioners
  - School psychologist, teachers
  - Provide information on disease-specific support group, attendance at a conference with age peers, or comparison to other similar situations familiar to the child and family.

Consider the Genetic Information in Stages with Each Stage Having Different Implications for the Child

- Explore different orders in the stages to help identify what might work best for a particular family.
- Develop a plan for talking with the children:
  - Consider who the conversation should include, what type or stage of information, and the appropriate time.
- Revise and adjust based on child's and parents' response to the information so that there is an open, dynamic, ongoing family discussion targeted to the
  - Age of the child
  - Stage of knowledge

Table 14.2 Tips for Parents

Have an Actual Conversation

- Make a plan about what information is to be shared and consider a setting that is conducive to a conversation.
- Allow for questions and develop an environment that is open and honest.

Consider Both Direct and Indirect Conversations

- Pay attention to how family members are talking about the diagnosis—both what is directly said as well as what is overheard.

Consider Framing the "Message" Being Conveyed to the Children in a Positive Manner

Positive framing includes:

- Focusing on what can be done
- Maintaining hope for the future
- Acknowledging what cannot be changed
- Normalizing the information
- Reassurance

Contextualize the Information

- Information does not exist in a vacuum.
- Think creatively to identify concrete examples from the child's own life experiences to help the child draw appropriate conclusions.

It Is Not Just One Conversation

- Talking about genetic risk does not have to happen all at once.
- Do not assume because it was discussed once that the process will not need to be repeated; children's needs and understanding change over time.

Be Aware of Their Own As Well As Their Children's Emotional Reaction to the Information

- Communication is more than what is said; it is also what is felt and seen. Children, especially young children, easily remember situation-specific emotion.
- Children may or may not attach the same emotion to the information as the adults in the family.

Be Honest (with Themselves and Their Children) about Their Understanding

- Get the facts straight
- Be honest about what you do not know, but offer a way to find out.

Make a Plan

- If you feel ready to have a conversation with your child, then practice what you are going to say.
- Make sure you feel comfortable with the information.
- Try to anticipate questions your child might ask.

Table 14.2 for families to use to help develop a positive communication pattern. Working together, practitioners and parents can overcome barriers to communication to facilitate resiliency and foster positive communication with the children.

NOTES

1. We are using "parent" as an inclusive term for biological parents, step-parents, guardians, and so on.
2. We are using the terms "child" or "children" to refer to individuals under the age of 18 years.

REFERENCES

1. Hodgkinson R, Lester H. Stresses and coping strategies of mothers living with a child with cystic fibrosis: Implications for nursing professionals. *Journal of Advanced Nursing* 2002;39(4):377–383.
2. McConkie-Rosell A, Heise EM, Spiridigliozzi GA. Genetic risk communication: Experiences of adolescent and young adults from families with fragile X syndrome. *Journal of Genetic Counseling,* 2009. 18(4):313–25.
3. Metcalfe A, Coad J, Plumridge GM, Gill P, Farndon P. Family communication between children and their parents about inherited genetic conditions: A meta-synthesis of the research. *European Journal of Human Genetics* 2008;16:1193–1200.
4. McCubbin HI, Thompson AI, McCubbin MA. *FPSC: Family Problem Solving Communication. Family Assessment: Resiliency, Coping and Adaptation.* Madison: University of Wisconsin Publishers; 1996.
5. Boss P. *Family Stress Management.* Newbury Park, CA: Sage Publications; 1988.
6. Forrest LE, Curnow L, Martin B, Delatycki, Skene L, Aitken M. Health first, genetics second: Exploring families' experiences of communicating genetic information. *European Journal of Human Genetics* 2008;16: 1329–1335.
7. Holt K. What do we tell the children? Contrasting the disclosure choices of two HD families regarding risk status and predictive genetic testing. *Journal of Genetic Counseling* 2006;15(4):253–265.
8. Bradbury AR, Patrick-Miller L, Pawlowski K, Ibe CN, Cummings SA, Hlubocky F, et al. Learning your parent's BRCA mutation during adolescence or early adulthood: A study of offspring experiences. *Psycho-Oncology* 2009;18(2):200–208.
9. Fanos JH. Developmental tasks of childhood and adolescence: Implications for genetic testing. *American Journal of Medical Genetics* 1997;71:22–28.
10. Fanos JH, Davis J, Puck JM. Sib understanding of genetics and attitudes toward carrier testing for X-linked severe combined immunodeficiency. *American Journal of Medical Genetics* 2001;98(1):46–56.
11. Fanos JH, Gatti RA. A mark on the arm: Myths of carrier status in sibs of individuals with ataxia-telangiectasia. *American Journal of Medical Genetics* 1999;86:338–346.
12. Sparbel KJH, Driessnack M, Williams JK, Schutte DL, Tripp-Reimer T, McGonigal-Kenney M, et al. Experiences of teens living in the shadow of Huntington disease. *Journal of Genetic Counseling* 2008;17(4):327–335
13. Wehbe RM, Spiridigliozzi GA, Heise EM, Dawson, DV, McConkie-Rosell A. When to tell and test for genetic carrier status: Perspectives from adolescents and young adults from families with fragile X syndrome. *American Journal of Medical Genetics,*2009; 149A (6) 1190–1199.

14. Forrest K, Simpson S, Wilson B, Teijingen Ev, McKee L, Haites N, et al. To tell or not to tell: Barriers and facilitators in family communication about genetic risk. *Clinical Genetics* 2003;64:317–326.

15. McConkie-Rosell A, Robinson H, Wake S, Staley L, Heller K, Cronister A. The dissemination of genetic risk information to relatives in the fragile X syndrome: Guidelines for genetic counselors. *American Journal of Medical Genetics* 1995;59:426–430.

16. Tercyak K, Peshkin B, DeMarco T, Brogan B, Lerman C. Parent-child factors and their effect on communicating BRCA1/2 test results to children. *Patient Education and Counseling* 2002;47(2):145–153.

17. Tercyak K, Peshkin B, Demarco T, Patenaude A, Schneider K, Garber J, et al. Information needs of mothers regarding communicating BRCA1/2 cancer genetic test results to their children. *Genetic Testing* 2007;11(3):249–255.

18. Brown-Smith N. Family secrets. *Journal of Family Issues* 1998;19(1):20–23.

19. Hilden JM, Watterson J, Charastek J. Tell the children. *Journal of Clinical Oncology* 2000;18(17):3193–3195.

20. Spinetta JJ, Jankovic M, Eden T, Green D, Martins AG, Wandzura C, et al. Guidelines for assistance to siblings of children with cancer: Report of the SIOP Working Committee on Psychosocial Issues in Pediatric Oncology. *Medical and Pediatric Oncology* 1999;33:395–398.

21. Walsh F. *Strengthening Family Resilience* (2nd ed.). New York: The Guilford Press; 2006.

22. Miller IW, Ryan CE, Keitner GI, Bishop DS, Epstein NB. The McMaster Approach to families: Theory, assessment, treatment and research. *Journal of Family Therapy* 2000;22:168–189.

23. Tercyak K, Hughes C, Main D, Snyder C, Lynch J, Lynch H, et al. Parental communication of BRCA1/2 genetic test results to children. *Patient Education and Counseling* 2001;42:213–224.

24. Walsh F. Family resilience: A framework for clinical practice. *Family Process* 2003;42(1):2–18.

25. Koopman HM, Baars RM, Chaplin J, Zwinderman KH. Illness through the eyes of the child: The development of children's understanding of the causes of illness. *Patient Education and Counseling* 2004;55:363–370.

26. Raman L, Gelman SA. Children's understanding of the transmission of genetic disorders and contagious illnesses. *Developmental Psychology* 2005;41(1):171–182.

27. Springer K. Children's awareness of the biological implications of kinship. *Child Development* 1992;63:950–959.

28. McConkie-Rosell A, O'Daniel J. Beyond the diagnosis: The process of genetic counseling. In: Mazzocco MMM, Ross JL, eds. *Neurogenetic Developmental Disorders: Variation of Manifestation in Childhood*. Cambridge, MA: The MIT Press; 2007:367–389.

29. Jack F, Hayne H. Eliciting adults' earliest memories: Does it matter how we ask the question? *Memory* 2007;6:647–663

30. Dunst CJ, Paget KD. Parent-professional partnerships and family empowerment. In: Fine M, ed. *Collaboration with Parents of Exceptional Children*. Brandon, VT: Clinical Psychology Publishing; 1991:25–44.

31. McConkie-Rosell A, Spiridigliozzi GA. "Family matters": A conceptual framework for genetic testing in children. *Journal of Genetic Counseling* 2004;13(1):9–29.

32. Weil J. *Psychosocial Genetic Counseling.* New York: Oxford University Press; 2000.
33. Opperman S, Alant E. The coping response of the adolescent siblings of children with severe disabilities. *Disability and Rehabilitation* 2003;25(9):441–454.
34. Langellier KM, Peterson EE. Narrative performance theory: Telling stories, doing family. In: Braithwaite DO, Baxter LA, eds. *Communication Privacy Management Theory: Understanding Families.* Thousand Oaks, CA: Sage; 2006:99–114.
35. McCubbin HI, Thompson AI, McCubbin MA. *Family Assessment: Resiliency, Coping, and Adaptation.* Madison: University of Wisconsin Publishers; 1996.
36. McConkie-Rosell A, Spiridigliozzi G, Melvin E, Dawson D, Lachiewicz A. Living with genetic risk: Effect on adolescent self-concept. *American Journal of Medical Genetics* 2008;148C:56–69.
37. McConkie-Rosell A, DeVellis BM. Threat to parental role: A possible mechanism of altered self-concept related to carrier knowledge. *Journal of Genetic Counseling* 2000;9(4):285–302.
38. Sutton EJ, Jessica Young J, McInerney-Leo A, Bondy CA, Gollust SE, Biesecker BB. Truth-telling and Turner syndrome: The importance of diagnostic disclosure. *Journal of Pediatrics* 2006;148(1):102–107.

15

FACILITATING FAMILY COMMUNICATION ABOUT GENETICS IN PRACTICE

Clara L. Gaff, Kathleen M. Galvin, & Carma L. Bylund

The preceding chapters have presented different perspectives and theories on family communication about genetics. This chapter serves as an epilogue, drawing on the preceding chapters to consider how to integrate these perspectives and theories into everyday practice in genetic counseling and health care.

A review of English-language guidelines and position papers related to the communication of genetic information in families identified a general consensus that genetics practitioners have a responsibility to, at minimum, inform their clients about the implications that genetic information holds for their family members [1]. It appears that this is in fact standard practice, with an international survey revealing that 98% of genetics practitioners always explain how family members could also have inherited the condition [2]. However, the same study found considerably fewer genetics practitioners always explore the family's current communication patterns (33%–60%, depending on the genetic condition) and family relationships (48%–74%). The theories and perspectives on family communication presented in earlier chapters provide an opportunity to consider the ways in which health-care practitioners might move beyond simply "informing" clients to work in a more sophisticated way that recognizes the complexity of communication within families. Our colleagues offer ways of *gaining insight* into a family's communication patterns and *strategies* for practitioners to assist families to make informed decisions about communicating and to act on these. In this chapter, we draw these threads together and consider how they may be woven into clinical practice.[1] In doing so, we have found it necessary to contextualize by documenting current clinical practice with respect to family communication.

Although this chapter refers predominantly to the documented practice of genetics practitioners and focuses on genetics consultations, there are similarities between good practice in genetic counseling interactions and in "nongenetic" health care, as pointed out by Smets et al. [3]. Specifically, in both a patient-centered approach is advocated, good information-giving skills are crucial, there is an emphasis on patient involvement in the decision-making processes, and discussion of health-related behavior is recommended. These similarities suggest that, where relevant, exploration of family communication may be incorporated into discussions regardless of the service context in which they occur. Smets and colleagues suggest the salient difference between genetics and other health-care practice is in the form and degree of family involvement. We recognize that other health-care practitioners have different primary responsibilities and duties of care with respect to a patient's family. Furthermore, any practitioner's capacity to incorporate new approaches to discussing family communication depends on the resources available (such as time and privacy) and the communication skills of the practitioner.

Exploration—as distinct from informing—is aided by well-developed communication skills, such as active listening and questioning. In Table 15.1 we provide a summary of skills that may be useful when discussing genetics. To compile this, we have drawn on widely used skills and also specific communication skills frameworks developed for health-care practitioners [4, 5]. These skills are evident in and important for genetic counseling practice [6, 7], although more work is required to fully explicate the ways in which they relate to a model of practice [8]. The skills summary serves as an introduction or refresher to common communication skills and is simply a list, not a chronology or recipe to be followed. Elaborating on these is beyond the scope of this chapter. Readers who wish to develop their communication skills further are encouraged to consult one of the many texts on communication or to consider participating in communication skills workshops or classes.

CURRENT PRACTICE

Guidelines on family communication diverge on how actively genetics practitioners should encourage clients to disclose genetic information to their family members. At one end of the spectrum is the stance that active encouragement violates patient autonomy, while at the other end is the view that the practitioner should do everything within his or her power to encourage disclosure [1]. In practice, when asked about four conditions with variable onset, inheritance, treatability, and health consequences (Huntington disease, familial adenomatous polyposis, chromosome

Table 15.1 Summary of Common Communication Skills

Skills	Definition	Examples
Establish a framework for the consultation		
Invite client agenda	At the beginning of the consultation, ask the client(s) what she or he would like to happen in today's visit.	"Could you tell me what you hope to get from this consultation today?" "What is your understanding of why Dr James has referred you? What would you like to be sure we talk about today?"
Establish agreed agenda	State what you are hoping to accomplish	"In order to answer your questions, I need to find out first about your family history, then talk with you about the genes that can cause this condition. I would also like to discuss your options with you."
Responding empathically		
Encourage expression of feelings (open questions)	Ask the client to tell you about how he or she is feeling.	"How are you feeling about all of this?" "It would be helpful for me to better understand how this news has impacted you."
Acknowledge or reflect	Verbally or nonverbally demonstrate that you have heard what the client is saying.	"It seems that you are confused by your mother's response." "I can tell that this has been a very stressful experience for you."
Normalize	Let the client know that what he or she is feeling or experiencing is normal.	"Many of the people I see in your situation also describe feeling anxious—it can be very difficult to pass this information on when you're worried it might make your daughter worry more." "It's perfectly natural to feel........."
Recognize client's strengths	Identify and commend coping, positive actions	"Even though it was really difficult, you did as you planned and made sure your brother knows about this condition." "You've had so much to deal with recently, but you still seem very committed to helping your relatives too."
Connecting		
Involving all participants in the room	Work to involve others, especially when one person dominates.	"Nancy, how are you responding to what Maria is saying?" "Mark, what do you think about this?"

Table 15.1 (*Continued*)

Skills	Definition	Examples
Metacommunication		
Preview	Give the client a short overview of what you are going to talk about	"As well as the way this affects you, there are also implications for your relatives that I would like to discuss with you." "There are two options that we can discuss at this point."
Check understanding	Ask the client what she or he understands. This can be done before or after you have given information.	"Tell me what you know about Huntington disease." "I want to make sure I've explained things clearly. Would you mind telling me what you understand about the chances your relatives will be affected by this condition?" "I've covered a lot of information. How do you think you will explain this to your relatives?"
Talk about the consultation talk	Ensure that the clients' needs and preferences for information are being met.	"Would you like me to explain more about how we look to see if other members of your family have the gene change causing this condition?" "I have just given you a lot of new information, so I'd like to stop here and see if you have any questions."
Endorse question asking	Make it clear to the client that you think his or her questions are important.	"While I'm talking, please feel free to interrupt and ask questions or request more detail." "I'd be happy to answer any questions that you have."
Establishing credibility		
Establish counselor's competence	Describing years of experience, any previous experience with the particular genetic disorder while avoiding minimizing the client's unique experiences	"During the past several years, I've worked with hundreds of families who have requested genetic testing." "I've seen many families in similar situations to yours and, though everyone's circumstances are different, from them I've learned . . . . ."
Demonstrate caring	Indicating concern for clients and the anxiety (if appropriate) they may be experiencing	"You all seem to be feeling a bit nervous about telling your mother. That's a perfectly natural thing to be feeling right now." "It seems that this has been really hard for you to think about."
Reframing		
Restructure a client's thoughts	Helping the patient to see something from a different perspective	Client: "My father lied. He kept this secret from me!" Practitioner: "It seems your father thought he could protect you." Client: "My brother was furious with me when I told him he could have genetic testing." Practitioner: "You were wanting to help him, but sometimes people see this as bad news and take their anger at the situation out on the messenger."

translocation, and hereditary hemochromatosis), the vast majority of genetics practitioners (93%) said they always encourage their clients to communicate information about these conditions to their families during the consultation. There was no evidence to suggest that the practice was variable between conditions [2].

As pointed out by Leonard and Newson in Chapter 12, much of the literature on genetic counseling practice and family communication focuses on genetics practitioners' responses to nondisclosure by clients and their "duty to warn." Surveys of genetics practitioners suggest that a significant proportion have faced this dilemma [9, 10]. However, while it is important to consider this challenging situation, focusing predominantly on this expressed "active" nondisclosure seems disproportionate when one considers that in practice refusal to inform specific relatives is a relatively rare occurrence [11]. Most people do communicate with at least some of their at-risk relatives [12, 13], although there is a gap between the intention to communicate to "all" relatives and the reality that a significant proportion of relatives are not in fact informed directly [14]. Closing this gaps seems to be the aim of research studies that are predicated on the need to *encourage* family communication, for example, by sending letters to at-risk relatives [15] or providing among other things "guidance about how to approach relatives" during follow-up telephone calls [16]. In contrast, the reciprocal engagement model of genetic counseling (see Chapter 11 and Veach et al. [8]) has as one of its key tenets that "patient autonomy must be supported' (Box 15.1). That is, rather than determine what the outcome of an individual or family "decision" about communication should be, the genetic counselor adopts a collaborative role and promotes individual- and family-directed decisions. In general, the client knows best about what he or she should do. The role of the genetic counselor is, in part, to help the client understand how his or her emotions may influence decision making. Caveats to this are the client with a personality disorder or whose cognitive ability has been compromised, for example by onset of the genetic condition.

There seems, then, to be a need to reconcile genetics practitioners' belief that it is better for people to be informed than uninformed [8] with the genetic counseling tenet that patient autonomy must be supported. Although the parallels are imperfect, Motivational Interviewing may be helpful in this regard. Motivational Interviewing "begins with the assumption and honouring of personal autonomy: that people make their own behavioral choices and that such power of choice cannot be appropriated by another" but is nonetheless goal oriented, "a collaborative, person-centered form of guiding to elicit and strengthen motivation for change"[17]. Critically, the goal or change desired must be that identified by the client rather than the practitioner. In the context of family communication, the client must have a desire to pass genetic information on to relatives. Intervention studies in genetics, such as those mentioned earlier, which aim to increase relatives' awareness of the availability of genetic testing, imply that the outcome (goal) sought by the service or

---

Box 15.1 Tenets and Supporting Goals of Genetic Counseling

Tenet: Genetic information is key (*being informed is better than being uninformed*)
    Patient is informed
    Counselor knows what information to impart
    Counselor presents genetic information
    Patient gains new perspectives
Tenet: Relationship is integral to genetic counseling
    Counselor and patient establish a bond
    Good counselor–patient communication
    Counselor characteristics positively influence process
Tenet: Patient autonomy must be supported
    Establish working contract
    Integrate familial and cultural context into counseling relationship and decisions
    Patient feels empowered and more in control
    Facilitate collaborative decisions
    Tenet: Patients are resilient
    Recognize patient's strengths
    Adaptation
    Empowerment
Tenet: Patient's emotions make a difference
    Counselor and patient know patient's concerns
    Patient's family dynamics are understood by counselor and patient
    Patient's self-esteem is maintained or increased

Adapted from: Veach PM, Bartels DM, Leroy BS. Coming full circle: A reciprocal-engagement model of genetic counseling practice. *Journal of Genetic Counseling* 2007;16(6):713–728.

---

practitioner is that "the client communicates with their family" or "the family is informed." The danger here is of course that this may undermine autonomy if the outcome of an informed family is at odds with the person's own conscious or instinctive preferences, for example, to protect relatives. A goal more consistent with the tenets of genetic counseling is *process* related, for example, that the counselor "has facilitated the person's ability to make a conscious decision about communication, with an awareness of the influences on that decision." If that person's decision (desired change or goal) is to communicate, only then does the goal of the counselor become to facilitate the person's ability to pass information on to relatives. To quote Miller and Rollnick, "It is not the communication of an expert who assumes that 'I have what you need,' but rather the facilitative style of a companion whose manner says, 'You have what you need, and together we'll find it'" [17]. This returns us to the need to gain insight into the client's family communication context and for practitioners to have strategies by which they can assist the people to consider their options, identify their preferences, and understand the basis of any intrinsic or instinctive reactions, whether they be to communicate or not.

It is difficult to know how issues relating to family communication are handled in genetics consultations because there are no published observational studies of genetic counseling addressing family communication specifically [18, 19]. As mentioned earlier, genetics practitioners themselves indicate that they do not always try to gain insight into family communication. There is even less information available on the strategies used in practice. One study of physicians collecting family history information about hereditary cancer demonstrated coercion and the use of the persuasive strategy, with the physician involved generating new options for contacting relatives, after the previous suggestion has been rejected by the person attending the consultation [20]. It is impossible to know how commonly this strategy is used. Our impression, gleaned through clinical work, case discussion, and research analysis of consultation transcripts, is that persuasion by repeatedly generating solutions is not uncommon in genetics practice. Persuasion (or "compliance-gaining") strategies were recognized early in the field of communication studies, which traditionally focused on the messages that a sender gives to a receiver in order to achieve a behavioral or attitudinal change. The field has more recently taken new perspectives on persuasion, including what Baxter and Bylund [21] call the "social-meaning perspective." This perspective on persuasion considers the social and interpersonal contexts within which the persuasion is taking place. For example, the process of persuasion will differ depending on a family's communication patterns (see Chapter 11). In a family characterized by conversation orientation, persuasion may be a mutual negotiation over time. In a family characterized by conformity orientation, persuasion may be a set of repeated messages that are complied with or not complied with. We suggest that in communication with families about genetics, a singular focus on persuasion is ultimately unproductive. Persuasion does not necessarily address the person's underlying concerns about communicating; it leads at best to unwilling acceptance rather than strong commitment, and it does not support the person's autonomy or resilience. In fact, there is evidence that an approach which seeks to persuade can instead increase client resistance [22]. Alternative communication strategies are required, ones that focus on the person who might act—his or her social and personal context—rather than on the action itself. The most effective communicators are those who have a repertoire of skills and who select the appropriate skill in relation to the context and other individuals. As we hope has been demonstrated through previous chapters, theoretical insights can assist the practitioner in gaining insights into a family's communication patterns and developing further strategies to work effectively with them. However, before exploring these further, we first discuss the opportunities genetics practitioners have to explore family communication as part of their regular practice.

CONTEXT

Although the milieu of genetics services will be very familiar to those working in one, the nature of genetics professionals' contact with their clients requires some explanation for academics or health-care practitioners unfamiliar with genetic services. The nature, purpose, and context of genetics practitioners' contacts with their clients define both the opportunities to identify and to address issues of family communication and also the constraints on practitioners' ability to do this well. Although the focus here is on genetics practitioners' interactions with their clients, we encourage other health-care practitioners to consider their own milieu and the extent to which there are similar opportunities and limitations.

It is difficult to be definitive about how genetic counseling is delivered internationally because little descriptive or comparative information on the delivery of services exists. It can be reasonably assumed that virtually all genetics services, or clinics, based in a medical setting have outpatient consultations where either one person or multiple family members simultaneously may be seen. Genetics practitioners pride themselves on the time that they spend with families, particularly in comparison to other medical specializations: consultations are commonly up to an hour in length, and this time to talk is also valued by people who attend these services [23]. Many people are seen only once, while others may require several appointments, depending on the needs of the client, the condition involved, and the scope of services provided by the genetics service. Predictive testing consultations, for example, have a focus on "fostering emotional insight and understanding that will help clients in their....subsequent adjustment to the result" [24] (p. 18) in addition to the provision of relevant medical and genetic information. As a result, protocols for predictive testing suggest several appointments separated by a period of time for reflection [25, 26]. Exploration of family relationships and coping is recommended as part of this predictive testing process. In contrast, an adult or parents of a child may be seen by a genetics service only once in order to for a genetic diagnosis to be made, with ongoing care provided by the referring practitioner or department. Even if a person is seen only once, there is an opportunity to explore family communication as information about family members and their relationships—biological if not social—is gathered during the construction or review of a (three-generation) family tree that is central to the clinical evaluation. This is discussed in more detail below.

Flanking the consultation are the processes of intake and follow up [27]. Intake processes occur prior to the consultation and are highly variable. Indeed, one service may have different practices at different sites depending on staff skill mix and support [28]. Intake may be as simple as receipt of a referral letter, or it may (also) involve contact by telephone. In some countries, a home visit by the genetic (nurse) counselor may precede the consultation [29]. Similarly, multiple options exist for follow-up support after a consultation for clients communicating to relatives [2]. Some genetic services purposefully aim to increase the uptake of genetic services by relatives by promoting communication with other family members via post-consultation letters [15] or telephone calls [16]. The vast majority of genetics professionals (92%) in an international study offered some form of follow-up support for family communication at the time of the study, and 72% thought ideally there would be "adequate staff to allow for review appointments, continuity and maintenance of long-term engagement with families" when asked about preferences for options to assist family communication [2]. Again, follow up is valued by people attending genetics services [23], and family communication is an issue raised by clients in follow-up contact [30].

Although one person may be seen only a few (or less) times, in total there may be many contacts with their family over time as other family members are seen by the service to discuss the personal implications of a familial condition. As the following example illustrates, contact with a family may extend over generations as children grow up and seek information for themselves. Mary and John were seen after their young son was diagnosed with the progressive muscle wasting condition Duchenne muscular dystrophy. The discussion focused on the meaning of this diagnosis for their son, their plans to have more children, and their reproductive options (see also Table 2.2 in Chapter 2). Twenty years later, their daughter Liz attended the clinic to learn whether she was a carrier because she and her partner were considering children. This is reminiscent of the issues raised in Chapter 5: social and biological turning points in an individual's and family's life course promote engagement again with the genetics service. During these contacts, genetics practitioners may increase their understanding of the family, and its communication, as they listen to the perspectives of different family members and unfolding of the family story over time. In contrast to individual medical files, genetics records are usually family files, with all the information on each family member and their contact with the service stored in one record.

In summary then, there are potentially several points of contact between the genetics practitioner and the client after referral or self-referral: at the intake, the consultation(s), and the follow up. The needs of the client and the family, and the resources available within the genetics service, will determine the form and content of each these contacts. However, across this chronology are common elements of genetics practice [31], which include gathering a medical and family history, assessing risk, inheritance/risk counseling, testing, psychosocial assessment and support, planning, and referral to other professionals and agencies. Directly or indirectly, performing many of these tasks can serve to enhance practitioners' exploration of family communication and their ability to effectively address family communication issues that are identified, even if this is not the primary purpose of the activity.

WORKING WITH FAMILIES

All families communicate: the family system and its dynamics, the family's communication patterns and rules, the attributions they make, the narrative they tell about themselves, as well as their beliefs about privacy (elaborated in Chapters 6, 11, 1, 4, and 7, respectively), all influence the content and ebb and flow of daily family conversations and interactions. Working effectively with clients means learning about the clients' and families' communication processes generally, as well as in relation to genetics specifically. This is captured by the genetic counseling goal: "patient family dynamics are understood by counselor and patient" (see Box 15.1) [8]. We now look at some of the ways that these insights can be gained during genetics practitioners' contact with individuals and their families and strategies for working, based on the theories presented throughout this book. Counseling should, as always, be tailored to the client and be congruent with the practitioner's own competence and context. Consequently, we encourage health-care practitioners to consider these ways of viewing families and incorporating some that seem natural for their own context. These suggestions are not exhaustive, and we hope to stimulate further dialogue and exploration of ways the theoretical insights can be incorporated into practice.

Family History

Family history is the cornerstone of genetics practice. Drawn in the form of a family tree or pedigree, it documents the relevant medical information and is used as a diagnostic tool to establish the pattern of inheritance and risks, to identify at-risk family members, and sometimes to determine their medical screening needs [32]. At the same time, the process of collecting a family's history can also help the health-care practitioner establish rapport with a client, identify family dynamics, and learn of the impact of the condition and related events on the individual and his or her family. Done with sensitivity and empathy, questions about a person's medical or family history can naturally lead to observations of, or questions about, the impact of these events and insights into a family's communication patterns. Jane, for example, attended a genetic service because she wanted to know whether she was a carrier of fragile X syndrome. Her elder sister's child had recently been diagnosed with this condition. While the genetics practitioner was asking about this child's condition, she asked Jane how she found out about the diagnosis. Jane replied that she had noticed that something was wrong but that her elder sister never spoke about this with her or acknowledged any problem. She had in fact been told about the diagnosis by her younger sister. When the practitioner observed that she seemed not to be so close to the elder sister, Jane replied that they saw each other a few times a year but had always been a bit competitive with each other. When invited to say a bit more about this, Jane's response suggested she was cautious of giving her elder sister "fuel" for further bickering, so their conversations were fairly superficial, while she spoke regularly and more openly to her younger sister. From this, the practitioner made some mental notes for later exploration on the family system and privacy boundaries present in this family.

In contrast, Kenen and Peters [33] take a somewhat different approach to the standard family tree documented by the practitioner. They suggest constructing a "colored ecological and genetic relational map" in partnership with the client. This map can be used to document interactions, such as the ones Jane described in her family. It also records social exchanges of information, "services" (such as baby-sitting), and emotions or social support, as well as identifying those family members who disseminate or block genetic information.

Collecting the family history is also an opportunity to listen for family narratives and thereby gain insights into peoples' perspectives, their socio-cultural backgrounds, their emotional needs, and the experiences they identify as important and relevant (Chapter 4). Drawing a family tree usually requires structured questioning by the health-care practitioner to be sure of accurately documenting all the relevant family members and their relationships to each other, but strict adherence to this approach can limit clients' scope to tell the stories that are important to them. Adelsward and Sachs [20] observed a "narrative contest" between a doctor who wished to construct a medical account of the family history and the client who wanted to tell her story about the family's problems. However, the thought of allowing people complete freedom to tell their own story at the outset is daunting for practitioners operating under time constraints and with a need to be certain of obtaining the information most relevant for genetic diagnosis and risk assessment. One approach may be to encourage people to tell their own story while providing some indication of what kind of medical events may be relevant. Once the story has been told by the client and actively heard by the practitioner, it is possible to return to the family tree to fill in any gaps or note any inconsistencies. An alternative is to collect the factual information using a questionnaire and draw the family tree prior to a consultation. The practitioner has the necessary information and, acknowledging this and the person's contribution before the consultation, can encourage the person to then tell the family's story as he or she wishes. Cancer genetics, where verification of diagnoses is often performed prior to the consultation, particularly lends itself to this approach, which has the additional benefit of allowing inconsistencies between the client's narrative and the medical "facts" to be identified. For instance, Greg reported prior to the consultation that his deceased father had bowel cancer and provided consent for this to be verified, but cancer registry documents conclusively showed that the diagnosis was in fact prostate cancer. Learning this at the consultation, Greg commented that his father was a very private man and would have been too embarrassed to tell Greg and his sister that he had prostate cancer. Greg was readily able to change his narrative from one of increased colorectal cancer risk to the population risk indicated by his family history.

Encompassed within the family narrative or story are attributions and personal theories (Chapter 9). For example, John was referred to a genetics service after a diagnosis of a spinocerebellar ataxia, which causes, among other things, a progressive lack of physical control over gait and speech. When talking about his diagnosis and the difficulties caused by the condition, John commented that his two adult children had noticed his deterioration. However, they made comments suggesting that they believe the symptoms are due to alcohol abuse and that he is trying to cover up a drinking problem. The genetics practitioner responded empathically—on the difficulty of not being believed or understood—but also noted the attribution with the intention of returning to the impact of it on family communication about the condition later in the consultation.

Although clients of genetic services may be self-selecting for beliefs consistent with genetic causation—by virtue of being willing to attend a genetics service—this cannot be assumed and in other health-care services attributions and personal theories may affect the person's acceptance of a referral to a genetics service. If these have not become apparent while drawing the family tree, it can be illuminating to ask about the person's own assessment of the family history. This can readily be done once the health-care practitioner has completed the family tree and before a genetic assessment of it is provided. For example, Ruby had given a detailed account of her own diagnoses of bilateral breast cancer and those of all three of her sisters. When asked what she thought had caused these, Ruby noted that all had occurred post menopause and stated somewhat emphatically that they were due to hormone replacement therapy. Knowing this attribution, the practitioner was able to incorporate these beliefs in her presentation of the "genetic" explanation of the family history.

Family communication can also affect the client's willingness to gather medical information [20] and the accuracy of information provided. Privacy boundaries (Chapter 7) affect what people believe they can ask relatives about and also assumptions about the extent of their own knowledge of the family history. A person may erroneously assume that he or she would be told about relatives' conditions and therefore has complete family history information. This is evident in the account of Greg, where his father's privacy boundaries—and Greg's assumptions about these—affected the accuracy of the information Greg was able to provide.

Psychosocial Concerns

The diagnosis of a genetic condition or risk can act as a psychological stressor, requiring the individual (and family) to adjust to new circumstances. The psychosocial sequelae of a genetic condition or risk have been widely explored, with people facing grief and loss, guilt and blame, uncertainty, stigma and discrimination, changed family/relationship dynamics, and chronic disability. "Adjustment requires the individual to resolve the issue by acknowledging, processing, accepting and adapting to the changes" [29] (p. 23). Depending on a health-care practitioner's scope of practice and discipline-related goals and skills, adjustment can be promoted in the course of health-care consultations. Certainly, facilitating adaptation to a genetic risk or condition is a core component of genetic counseling, according to the (U.S.) National Society of Genetic Counselors' definition of this activity [34]. McConkie-Rosell and Sullivan have explored stress and coping in the context of genetic disease and argue that genetic counseling interventions based on empowerment can enhance individual coping and adjustment [35]. Here we take a small step beyond the individual, looking at family adjustment as a dimension of individual adjustment and the ways in which this may be addressed during genetic counseling.

An individual's social environment impacts on the ability to cope with changed circumstances; family is often an important component of a person's social environment. After the diagnosis of a genetic condition, many people turn to their families for support, and a family's ability to communicate in a direct and supportive manner can directly and positively influence the coping process [36]. However, the often unexpected diagnosis of a genetic condition is likely to disrupt the family system (see Chapter 6). Crisis can result if a family lacks sufficient resources (including social support, cohesion, ability to adapt) and/or the condition is perceived as life altering. As the family responds to the crisis, stages of shock, recoil, depression, and reorganization resulting in acceptance and recovery are apparent [36]. Thus, as an individual family member attempts to adjust, the family is inextricably trying to do the same. As a consequence, the support available from the family varies greatly.

While some people do experience at least some family members as supportive and communicative, others experience frustration or even conflict as expectations are not met or needs are not satisfied. This is a consequence of "disturbances in equilibrium [which] lead to conditions in which groups or individuals no longer do willingly what they are expected to do"[36] (p. 221), such as provide support, or discuss the issue. It is of particular relevance to genetic counselors that conflict in *response* to genetic information is not necessarily *caused* by it; conflict is based in the history of the relationship(s), and cracks become apparent under pressure. It is also important to bear in mind that not all conflict is destructive. Conflict can be managed constructively by recognizing both individual needs and the responsibility to further maintain and support the family system. This often takes compromise. However, genetic counselors often have limited access to the wider family network, and so they need to work with the individual to promote that person's adjustment while bearing in mind the process that the wider family may be experiencing and consequences of this for the client. As suggested in Chapter 10, this can be done prospectively as part of planning for disclosure—working with the client to consider the current family dynamics, availability of good family support, and possibility of future conflict—as well as in response to conflicts the client may have already experienced in relation to genetics.

Clients experiencing frustration or overt conflict with family members after talking to them about a genetic condition or risk may be helped by constructive exploration of this experience. This entails the genetic counselor listening to the person's description of what happened and helping the client identify what he or she hoped would have happened and what expectations may have been held, consciously or unconsciously. It is then possible to identify and validate the needs underpinning these expectations. People who are "stuck" in repeating their story and grievances are not constructively exploring the conflict and may need some assistance to move from this point. It may also be helpful to explore past conflicts with family members, whether these were resolved, and if so how. This may assist the client to understand how relatives respond to conflict, the client's own role in the conflict, and how realistic it is to expect a different outcome in the current situation. In some cases, people may benefit from a referral to a family therapist, individual therapist, or psychologist to address long-standing issues or problems with coping styles.

In some situations the genetic counselor is in a position to work with multiple family members. This usually arises when several family members wish to attend a genetic consultation together. This may be prompted by efficiency—family members wishing to learn about their situation(s) at the same time, by a desire to receive or provide support, by obligation a family member is necessary to provide information or samples to assist another person, or a combination of these. The counselor may learn much about a family's dynamics by careful observation and questioning of those attending the consultation [29]. The presence of several family members in the room is an opportunity to facilitate shared exploration of the family members' differing perspectives on their family, uncover assumptions that are not shared, and thereby broaden each member's view of the implications of a genetic condition or testing. For example, siblings at risk of hereditary hemochromatosis may be able to explore together the attributions they have made about their affected brother's fatigue prior to his diagnosis, the way their interactions with him were affected by these, and the implications of these for their own genetic testing.

However, there are also potential pitfalls in shared consultations. A family member may not feel able to say what he or she really thinks in the presence of other family members. Family members may feel constrained from sharing relevant information by privacy boundaries that exclude other family members [37]. For example, most genetic counselors will be familiar with women (of any age) who are not comfortable discussing their contraceptive use or reproductive plans with a parent present. There are particular hazards in two or more relatives undertaking predictive testing at the same time being seen in the same consultations, particularly if they intend to provide support for each other when receiving results. While they may in fact be well placed to do this, it is also possible that their needs upon receiving results are in fact so different that one person is not in a position to support the other. Frustration and conflict may arise as a result. Of course, having multiple family members in the session together is an opportunity for the genetic counselor to identify these expectations and encourage the family members present to consider how realistic they may be. However, this strategy may not be successful if they have a strong need to preserve the family dynamics (e.g., supporter, supported) and so are unwilling to consider that testing may disrupt the existing family dynamics. Nonetheless, it is important not to take statements of support or agreement at face value, but to explore what this support or agreement means to each person, to understand their need to be seen together, and to encourage some time spent individually with the genetic counselor to explore their distinct needs.

In summary, adaptation to the risk or condition potentially has two interdependent facets: the internal adaptation of the affected or at-risk individual and the adaptation of the client's family. Often the genetics practitioner is only in a position to work directly with the client but can do so while keeping the broader family context and implications in mind. Referral to a family therapist is suggested if entrenched, unhelpful family communication patterns are apparent or there is ongoing conflict.

Plans and Follow Up

Skene and Forrest (Chapter 13) suggest that genetics practitioners have an obligation to at least make clients aware of the implications of a genetic condition for other relatives and discuss how these people may be made aware of the genetic information. When there is a well-established family history of a condition, experience suggests that clients usually are willing to pass information on to their relatives, particularly about the availability of genetic testing. In fact, helping other family members is a common reason given for undergoing genetic testing [38–44]. When a new or unexpected diagnosis has been made, the situation is less clear and the intention to talk to family members may be primarily to obtain family support rather than convey risk information [45, 46]. Thus, as discussed in Chapter 10, exploring the goals that underpin the client's intention to communicate will assist the practitioner to facilitate the formulation of a plan by the client that is consistent with these goals. For example, a plan developed with Georgia to tell her family that her newborn son has been diagnosed with cystic fibrosis in order to get the family's practical and emotional support may be different to Liam's plan to ensure that his siblings are aware that they have a risk of hereditary hemochromatosis.

Developing a plan for communication can naturally form part of the discussion about "what happens next" that occurs toward the end of the consultation and may support the genetic counseling goal of the person feeling empowered, thereby promoting resilience (Box 15.1) [8]. However, there is also a risk that people may feel patronized by such a discussion. In one small study exploring the perceived utility of genetic counseling and other strategies to facilitate communication with at-risk relatives, female (but not male) respondents seemed affronted that genetics practitioners thought it necessary to discuss who in the family should be informed and how they might do this, the implication being that practitioners did not consider the women capable [14]. Nonetheless, accounts suggest that communicating with relatives about genetic risks can present people with unexpected difficulties and negative responses [18, 46]. As discussed earlier, there is potential for conflict which may be minimized if considered in advance. Although some people see conveying information as simply

Table 15.2   Elements of Family Communication and Relevant Theories

Element	*Relevant Theories (Chapter Number)*
Who will be told	Family Systems Theory (ch. 6), Family Communication Pattern Theory (ch. 11), Communication Privacy Management (ch. 7), Attributions and Personal Theories (ch. 9), Goals-plans-action theories (ch. 10)
What will be told	Family Narratives (ch. 4), Communication Privacy Management (ch. 7), Attributions and Personal Theories (ch. 9)
When this will happen	Time Theory (ch. 5), Uncertainty Management Theory (ch. 8)
Possible reactions	Societal Narratives (ch. 3), Family Systems Theory (ch. 6), Family Communication Pattern Theory (ch. 11), Communication Privacy Management (ch. 7), Attributions and Personal Theories (ch. 9), Time Theory (ch. 5), Uncertainty Management Theory (ch. 8)

providing their relatives with options [14], a sense of responsibility to inform family members can also be accompanied by a belief that their relatives have a responsibility to act on the information [43]. Perhaps consequently, people have reported being disappointed by even neutral or disinterested responses to the news that predictive genetic testing is available [14]—one or more of their goals has not been achieved. As described in Chapter 10, a person who has not achieved a goal may continue to pursue it, for example, by "active and consistent persuasion" [47] arising from a sense of responsibility to ensure relatives act. Alternatively the person may be discouraged by failure to achieve the goal(s) and therefore less inclined to talk with other family members (i.e., disengaged).

If people do not immediately pass new information on to relatives, they may be engaging in a deliberative process that contains elements of planning within it, namely deciding who will be told, what will they be told, and when this will happen [18, 48]. The mode of communication may also be considered [49]. These decisions, and the possible reactions of relatives, can be seen to be related to the theories presented in this book (Table 15.2). Arguably there is value in health-care practitioners making these elements explicit during discussions with clients about family communication and asking for the clients' thoughts on these in relation to their own communication with relatives. This approach has several functions: *(1)* it serves to make plans to communicate more specific; *(2)* it makes it clear that the client has the answers and the practitioner is eliciting these, not providing them; *(3)* it encourages the client to be aware that this is an achievable but not necessarily simple task. If the practitioner observed earlier that the client's narrative was lacking in coherence or consistency, or if the client had attributions that were at odds with genetic causation, the practitioner may enquire further about what the client plans to say and help in the development of a clear narrative.

Written information may assist clear communication, either in isolation or as an adjunct to verbal communication. It is common practice for the summary letters provided by genetics practitioners after a consultation to contain information about the risks for other family members and to encourage communication, but much less common to write a letter for the at-risk relatives [2]. Relatives may also be directed to well-respected Web sites. Some evidence suggests that relatives who receive both direct communication from the person seen in clinic and a letter from a genetic service are most likely to contact the genetic service [15].

Daly et al. [50] identified a need for a protocol for women to use when communicating genetic risk information about hereditary breast and ovarian cancer to relatives and developed a six-step strategy based on Buckman's text on breaking bad news [51]. The protocol covers preparing the physical location of the discussion, finding out how much the recipient knows already, how much he or she wants to know, sharing the information, responding to the recipient's feelings in response to the information, and planning in the form of referral and provision of written information.

Planning for communication can include encouraging the client to anticipate family members' reactions to the information. Situations in which the family member may be more likely to respond adversely can be predicted from the list of relevant theories in Table 15.2. For example, differing beliefs held about the cause or inheritance of a condition; divergent ideas about what is private and shared information; past or present conflict or strained family systems; communication that challenges existing family rules or communication patterns; and/or difficulties living with uncertainty. The process of anticipation can be particularly useful if the client believes he or she is acting in the best interests of relatives and has not considered the possibility that these relatives may not feel the same way. The intent is not to discourage communication of course but to prepare the person for otherwise unexpected reactions and possible ways of responding to these. If time allows or the client is concerned, then rehearsal of these situations may be beneficial; presenting the argument out loud or to another person serves to clarify and refine a message [52].

Leonard and Newson (Chapter 12) suggest that ideally the client should have maximal time to consider, adjust, and plan. Therefore, when genetic testing is being considered, the possible implications for family members should be raised as early as is reasonable, and the means by which they may be informed of these should be discussed. In this way, people have the opportunity to consider their options without the pressure of conveying a test result. They can discuss the situation with their relatives in advance, learn what the relatives wish to know, and get a clearer idea of how they might react. An additional benefit is that the person does not have to think about family communication for the first time while adjusting to bad news.

Once clients have had some time to communicate with their relatives, follow-up contact from health-care practitioners can be beneficial. This allows clients to convey the evolving story or narrative of communication with their family members and practitioners to identify any areas where clients' coping and capacity to achieve their goal(s) may be recognized or strengthened. The general approach here is the same as earlier: continuing to gain insight into clients' situations and working with them to assess if their goals have been achieved, if any of these need to be modified or abandoned, and what they plan to do next. For example, after discovering that their baby had cystic fibrosis, Sally and Jim planned to tell their families about the diagnosis so that their siblings could have carrier testing. When contacted some months after the appointment, Sally said that her family members were aware and interested in testing. However, it had proved difficult to make sure that Jim's sisters knew that they could have carrier testing because Jim's mother wanted to tell them but did not seem to have acted on this yet. The practitioner explored the situation with Sally, who reiterated that she wanted to make sure that her sister-in-law were informed and decided to raise the issue again with her mother-in-law. The practitioner can then make a second call some months hence to follow up with Sally. Working with clients around issues of family communication can, therefore, be an iterative process, with new issues arising and others diminishing as circumstances evolve over time (Chapter 5).

Nondisclosure

Although most individuals talk to some or most family members, some reveal nothing about a diagnosis. Hallowell et al. [53] found that people used three different communication strategies when faced with informing relatives of genetic risk and test results: complete openness, limited disclosure, and total secrecy. Secrecy provides both a practical and ethical challenge to the health-care practitioner. Skene and Forrest (Chapter 13) consider health-care practitioners' duties with respect to the law in this situation and provide a structured approach based on these—balancing the duty to warn relatives with maintaining the client's confidentiality. Leonard and Newson (Chapter 12) suggest there are ethical justifications in taking a proactive approach to working with the family and promoting sharing of information under a "family comity" model if the information will bring benefit to family members. We believe there is a need to complement these approaches with counseling that remains centered on the client.

For the purposes of this chapter, we take a broad interpretation of nondisclosure and consider it to encompass the following: a client who states that he or she will not inform a relative(s) about relevant genetic information; a client who plans to tell "all" relatives but does not consider this to include all those at biological risk; and the client who intends to tell another relative but has not yet done so or intends to wait until "later." Although the sense of responsibility or concern felt by health-care practitioners may be very different in each of these situations, we suggest that a similar counseling framework can be applied to each. Of course, it is rather naive to suggest that the "solution" to nondisclosure is simply better counseling, but an approach grounded in counseling recognizes the social and interpersonal context of the client in decision making and is more consistent with good health care and genetics practice than one based on coercion and the persuasive strategies mentioned above. Arguably, it is more likely to facilitate the successful achievement of outcomes that the client considers important.

When a health-care practitioner attempts persuasion (i.e., pursues the practitioner's own goals) and faces resistance from the client, the center of the consultation moves from being the client to being either the "act" of communication or the potential recipient of the information. This is evident in a dialogue observed by Adelsward and Sachs between a doctor and a woman who does not wish to inform relatives of their hereditary cancer risk [20]. The doctor first attempts to emphasize the relative's high risk of cancer and the possible consequences of not considering prophylactic mastectomy. Shortly thereafter the doctor suggests that the information is "good" because it enables the relative to make decisions. Next he suggests a letter could be sent to inform the relatives. Finally, the doctor returns to the suggestion that the woman talk with her relatives. This emphasis on the needs of the "other" can compromise the counselor–patient relationship, as well as patient autonomy [8]. One might imagine that the woman in this consultation felt that her personal situation—complete lack of contact with the relatives—and concerns were given scant attention. Working effectively with the client requires the practitioner to keep the client at the center of his or her focus. When a practitioner recognizes that he or she is using sequential persuasion strategies and the client is unconvinced, it can be helpful to note what is occurring. For example, the counselor could use metacommunication, such as: "I seem to be pushing you to do something you don't want to do and ignoring your concerns about telling your relatives when you don't have contact with them." This use of "immediacy" (stating what the counselor perceives to be occurring then and there) enables the practitioner to acknowledge the difficulty in communication and move forward with the client as the focus of the consultation rather than her relatives.

The first step, when encountering nondisclosure in any of its forms, is to remain focused on gaining insight into the client's situation and exploring the client's reluctance to share the information. That is, identifying the goal the client is pursuing by not communicating. It is important that this is done with a true desire for understanding, rather than the intention of providing counter-arguments to "flaws" in the person's logic. A client-centered approach is to accept what is presented as the client's reality and explore this reality with the client; the attention remains firmly on understanding the client, rather than encouraging him or her to act in a particular way. The practitioner can work with the client to illuminate "blind spots" in thought or behavior and assist them to find ways of managing their situation effectively [54] (p. 177).

A reluctance to tell any relatives may indicate that the person is still adjusting to the news he or she has received and is not yet ready to talk with relatives. Forrest and colleagues observed that people need to make sense of their own risk before being able to tell others; those who continue to perceive their risk as uncertain or ambiguous are more likely to have problems knowing what to tell their relatives [55]. These people may have trouble forming a coherent story to give relatives and may benefit both from genetic counseling aimed at facilitating adjustment and also from some assistance from the practitioner in helping them to develop a narrative. Simply asking people what they have said—or plan to say—to their relatives can give some indication of the coherence and ease with which they may tell their story.

There are numerous reasons people give for not passing genetic information on to one or more relatives. Forrest et al. [55] suggest that these can be broadly categorized into the following: acting to produce benefit for their relative (acting "positively"), perceiving that there is no need to communicate (neutral), or failing to overcome barriers (negative). These are quite different situations and are likely to require very different responses. An example of each is given below with some discussion of counseling approaches that may be helpful for each of these types of nondisclosure.

Case Study 1: Nondisclosure to Benefit Relatives

Cindy was recently found to have early symptoms of the neurodegenerative condition Huntington disease (HD). She has two teenage children and is estranged from their father. She had known little about the condition because her own father had died young in a car accident and she had little contact with his family. Although HD is ultimately fatal, it progresses slowly over 15–20 years. She told her family physician that she does not intend on telling her children. When asked about how she came to this decision, she says that they are still in high school and she does not want to give them information that may be upsetting at a critical point in their lives. In addition, she is concerned that her ex-husband may use this information to gain custody. Cindy feels she is protecting her children from these potential harms.

When people are acting to benefit others by concealing information, we suggest that this positive attribute—their caring for their relatives—be acknowledged. This is in keeping with promoting client resilience and recognizing strengths (Box 15.1) and may be undermined in the case of Cindy if her family physician suggests that Cindy is not in fact acting in their interests. If the client clearly understands the technical information about implications for relatives, then she has assessed the various consequences and, within her frame of reference, decided the potential harms to her relative(s) outweigh the benefits [18].

The belief that harm may occur through disclosure may be an accurate assessment of the relative's vulnerability and/or receptiveness to genetic information. A person who has recently lost a spouse may not be well placed to receive news of a high risk of developing cancer or a neurodegenerative condition. However, it is also possible that psychological harms being experienced by the client in response to the condition or genetic test result may be projected onto family members; projection is an unconscious defence mechanism in which the client attempts to displace unacceptable or burdensome feelings onto another person [56]. If the person seems to be highly protective of a relative, then the practitioner might choose to empathically explore the extent to which the client feels that she has been harmed or hurt by learning of her condition. To quote Evans, the practitioner acts as a facilitator who "has questions, not answers and is a companion to a patient who is struggling to find a path through emotional experience" [29] (p. 154).

Clients who delay communicating with relatives until an unspecified "right time" and those who decide not to tell others are in effect creating a secret. The means by which the secret will be kept and the consequences of carrying a secret for the bearer form areas for exploration by the practitioner and may encourage the client to realistically assess whether this strategy will serve her goals and plan accordingly. Using the example of Cindy above, dimensions of this include the extent to which Cindy will keep the information strictly to herself or will share it with someone; under what conditions Cindy will share the secret with another person and whether these conditions will be made explicit so that her privacy rules are respected; what situations may arise where Cindy's desire to protect her relatives will be challenged and how will these be managed; when or under what circumstances she will tell her children; what might it be like for her to live with this secret; and whether she envisages any changes occurring over time. Secrets are notoriously difficult to keep and, when kept, the impact is often to transform the relationship. This may reveal itself in avoidance, distancing, or limited conversational topics. According to the family therapist Imber-Black, "Relationships that would ordinarily change and grow become frozen in time, as the presence of a secret locks people in place" [57] (p. 10). Keeping a secret also extracts a cost by limiting the sources of social support.

Case Study 2: Nondisclosure by Failing to Overcome Barriers

Jeff also has HD. His wife and children are aware of this, but his younger brother, Steve, is not. After a falling out many years ago, Steve and Jeff have not spoken or had any contact with each other. This situation is made somewhat easier for all involved because Steve moved a considerable distance away some time ago. Jeff has stated that he does not plan to tell Steve because they have no contact.

The nature and significance of barriers to disclosure perceived by the client need to be explored when encountered. In a situation like Jeff's, where the person seems unable to overcome social barriers such as estrangement, it may be helpful to explore the person's goals and privacy boundaries in greater detail. Again it should be stressed that care must be taken that the purpose of this is to learn more about the client rather than to find a way of persuading the client to act. By focusing on the client's privacy boundaries, the health-care practitioner may get some insight into his goals while avoiding a detailed history of the conflict and associated events, the retelling of which may serve to reinforce the client's grievances and restrict the time available for the consultation. The practitioner may learn if the client's primary goal is to keep the information from the relative(s) or if it is to avoid contact with him or her. If the client wishes to withhold information, it can be helpful to clarify whether this means all of the available information (i.e., the presence of the condition in the family) or only personal information (i.e., Jeff's own health and genetic status). Exploring this further, the practitioner learns that Jeff is not in fact opposed to Steve knowing that there is HD in the family, but he does not want to make contact or have his personal information conveyed. The practitioner can then ask if Jeff has any thoughts on how the news of the condition might be conveyed to Steve in a way that Jeff is comfortable with. In situations where the person feels uncomfortable communicating or requires support, intermediaries may be used to convey the information [14, 58].

When a person plans to withhold information, exploring the impact of this decision on the client and what the client feels he or she will gain and lose may be useful. However, ultimately, when a family relationship is conflicted, it is likely that the genetic information may provide a new ground for the existing tensions and estrangement to play out.

Case Study 3: Nondisclosure as a Result of Perceiving That Communication Is Not Required

Nisa migrated to Canada from Turkey at 22 years of age. Twenty years on, she has been diagnosed with endometrial cancer and found to have the hereditary cancer condition Lynch syndrome. She has a 21-year-old nephew in Canada and numerous relatives living in Turkey. She has not told her relatives about Lynch syndrome for two reasons. First, she believes that relatives in Turkey will not have access to genetic testing or surveillance services. Secondly, her nephew in Canada is not yet old enough to participate in colonscopic screening for bowel cancer. Therefore, she sees no reason to pass the information on.

Sometimes a client holds a strong perception that it is not necessary to tell relatives about a diagnosis, even in the case of genetic conditions. A perception such as Nisa's that relatives do not (yet) have access to the necessary health-care services may be accurate and the decision to tell or not comes down to the way in which the person—or the person's family—values information that cannot be acted on. Alternatively, if the person is laboring under a misconception, providing her with the correct information is entirely appropriate. It is also possible that, with misconceptions corrected, the client may remain reluctant to disclose. This may suggest that she feels that her relatives may benefit by not being informed or that she has not overcome other barriers, such as social or geographical.

Our experience suggests that nondisclosure can be perceived by the genetics practitioner or their colleagues as a form of failure, that is, that with "better" counseling the client would have disclosed. This does not take into account the fact that disclosure is a process that occurs over time—what is not communicated today may be communicated next year, or the year after—and, most importantly that ultimately, communication is the client's decision. The role of the counselor is to facilitate this decision-making process, ensure that the client is aware of the factors that have influenced this decision, and considered its potential impact - regardless of whether this was to communicate or not.

REFLECTIVE PROFESSIONAL PRACTICE AND FAMILY COMMUNICATION

In its broadest sense reflective practice involves the critical analysis of everyday working practices to improve competence and promote professional development. [59]

Every human interaction has its own dynamics, regardless of whether it is an interaction between family members or between health-care practitioners and their patients. These dynamics both affect and are affected by the relationship between the participants in the interaction. Veach and colleagues point out that "to be an effective genetic counselor you must be aware of the issues that impact your relationship with clients" [7] (p. 242). There are numerous issues that can impact on the client–practitioner relationship; family communication is clearly one of these. An individual's beliefs about what is private, as well as his or her family story, attributions, family dynamics, and pattern of communicating and managing conflict with family members, will all affect a person's relationship with others, including with health-care practitioners and therefore the working relationship with them. In Chapter 11, Koerner and colleagues demonstrate the ways in which a family's communication patterns affect the genetics consultation. The "unconscious way that a client relates to practitioner based on her or his history of relating to others" is known as transference [7] (p. 242).

However, the client's reactions are only one half of the equation. The practitioner also brings to the consultation his or her own history, which can affect the way he or she feels in response to a client or the client's situation. This is referred to as counter-transference, a term which encompasses re-experiencing of a previous personal experience being triggered by the client [29]. Again, this may not be a conscious process. For example, John is a recently graduated genetic counselor whose own family has a laissez-faire pattern of communication. He makes his decisions separately from his own family but values the views of external authority figures such as his family physician. He gets frustrated with counseling clients who seem to be "overly" influenced by family members, particularly when someone appears to be making progress and John's work is "undone" by further discussions with authoritative family members. By recognizing the ways in which his own family-of-origin communication patterns have unconsciously shaped his expectations of other families, he can develop a respectful working relationship with clients from families very different to his own. Of course, sharing a similar pattern of family communication with a client can also impact on a practitioners' perception of the client and counseling. Supervision is a central part of gaining such insights and ways of counseling effectively in these situations.

Although the term *supervision* for many health-care practitioners has implications of hierarchy and "being watched, trained, or critiqued" or "directed and evaluated," in counseling professions the focus is on professionals in practice "receiving diverse and varied perspectives on their work as well as guidance at their own individual level of proficiency" [60]. Supervision provides support and a place for reflection that helps the practitioner develop self-awareness, and thereby facilitate professional development [29]. Supervision can help practitioners develop an "internal supervisor" that allows them to concurrently take note of clients' verbal and nonverbal communication, identify the underlying messages and patterns, and also monitor their own feelings and responses [61]. While there is much to be gained by reading textbooks that encourage readers to consider their own family communication, this does not replace the "thinking space" provided by a professional supervisor or peer supervision.

TEAMWORK

Multidisciplinary and interdisciplinary models of teamwork are increasingly common in health care. Both involve professionals from different disciplines working together to provide patient care. In a multidisciplinary approach each discipline approaches the patient from its own perspective and works toward discipline-specific goals. Usually this involves separate individual consultations, which may be coordinated at a "one stop shop," where all the relevant practitioners are available at the same time to see the person, rather than requiring multiple visits. In this model shared communication occurs via multidisciplinary team meetings.

In contrast, interdisciplinary teams integrate the perspectives of different disciplines into a single approach, with a collaboratively developed team plan and collaborative communication. This may involve a single consultation or a series of meetings that involve the whole team.

Genetic services usually entail medically trained geneticists and genetic counselors working closely together, and some services also employ social workers or clinical psychologists. In oncology, genetic counselors may work with teams that provide cancer care; similarly genetic counselors may work in obstetric services with obstetricians, midwives, and social workers. As genetics becomes more integrated into the health care of people with many different conditions, new multidisciplinary or interdisciplinary teams will form accordingly to address the medical management, genetic, and psychosocial care of both the person and family.

When considering family communication, there are opportunities to partner with family therapists. The emerging field of medical family therapy "has as its focus the interactions of patients, families, healthcare professionals, and illness" [62] (p. 124). McDaniel discusses how some patients and families struggle with genetic problems that are "directly relevant to family therapists" [63] (p. 29); these include cognitive-behavioral stress reduction and decision making, sibling-focused family therapy, and extended family psychoeducation. Currently some family therapists are developing specializations in genetics, and already some genetic counselors are choosing to undergo additional training in psychotherapy or family therapy to enhance their work with clients.

Models of genetics practitioners working with family therapists are evident in two group interventions for women with *BRCA1/2* mutations. McDaniel [63] describes an emotionally intense 6-week, 90-minute, systemically oriented psychoeducational group for women who tested positive for *BRCA1/2* mutations. A medical geneticist and a genetic counselor answered questions for 15 minutes and communicated any new information. The next 75 minutes, led by family therapists, were spent on topics developed by the women themselves. Topics included family reactions to testing, disclosure issues, and emotional reactions and coping strategies. These family therapists, plus a medical geneticist, also conducted large family sessions with as many as 37 members. Esplen and colleagues [64, 65] describe a supportive-expressive group therapy intervention of 70 women who participated in 12 sessions of supportive-expressive group therapy over 6 months. Groups were conducted by a genetic counselor and psychologist or social worker and included notification of test results, along with many other issues. The supportive-expressive group therapy resulted in significant decreases in cancer worry, anxiety, and depression, although its impact on family communication is not known. These may serve as models for other group interventions and suggest the value of working in partnership to address issues of family dynamics and communication in ongoing support groups.

In discussing the ways in which health-care practitioners may address family communication as part of their practice, we have taken it for granted that information is likely to impact a family system but that the family and its members are sufficiently resilient to adjust to this and reach some functional equilibrium again. In fact, this is not always the case. A practitioner may become aware that a client has serious concerns about the impact of a genetic condition or testing on family functioning. For example, recommendations that other family members are informed about their risk of a genetic condition may bring family secrets to the surface. Such secrets may involve the unspoken use of in vitro fertilization involving donor eggs, a never-revealed step-parent, or intrafamilial adoption. The communication of test results to siblings or other relatives can cause resentment, distancing, or altered family dynamics as people react to the changed circumstances [66]. Finally, partners may struggle with changes in marital dynamics [67, 68]. In such cases, the family may benefit from the involvement of a family therapist. A family therapist always attempts to include all the key players in a family system. An initial meeting might involve both professionals in order to ensure that the family therapist and the family members understood the diagnosis and its potential ramifications; subsequent meetings may involve only the family therapist. The aims of the family therapist would be to stabilize the family system, to assist family members to find ways to talk about the diagnosis and ongoing effects on all members of the family, to help the family adapt to critical changes, and to teach members how to support the affected individual and each other.

CONCLUSION

Although addressing "family communication issues" is a significant and common task in genetic counseling practice [31], there has been little to no exploration of what this actually entails prior to this book. Discussion has centered on the role and responsibilities of the genetics practitioner, while research studies have focused on family experiences and quantification of the relatives informed. If there is little certainty about professional roles and the process of family communication about genetics, there is even less about the ways these issues are currently explored and addressed by practitioners. Our suggestions for practice are grounded in theory, clinical experience, common sense, and to an extent speculation. They are by no means exhaustive, nor are they a guarantee of success. There is a need to critically observe the ways in which practitioners currently explore family communication and the outcomes of this counseling. On the basis of these observations, feasible counseling strategies with robust theoretical frameworks can be developed and tested for their acceptability to families and their impact on family communication patterns. These strategies need to be clearly articulated and reproducible, while also respecting that counseling is tailored to the individual needs of the client and his or her family context and cannot therefore be delivered as a "one-size-fits-all" script.

In this chapter we have attempted to broaden horizons by illustrating the ways in which the theories relating to family communication can complement the findings of genetics research and be incorporated into the care of families with genetics conditions. We hope this will encourage practitioners to view their clients' family communication through a range of theoretical lenses and, as a consequence, to test out new approaches to working with individuals and families.

NOTE

1. This chapter is written about working with clients without personality disorders. However, practitioners should be aware of the range of personality dysfunction and be able to address these or make referrals as appropriate.

REFERENCES

1. Forrest LE, Delatycki MB, Skene L, Aitken M. Communicating genetic information in families—A review of guidelines and position papers. *European Journal of Human Genetics* 2007;15(6):612–618.
2. Forrest LE. *Communicating Genetic Information in Families.* Melbourne, Australia: Melbourne University; 2009.
3. Smets E, van Zwieten M, Michie S. Comparing genetic counseling with non-genetic health care interactions: Two of a kind? *Patient Education and Counseling* 2007;68(3):225–234.
4. Brown RF, Bylund CL. Communication skills training: Describing a new conceptual model. *Academic Medicine* 2008;83(1):37–44.
5. Rowan KE, Sparks L, Pecchioni L, Villagran MM. The CAUSE model: A research-supported aid for physicians communicating with patients about cancer risk. *Health Communication* 2003;15(2):235–248.
6. Weil J. *Psychosocial Genetic Counseling.* New York: Oxford University Press; 2000.
7. Veach PM, Leroy BS, Bartels DM. *Facilitating the Genetic Counseling Process* (1st ed.). New York: Springer-Verlag; 2003.
8. Veach PM, Bartels DM, Leroy BS. Coming full circle: A reciprocal-engagement model of genetic counseling practice. *Journal of Genetic Counseling* 2007;16(6):713–728.
9. Dugan RB, Wiesner GL, Juengst ET, O'Riordan M, Matthews AL, Robin NH. Duty to warn at-risk relatives for genetic disease: Genetic counselors' clinical experience. *American Journal of Medical Genetics* 2003;119C(1):27–34.
10. Falk MJ, Dugan RB, O'Riordan MA, Matthews AL, Robin NH. Medical geneticists' duty to warn at-risk relatives for genetic disease. *American Journal of Medical Genetics* 2003;120A(3):374–380.
11. Clarke A, Richards M, Kerzin-Storrar L, Halliday J, Young MA, Simpson SA, et al. Genetic professionals' reports of nondisclosure of genetic risk information within families. *European Journal of Human Genetics* 2005;13(5):556–562.
12. Costalas JW, Itzen M, Malick J, Babb JS, Bove B, Godwin AK, et al. Communication of BRCA1 and BRCA2 results to at-risk relatives: A cancer risk assessment program's experience. *American Journal of Medical Genetics* 2003;119 C(1):11–18.
13. Stoffel EM, Ford B, Mercado RC, Punglia D, Kohlmann W, Conrad P, et al. Sharing genetic test results in Lynch syndrome: Communication with close and distant relatives. *Clinical Gastroenterology and Hepatology* 2008;6(3):333–338.
14. Gaff CL, Collins V, Symes T, Halliday J. Facilitating family communication about predictive genetic testing: Probands' perceptions. *Journal of Genetic Counseling* 2005;14(2):133–140.

15. Suthers GK, Armstrong J, McCormack J, Trott D. Letting the family know: Balancing ethics and effectiveness when notifying relatives about genetic testing for a familial disorder. *Journal of Medical Genetics* 2006;43(8):665–670.

16. Forrest LE, Burke J, Bacic S, Amor DJ. Increased genetic counseling support improves communication of genetic information in families. *Genetics in Medicine.* 2008;10(3):167–172.

17. Miller WR, Rollnick S. Ten things that motivational interviewing is not. *Behavioural and Cognitive Psychotherapy* 2009;37(2):129–140.

18. Gaff CL, Clarke AJ, Atkinson P, Sivell S, Elwyn G, Iredale R, et al. Process and outcome in communication of genetic information within families: A systematic review. *European Journal of Human Genetics* 2007;15(10):999–1011.

19. Meiser B, Irle J, Lobb E, Barlow-Stewart K. Assessment of the content and process of genetic counseling: A critical review of empirical studies. *Journal of Genetic Counseling* 2008;17(5):434–451.

20. Adelsward V, Sachs L. The messenger's dilemmas—Giving and getting information in genealogical mapping for hereditary cancer. *Health, Risk and Society* 2003;5(2):125–138.

21. Baxter LA, C.L. B. Social influence in close relationships. In: Seiter J, Gass RH, eds. *Perspectives on Persuasion, Social Influence, and Compliance Gaining* Boston: Allyn & Bacon; 2004:317–336.

22. Miller WR, Benefield RG, Tonigan JS. Enhancing motivation for change in problem drinking: A controlled comparison of two therapist styles. *Journal of Consulting and Clinical Psychology* 1993;61(3):455–461.

23. McAllister M, Payne K, Macleod R, Nicholls S, Donnai D, Davies L. What process attributes of clinical genetics services could maximise patient benefits? *European Journal of Human Genetics* 2008;16(12):1467–1476.

24. Soldan J, Street E, Gray J, Binedell J, Harper PS. Psychological model for presymptomatic test interviews: Lessons learned from Huntington disease. *Journal of Genetic Counseling* 2000;9(1):15–31.

25. Brain K, Soldan J, Sampson J, Gray J. Genetic counselling protocols for hereditary non-polyposis colorectal cancer: A survey of UK regional genetics centres. *Clinical Genetics* 2003;63(3):198–204.

26. Craufurd D, Tyler A. Predictive testing for Huntington's disease: Protocol of the UK Huntington's Prediction Consortium. *Journal of Medical Genetics* 1992;29(12):915–918.

27. Uhlmann WR. A guide to case management. In: Baker DL, Scheuette JL, Uhlmann WR, eds. *A Guide to Genetic Counseling.* New York: Wiley-Liss; 1998:1–26

28. McCann E, Baines EA, Gray JR, Procter AM. Improving service delivery by evaluation of the referral pattern and capacity in a clinical genetics setting. *American Journal of Medical Genetics* 2009 Aug 15;151C(3):200–6.

29. Evans C. *Genetic Counselling: A Psychological Approach.* Cambridge, England: Cambridge University Press; 2004.

30. Hodgkin L, Kentwell M, Bogwitz M, Bylstra Y, D'Souza R, Macrae F, et al. Long-term follow up of carriers of a cancer predisposition gene: An alternative model for clinical follow up. *Familial Cancer Research and Practice Conference.* Couran Cove, Australia 2008.

31. Hampel H, Grubs RE, Walton CS, Nguyen E, Breidenbach DH, Nettles S, et al. Genetic counseling practice analysis. *Journal of Genetic Counseling* 2009;18(3):205–216.

32. Bennett RL. *The Practical Guide to the Genetic Family History*. New York: Wiley-Liss; 1999.

33. Kenen R, Peters JA. The Colored, Eco-Genetic Relationship Map (CEGRM): A conceptual approach and tool for genetic counseling research. *Journal of Genetic Counseling* 2001;10(4):289–309.

34. Resta R, Biesecker BB, Bennett RL, Blum S, Hahn SE, Strecker MN, et al. A new definition of genetic counseling: National Society of Genetic Counselors' Task Force report. *Journal of Genetic Counseling* 2006;15(2):77–83.

35. McConkie-Rosell A, Sullivan J. Genetic counseling—Stress, coping and the empowerment perspective. *Journal of Genetic Counseling* 1999;8(6):345–357.

36. Galvin KM, Bylund CL, Bernard BJ. *Family Communication, Cohesion and Change* (8th ed.). Boston: Allyn & Bacon; 2008.

37. Gaff CL, Lynch E, Spencer L. Predictive testing of eighteen year olds: Counseling challenges. *Journal of Genetic Counseling* 2006;15(4):245–251.

38. Hallowell N. Doing the right thing: Genetic risk and responsibility. *Sociology of Health and Illness* 1999;21(5):597–621.

39. Hallowell N, Ardern-Jones A, Eeles R, Foster C, Lucassen A, Moynihan C, et al. Men's decision-making about predictive BRCA1/2 testing: The role of family. *Journal of Genetic Counseling* 2005;14(3):207–217.

40. Foster C, Evans DG, Eeles R, Eccles D, Ashley S, Brooks L, et al. Predictive testing for BRCA1/2: Attributes, risk perception and management in a multi-centre clinical cohort. *British Journal of Cancer* 2002;86(8):1209–1216.

41. d'Agincourt-Canning L. Genetic testing for hereditary breast and ovarian cancer: Responsibility and choice. *Qualitative Health Research* 2006;16(1):97–118.

42. Etchegary H. Genetic testing for Huntington's disease: How is the decision taken? *Genetic Testing* 2006;10(1):60–67.

43. Etchegary H, Miller F, deLaat S, Wilson B, Carroll J, Cappelli M. Decision-making about inherited cancer risk: Exploring dimensions of genetic responsibility. *Journal of Genetic Counseling* 2009;18(3):252–264.

44. Taylor SD. Predictive genetic test decisions for Huntington's disease: Context, appraisal and new moral imperatives. *Social Science and Medicine* 2004;58(1):137–149.

45. Coates N, Gregory M, Skirton H, Gaff C, Patch C, Clarke A, et al. Family communication about cystic fibrosis from the mother's perspective: An exploratory study. *Journal of Research in Nursing* 2006;12(6):619–634.

46. Forrest LE, Curnow L, Delatycki MB, Skene L, Aitken M. Health first, genetics second: Exploring families' experiences of communicating genetic information. *European Journal of Human Genetics* 2008;16(11):1329–1335.

47. Peterson SK, Watts BG, Koehly LM, Vernon SW, Baile WF, Kohlmann WK, et al. How families communicate about HNPCC genetic testing: Findings from a qualitative study. *American Journal of Medical Genetics* 2003;119C(1):78–86.

48. Hamilton RJ, Bowers BJ, Williams JK. Disclosing genetic test results to family members. *Journal of Nursing Scholarship* 2005;37(1):18–24.

49. Forrest K, Simpson S, Haites N, Van Teijlingen E, Wilson B, McKee L, et al. To tell or not to tell: The passing on of genetic knowledge to family members. *Journal of Medical Genetics* 2000;37:A15-A.

50. Daly M, Barsevick A, Miller S, Buckman R, Costalas J, Montgomery S, et al. Communicating genetic test results to the family: A six step, skills building strategy. *Family and Community Health* 2001;24(3):13–26.

51. Buckman R. *How to Break Bad News: A Guide for Health Care Professionals.* Baltimore: Johns Hopkins University Press; 1992.

52. Wood JT. *Communication in Our Lives.* Boston: Wadsworth: Cenage Learning; 2009.

53. Hallowell N, Ardern-Jones A, Eeles R, Foster C, Lucassen A, Moynihan C, et al. Communication about genetic testing in families of male BRCA1/2 carriers and non-carriers: Patterns, priorities and problems. *Clinical Genetics* 2005;67(6):492–502.

54. Egan G. *The Skilled Helper* (7th ed.). Pacific Grove, CA: Brookes/Cole; 2002.

55. Forrest K, Simpson SA, Wilson BJ, van Teijlingen ER, McKee L, Haites N, et al. To tell or not to tell: Barriers and facilitators in family communication about genetic risk. *Clinical Genetics* 2003;64(4):317–326.

56. Djurdjinovic L. *Psychosocial Counseling.* In: Baker DL, Scheuette JL, Uhlmann WR, eds. *A Guide to Genetic Counseling.* New York: Wiley-Liss; 1998:127–170

57. Imber-Black E. *The Secret Life of Families: How Secrets Shape Relationships—When and What to Tell.* New York: Bantam Books;1998.

58. Kenen R, Arden-Jones A, Eeles R. We are talking, but are they listening? Communication patterns in families with a history of breast/ovarian cancer (HBOC). *Psycho-oncology* 2004;13(5):335–345.

59. Clouder L. Reflective practice in physiotherapy education: A critical conversation. *Studies in Higher Education* 2000;25:211–223.

60. Kennedy AL. Supervision for practicing genetic counselors: An overview of models. *Journal of Genetic Counseling* 2000;9(5):379–390.

61. Casement P. *On Learning from the Patient.* Hove, England: Tavistock Publications; 1985.

62. Seaburn DB, McDaniel SH, Kim S, Bassen D. The role of the family in resolving bioethical dilemmas: Clinical insights from a family systems perspective. *The Journal of Clinical Ethics* 2004;15(2):123–134;discussion 35–38.

63. McDaniel S. The psychotherapy of genetics. *Family Process* 2005;44(1):25–44.

64. Esplen MJ, Hunter J, Leszcz M, Warner E, Narod S, Metcalfe K, et al. A multicenter study of supportive-expressive group therapy for women with BRCA1/BRCA2 mutations. *Cancer* 2004;101(10):2327–2340.

65. Esplen MJ, Toner B, Hunter J, Glendon G, Liede A, Narod S, et al. A supportive-expressive group intervention for women with a family history of breast cancer: Results of a phase II study. *Psycho-oncology* 2000;9(3):243–252.

66. Foster C, Eeles R, Ardern-Jones A, Moynihan C, Watson M. Juggling roles and expectations: Dilemmas faced by women talking to relatives about cancer and genetic testing. *Psychology and Health* 2004;19(4):439–455.

67. Decruyenaere M, Evers-Kiebooms G, Cloostermans T, Boogaerts A, Demyttenaere K, Dom R, et al. Predictive testing for Huntington's disease: Relationship with partners after testing. *Clinical Genetics* 2004;65(1):24–31.

68. Richards F, Williams K. Impact on couple relationships of predictive testing for Huntington disease: A longitudinal study. *American Journal of Medical Genetics* 2004;126A(2):161–169.

Appendix

GENETIC CONDITIONS

The following information highlights key features of genetic conditions mentioned in the text and provides an introduction to their implications. These are not meant to be comprehensive descriptions of the conditions. Readers interested in more detail may wish to consult information available through the Web sites of the Genetic Alliance (http://www. geneticalliance.org), genetics and rare conditions Web site (http://www. kumc.edu/gec/support/), and Centre for Genetic Education (http:// www.genetics.com.au). Explanations of inheritance patterns are given in Chapter 2.

Abbreviation	Name	Gene	Inheritance	Description
AATD	Alpha-1 antitrypsin deficiency	*SERPINA1*	Autosomal recessive	This condition is a predisposition rather than a disease in itself. Many people with this condition remain perfectly healthy, but some develop emphysema, especially if they smoke. A small number of babies with the condition develop a serious form of liver disease.
CF	Cystic fibrosis	*CFTR*	Autosomal recessive	Cystic fibrosis causes the production of a thick sticky mucus, which clogs the lungs and pancreas and causes problems in the function of these organs. The lungs are susceptible to infection, which can cause irreversible lung damage and death, and impaired pancreatic function can result in the malabsorption of food and in diabetes mellitus.
HD	Huntington disease	*HD (IT15)*	Autosomal dominant	Huntington disease causes brain cells to degenerate. It often begins in middle life and gets progressively worse over 10–25 years. The effects include incoordination made worse by involuntary, jerky movement s, impaired memory and ability to plan, and personality changes.
FAP	Familial adenomatous polyposis	*APC*	Autosomal dominant	A condition that causes hundreds or thousands of polyps to grow in the large bowel, often from adolescence onward. The bowel is usually removed to prevent the polyps developing into colorectal cancer.
FraX	Fragile X syndrome	*FMR1*	X-linked	Fragile X syndrome is an inherited condition causing developmental delay, attention deficit and hyperactivity, autism, and some characteristic facial and other physical features in those with a full mutation. Relatives with a premutation may develop an adult-onset neurodegenerative condition or experience a premature menopause.
HBOC	Hereditary breast and ovarian cancer	*BRCA1 and BRCA2*	Autosomal dominant	This is a hereditary cancer syndrome that greatly increases the risk of developing breast and ovarian cancers and, to a lesser extent, some other specific types of cancer.

HH	Hereditary hemochromatosis	*HFE*	Autosomal recessive	Hereditary hemochromatosis leads to the excessive absorption of iron. Like AATD (above) it is a predisposition; it predisposes the affected individual to iron overloading. A small proportion of those with the predisposition suffer ill effects from the excessive accumulation of iron that results in damage to organs, including the liver, heart, and pancreas. The effects can be prevented by regular blood donation.
	Lynch syndrome	*MLH1*, *MSH2*, *MSH6*, and *PMS2*	Autosomal dominant	Once known as hereditary nonpolyposis colorectal cancer, this inherited cancer syndrome mostly causes cancers of gastrointestinal organs, particularly the large bowel, and endometrial (uterine) cancer.
	Marfan syndrome	*FBN1*	Autosomal dominant	Marfan syndrome is a connective tissue disorder. Its features are very variable, but it typically leads to problems with the eyes, skeleton, and cardiovascular system. Many affected people are tall and/or have a risk of sudden death through rupture of the artery leading out of the heart.
NF	Neurofibromatosis	*NF1* and *NF2*	Autosomal dominant	Neurofibromatosistype 1 is a common condition characterized by pigmented (café-au-lait) patches of skin and the growth of benign tumors called neurofibromas. Some with this condition have serious medical problems from these tumors, but many have cosmetic problems as the major effect. Neurofibromatosis type 2 is a very different and very rare condition. In this condition, benign tumors typically develop in the brain or spinal cord and often cause deafness.
PKU	Phenylketonuria	*PAH*	Autosomal recessive	This is a disorder of the metabolism, which causes mental retardation in babies due to buildup in the brain and tissues of an amino acid (phenylalanine, Phe) found in many foods. It can be prevented by staying on a special diet throughout childhood and early adulthood.

INDEX

Note: Page numbers followed by "*f*" and "*t*" denote figures and tables, respectively.